The People's Pharmacy-2

by Joe Graedon
with Teresa Graedon

D0972986

AVON
PUBLISHERS OF BARD, CAMELOT AND DISCUS BOOKS

Other Avon Books

by Joe Graedon

THE PEOPLE'S PHARMACY   **76299 $5.95**

NOTICE

The medical and health procedures contained in this book are based on research and recommendations of responsible medical sources. But because each person is unique, the author and publisher *urge the reader to check with his physician before implementing any of them.*

The author and publisher disclaim responsibility for any adverse effects or consequences resulting from the suggestions or the use of any of the preparations or procedures contained herein. No one should ever commence taking drugs, or discontinue a prescribed drug regimen without first consulting a physician.

This book is dedicated to:

DAVID EMIL

Who patiently put up with an upstairs daddy
for far too long

ALENA BONNELL

Who displayed a marvelous sense of timing

SID AND HELEN

Whose unwavering enthusiasm, encouragement and love
gave us the energy to carry through

and those

HEALTH PROFESSIONALS

Who take the time to communicate clearly and help people
make responsible decisions about the drugs they use

ACKNOWLEDGEMENTS:

A great many people helped us put this book together. We never could have made it without the assistance of the following individuals:

R. Meade Christian, a superb pediatrician whose contribution to this book was invaluable,

Tom Ferguson, an extraordinary human being and a physician who is helping people practice informed self-care,

Susan Moldow, a fantastic editor who combined wisdom, patience and firmness to help make this book what it is,

Brian Weiss, a wonderful friend without whose dedication and perseverance the book never could have been completed,

Stanley B. Levy, a fine dermatologist who appreciates the value of clear communication,

Joseph Strayhorn, a psychiatrist with a heart and a clear head who really wants to help people prevent mental illness,

Doris Ledford, a super lady who more than any other single individual helped make this book a reality,

William P. Pinna, a tough cookie who really cares about his clients' best interests,

Sid Graedon, a great father and a bookman par excellence,

Helen Graedon, a wonderful mother who waded through an extraordinary amount of mail in order to find the pearls,

Lou Wolfe, numero uno in publishing and a man whose faith in *The People's Pharmacy* helped make it a success,

Diane Glynn, a kind and generous woman and the best publicity person in publishing,

Deborah Wright, an excellent researcher who uncovered lots of golden nuggets,

Cliff R. Butler, an exceptional pharmacist who always came through with key information in the nick of time,

Tad Smith, whose shortsightedness and cruel behavior unwittingly contributed to the conception and completion of *The People's Pharmacy*,

Betty King, a fine researcher who really understood what this book was all about,

Ruth Shipley, an able research assistant who provided much of the raw material for the vitamin chapter,

Warren Jones, a knowledgeable pharmacist who really believes in service to his clients,

the inspiration lent by:

Jere Goyan, the best damn Commissioner of the Food and Drug Administration this country has ever had!

Hugh Drummond, a psychiatrist with such clarity of thought it is breathtaking,

and most important of all, the extraordinary vote of confidence provided by thousands of people all over this country who offered kind words and encouragement.

The following friends have all contributed in one way or another to the idea of this work. Without their support the book could never have evolved:

Leo Ars, Jorge and Vilma Ayala, Pat Barry, John Barth, Molly and Frederick Bernheim, Maria Berumen, Peter and Louise Brown, Jim Burdine, Alice and Chuck Cambron, Betye Carey, Ed Cooke, Ila Cote, Ben and Mary Daitz, Polly Davenport, Gretchen Dery, Fred D'Ignazio, Martin and Vilunya Diskin, Henrie Eolis, Alice and Jorge Escobar, Izzy and Jill Figueroa, June Fisher, Fernando Galindo, Joseph Gardocki, Ken and Molly Glander, Leo and Luce Goldstein, Francis Goldstein, Kathe Gregory, Catherine Gutmann, Joanne Hall, Mike and Judy Hammond, Marcia, Jennifer, Amy and Ricardo Hofer, Georges Hufnagel, Tom Kaluzynski, Art Kaufman, Devva Kasnitz, Ed and Aleka Leydon, Cynthia and Dick Luke, Emma Mason, Lee and Kay Miller, Peggy and David Mohrman, Lorna and Bill Moore, Ada and Bernie Most, Dee and Paul Mundschenk, Barney, Judi and BJ Nietschmann, Katie Oppenheim, John-Henry Pfifferling, Allan Priaulx, Sam Putnam, Skip and Ann Rappaport, Ed and Mary Scheier, Bill Shinker, Tom and Barbara Smigel, Carol and Ron Smith, Susan and Allen Spalt, Carol and Kevin Stack, Kate Sullivan, Vicki Swain, Hector Tenorio, Ellie White, Nancy and Jim Woods.

CONTENTS

LIST OF TABLES

1

To Your Health
Introducing
The People's Pharmacy-2

The People's Pharmacy-2: WHY?—Poor doctor-patient communication...their handwriting is off the wall • First for the good news: fewer prescriptions are being filled, Patient Package Inserts are coming, the FDA is starting to move—Big bans on Zirconium, sequential birth control pills (ORACON, ORTHO NOVUM SQ, NORQUENS), and diabetes drugs (DBI, MELTROL) • Zapping Odious Advertising—LISTERINE forced to swallow own hogwash • The bad news: We're spending more and enjoying it less! Advertisers still pull our strings. Doctors indicted on drug awareness. The VALIUM and DES horror stories go on and on • How to protect yourself from adverse drug reactions—Our Rules of Thumb.

The People's Pharmacy was a book that never should have been written. There shouldn't have been a need for such a book and it never should have sold more than a few copies. While I know that many doctors, pharmacists, and drug company representatives couldn't agree more with such statements, they must seem heretical coming from the author. What I mean is that if the Food and Drug Administration (FDA) really regulated our medicines we wouldn't have to be so concerned about issues of safety and effectiveness. If doctors took more time to talk to their patients about the drugs being prescribed, there wouldn't be a dangerous communication gap. If the Federal Trade Commission (FTC) really cracked down on false and misleading advertising, no one would have to take up a slingshot against the drug companies. In other words, if the system worked, books like *The People's Pharmacy* would be unnecessary and would not sell.

Well, at last count, *The People's Pharmacy* had over 750,000 copies in print and the ridiculous term "bestseller" actually is appropriate. This is a sad commentary on the medical profession and the state of the pharmaceutical industry. While some doctors would have preferred that the book be banned or better yet be available by prescription only, the message won't go away. People have a right to information about the medications they are urged to use with such great regularity. And as long as there are so many deceptive drug commercials on television that mislead and manipulate consumers, an alternative perspective needs to be aired.

If the first book should never have been written, why write book number 2? Well, one trouble with learning about drugs is that it can be habit-forming. People want to know more. They have discovered that the modern-day medicine show is sending out a line of hypocritical hype that rivals anything put out by traveling snake-oil salesmen in Grandpa's day. If the FDA and FTC aren't protecting them, then people want the information to protect themselves. And now that folks understand that all drugs have risks as well as benefits they want the knowledge to make informed decisions about their health care.

A great many physicians welcome questioning and active involvement by their patients, but some tend to feel threatened by enlightened clients. They use terms like "myocardial infarction" for a heart attack, "alopecia" for baldness, "xerostomia" for a dry mouth, "hematoma" for a bruise, and "cervical acceleration extension injury" for a whiplash. These 50-dollar words may sound impressive but they neither accelerate nor facilitate communication or understanding with patients or colleagues. About all they do is create anxiety and confusion.

The fear that patients may learn too much about drugs may explain why so many prescriptions are still written illegibly with Latin abbreviations. It is rumored that there is a secret course in most medical schools called "Scribbling for Beginners," and word has it that most students score an A+. If you don't believe that just look at the following samples. These are real live prescriptions that pharmacists sent in to a journal called *Pharmacy Times*.[1-6] The editor of this fine professional publication gave us permission to reproduce these extraordinary examples of illegibility.

You may think that this chicken scratching is funny, and in a sense it is. But it is also dangerous and costly. An illegible scrawl and a secret Latin code set up a barrier between the doctor and the patient and can interfere with appropriate drug administration. Numerous investigations have shown that people often make serious mistakes

Erythromycin   250 mg #24
Sig.: One q.i.d.

Elixir Pyribenzamine Expectorant
with Ephedrine   3 oz.
Sig.: One teaspoonful q. 4 h. for cough

with prescribed medications—anywhere from 50 to 80 percent take their drugs at the wrong time, in the wrong dose or for the wrong purpose. It would be easy to label such individuals stupid or uncooperative but it turns out that much of the misunderstanding is caused by unclear prescription instructions.

A recent article in the *Journal of the American Medical Association* titled "A Study of Physicians' Handwriting as a Time Waster" produced some fascinating statistics:

> **The average writing skill performance is fair to average. This means that 50% of all orders written require extra time to interpret because of handwriting . . .**
> **One of six (16%) of the physicians evaluated**

[in a 500-bed hospital] had illegible handwriting. Another 17% had poor-to-fair [barely legible] handwriting. That there is a problem in communication caused by poor handwriting is commonly acknowledged. Its actual effect on the cost of medical care can be evaluated in terms of time expended by nurses, secretaries, other physicians, pharmacists, and other personnel . . .

A member of the resident staff who was questioned about his ability to read the consultation notes of a physician who wrote with a 0-1 rating [completely illegible] responded, "It's no problem, we can't read them, so we don't try. We wait until he comes around again and asks us if such-and-such has been done. Then we know what to order."[7]

If doctors have difficulty understanding other doctors you can imagine how the poor patients fare. And if physicians won't communicate, then darn it, people have the right to find out what they need to know on their own. If you want to be able to read those Latin abbreviations your doctor loves to write on his prescriptions here is a handy translation guide:

SOME COMMON PRESCRIPTION SYMBOLS[8]

Latin	Abbreviation	Meaning
ad libitum	ad lib.	freely, as needed
ante cibos	a.c.	before meals
bis in die	b.i.d.	twice a day
capsula	caps.	capsule
gutta	gtt.	drop
hora somni	h.s.	at bedtime
per os	P.O.	by mouth
quaque 4 hora	q.4h.	every 4 hours
quater in die	q.i.d.	4 times a day
signa	Sig.	write on label
ter in die	t.i.d.	3 times a day
ut dictum	Ut dict., UD	as directed

It is a shame people have to struggle to find out what they need to know about their medications. Because we have been swamped, deluged, and otherwise flooded with mail from people all over the

United States and Canada requesting drug information and supplying home remedies, the inescapable conclusion is that while another book like *The People's Pharmacy* shouldn't have to be written, there is a desperate need for one.

ON THE BRIGHT SIDE

There have been some signs of improvement since the original *People's Pharmacy* was published. Over the last five years the total number of prescriptions dispensed in pharmacies has declined. In 1973 over one-and-a-half billion prescriptions were sold in United States drugstores. That's right, 1,518,462,000.[9] Incredible—mind-boggling—bizarre! Without counting hospital-dispensed medications or over-the-counter (OTC) drugs, that represents almost forty billion pills each year—about two hundred for every man, woman, child, and infant in the country. If you add in the billions and billions of non-prescription drugs like aspirin, antacids, and laxatives the statistics are staggering.

The good news is that the numbers are coming down. In fact, over a hundred million fewer prescriptions are now being filled each year than in 1973. It is hoped this trend means that doctors are being more careful about the drugs they prescribe and people are becoming a little less enthusiastic about popping a pill for every ill. Another good sign is that generic prescribing (by the scientific name instead of the brand name) is on the upswing and growing faster each year. This means that many physicians have accepted the fact that most generic drugs are good drugs and can represent significant savings for consumers.

There is more good news. Some doctors are waking up to the needs of their patients. In a recent letter to his colleagues titled "Somebody *DO* Something ... About Rehumanizing the Patient-Physician Relationship," Dr. Donald Schreiber of Louisville, Kentucky, demonstrated an extraordinary sensitivity that is all too often missing:

> **Despite the recent trend toward taking the physician off his pedestal, the majority of patients are still intimidated by the patient-physician relationship. The reasons are many, but center around one theme: the doctor's tendency to treat the patient as an object instead of a person. ... How much more appropriate it would be to treat the person instead of the disease. The patient is looking for reassurance, trust, and concern. ... The simplest things go a**

> long way to show that we care, not only for, but
> about the person. Asking someone to call back
> if symptoms persist, and inquiring about his
> general well-being, irrespective of his chief
> complaint, are just a few examples of this. . . .
> Respect begets respect. The patient's awareness
> that he is going to be seen by and be treated like
> a person instead of a machine can make the
> wait, fears, and pain a lot easier to endure.[10]

Amen, brother, and right on! It's nice to know that doctors like Donald Schreiber really have their eyes on the ball. We need more like him.

HOORAY FOR PATIENT PACKAGE INSERTS

There are other reasons to rejoice. After years of sitting on their duffs, the bureaucrats at the Food and Drug Administration are slowly moving in the direction of requiring Patient Package Inserts (PPIs). So what's so hot about PPIs? Well, for one thing, it means that when people receive a prescription they will also receive a piece of paper with important information on how the drug works and what the dangers might be. Until now, the only folks who saw the package insert that comes with each prescription drug were the doctor and the pharmacist and they generally just threw it away. Even if the patient were aware of the existence of this elusive piece of paper and requested a copy, it was usually considered too hot to handle and the consumer was given the brush-off. FDA has documented what can happen when doctors are unwilling or uninterested in supplying drug information:

> "Our daughter before age eight received
> medication from one of the tetracyclines. The
> result of the taking of this drug is that she now
> has discolored teeth. If we had known the effects
> of this drug we would have asked the doctor to
> give her different medication."

> "(My son) has permanent gum hyperplasia
> [increased growth] from Dilantin. We were not
> told to institute a vigorous gum brushing
> regimen until it was too late."

> These and hundreds of similar reports of
> personal experiences were received by the Food
> and Drug Administration after the agency asked
> for comments on a petition requesting that

certain prescription drugs carry warning for consumers... In some cases these reactions were transitory, disappearing when the drug was discontinued; in others, the reactions were serious and long lasting. Some drugs produced physical symptoms such as rash, swelling, severe headache, nausea, or vomiting. Others had a mind-bending effect leaving the patient feeling "like a zombie," acting "addlepated," or having hallucinations... The common thread throughout these letters is the claim that no one warned the patients or their families of the possible side effects from the drugs prescribed for them. Had they known, many wrote, they could have been spared much anguish.[11]

Patient Package Inserts are no substitute for good doctor-patient communication, but if that is lacking then the information provided on the brochure may enable people to make informed decisions about their treatment program. If an unexpected side effect does occur, the patient or his family will hopefully be able to recognize it as related to the medication and contact the physician so that a different drug can be prescribed before the problem gets out of hand and causes harm. We have received hundreds of heartbreaking letters from people relating their personal tragedies with drugs when inadequate information was provided.

It should come as no surprise to learn that drug companies and even some pharmacists have been actively resisting PPIs. Actually, resisting is a kind word for what has been going on. These folks have been fighting, kicking and screaming every inch of the way. They mainly argue that it will cost too much money to provide customers with a piece of paper which gives data on precautions and side effects. They also imply that it could undermine people's confidence in the doctor if they were aware of all the risks and benefits of a particular medication. Well, we believe that the costs of *not* providing this information are much too high. Patients should be encouraged to participate in their drug-taking decisions and that means knowing about benefits and risks. If a doctor writes an irrational prescription then the patient should have some way to protect him- or herself.

Despite the intense lobbying campaign being waged by the pharmaceutical manufacturers and pharmacists to prevent Patient Package Inserts we all have one BIG ace in the hole. The head of the Food and Drug Administration is committed to improving drug information for patients. Dr. Jere Edwin Goyan has made some extraordinary statements that deserve quoting:

> I am committed, and always have been, both personally and professionally to the concept that patients are entitled to know as much about the drugs they take as anyone else. I believe that people should, indeed must, actively participate in making decisions about their own health care, including the selection of prescription drugs. I would not want to swallow a pill about which I knew nothing, and I would not expect anyone else to do so either.
>
> I have always regarded myself as a leader in the fight to get more information to patients about prescription drugs ... I believe the time has come for consumers to have that information ... Patient labeling can help people understand better why they are taking a medication and when they should not take a drug. Patient labeling can, quite simply, bring the patient more into health decision making.
>
> In addition, patient labeling will help accomplish another of my objectives, and that is to try and reduce the number of prescription and nonprescription drugs being taken by Americans. Drugs have the potential to do great good ... They also have the potential to do great harm, especially when people become addicted to them or take them unnecessarily. Too many people in this country are taking too many drugs without proper understanding of their potential harmful effects.
>
> Our society has become overmedicated; we've become too casual about the use of drugs, and here I'm referring to legitimate prescription and nonprescription drugs, not illicit drugs. I intend to pursue other avenues, in addition to Patient Package Inserts, to try to encourage more responsible use of drugs. Americans must learn there is not a pill for every ill, and that they need not get a prescription every time they visit their doctors.
>
> Dr. Jere Edwin Goyan, Commissioner, FDA
> National Press Club, November 6, 1979

Basically, I'm a therapeutic nihilist. My general philosophy is the fewer drugs people take, the better off they are . . . I have a strong belief in a patient's right to know. My philosophy on this makes doctors and some of my colleagues [pharmacists] uneasy, but in the best interests of public health, it should be mandated . . . Drug companies have a tendency to try to sell drugs and not to convey information . . . Too often the wrong drug has been given to the wrong patient, at the wrong time, and in the wrong amounts, with no consideration of costs. . .

I staunchly refuse to accept the notion that any physician merely because he graduated from medical school and is currently a card-carrying member of his or her county medical society, is great, or good, or even tolerably competent. Too much drug therapy has been atrociously irrational.

Dr. Jere Edwin Goyan, Commissioner, FDA
Science Magazine, **October 12, 1979**[12]

WOW! That wasn't Joe Graedon speaking. It wasn't Ralph Nader speaking. That *was* the number-one man at the FDA. Dr. Goyan is an exceptional person. If he can resist the industry lobbying and survive the bureaucratic red tape we may all see some important changes over the next few years.

At the time of this writing the FDA has required a patient brochure to be included with birth-control pills, IUDs (intrauterine devices), estrogen hormones used to treat menopausal symptoms, DES (the morning-after pill called diethylstilbestrol), and ISUPREL (isoproterenol, an aerosol asthma medication). It is likely that progestins (drugs used for menstrual disorders) and FLAGYL (metronidazole, a drug used for vaginal infections) will also come with Patient Package Inserts. We may hope there will be a rapid expansion of this list so that in the not too distant future most drugs will be accompanied with an informational brochure.

Now, PPIs are not a perfect solution to drug-taking problems, and they involve a few potential drawbacks. If the inserts are filled with too much technical gobbledygook they may overwhelm some folks or scare others into not taking needed medicine. PPIs may also allow the FDA and the drug companies a convenient escape hatch—a way to cover their A**. In more delicate words, the brochure may give them an excuse for not banning hazardous drugs. Instead of eliminating a dangerous chemical the patient is given a brochure that lists all the horrendous side effects that could occur. The FDA and the drug companies then throw up their hands and walk away, leaving the patient holding the bag (or the time bomb, as the case may be). Needless to say, this puts a patient squarely between a rock and a hard place. The doctor has prescribed a drug to relieve a problem, but the brochure lists some very frightening side effects. For example, birth-control pills have been associated with strokes and heart attacks, and estrogens with uterine cancer. If something bad does happen, who is responsible? It's a dilemma! But at least now people can make decisions from a position of knowledge, not ignorance. Overall, Patient Package Inserts are an advance in the right direction.

THE ZAPPING OF ZIRCONIUM

Fortunately, there is more good news. The Food and Drug Administration has taken some decisive action. It is now requiring more accurate labels, reviewing non-prescription medications, and proposing a drug-reform act which will speed the development of important new drugs and the withdrawal of dangerous ones. In addition, some hazardous ingredients in drugs and cosmetics have been taken off the market. For example, the FDA finally acted to get zirconium out of aerosol spray deodorants. SECRET ANTIPERSPIRANT, SURE SUPER DRY, and ARID XX used to contain it, but at last they have been reformulated.[13] Well, what was so disturbing about zirconium? Getting the baddie on your underarms was the pits, but breathing it into your lungs was even worse. For years there was concern that it might cause granulomas—little growths to appear on the skin of sensitive individuals.[14-17] Moreover, long-term inhalation (like every morning for years) might have led to lung damage.[18] Tests have shown "that Zirconium compounds have caused lung disease and other toxic effects in animals."[19] At least now you can't breathe it when you coat your underarms. But the darn stuff can still be found in SECRET CREAM and ROLL-ON, and SURE ROLL-ON. A number of poison-ivy and oak preparations also contain zirconium; they include POISON IVY CREAM, RHULI CREAM, RHULIHIST, and RHULI SPRAY.

Another victory of sorts was the banning of the flame-retardant Tris from children's sleepwear. Because this cancer-causing chemical could be absorbed through the skin and into the body, federal regulators moved to eliminate the substance entirely. As happy as we should all be to have another carcinogen bite the dust, it is infuriating that such a dangerous ingredient could have been put into our children's pajamas in the first place.

Birth-control pills also came under close scrutiny by the FDA. After a number of medical teams reported a startling association between sequential oral contraceptive use and cancer of the uterine lining in young women the recommendation was made to yank these drugs from the market.[20–24] With relatively little fanfare, ORACON, ORTHO-NOVUM SQ, and NORQUENS suddenly disappeared. Needless to say, it must have come as quite a shock to the millions of women who had used these contraceptives to discover so suddenly that the pills were no longer available because of a potential cancer risk. For those of us who have been monitoring the estrogen-cancer controversy over the years it was gratifying to see the FDA move so quickly to remove a potential hazard.

What made "sequential" oral contraceptives different from other birth-control pills? The basic difference is that sequentials contained estrogen all by itself for fourteen to sixteen days, then added progestin for the remaining five to seven days of the pill-taking cycle. It has been suggested that estrogen alone changes the lining of the uterus to allow cancerous growth. The majority of the oral contraceptives on the market today are "combined" birth-control pills with both estrogen and progestin given simultaneously for the full three-week cycle. Only time will tell whether or not these drugs will also come under close scrutiny by the FDA.

Diabetics are another group that can breathe a little easier because of some good news. DBI, DBI-TD, and MELTROL (phenformin) were all zapped by the past commissioner of Food and Drugs, Dr. Donald Kennedy. It was discovered (after many years on the market) that phenformin could cause a fatal biochemical imbalance at relatively low doses. At the time these diabetes medications were banned approximately 336,000 people were using the drugs in the United States and the FDA estimated that as many as 700 patients could have died each year from a toxic reaction.[25] At least now diabetics have one less thing to worry about since phenformin has disappeared.

While it is a great relief to see a dangerous drug removed from the market, it is distressing to learn that it took the regulators so long to recognize the severity of the situation. Adverse reactions to drugs have occurred ever since man started looking around for medicinal plants and herbs. Many were beneficial, but some were poisonous and a few poor souls paid a high price for their experimentation. With the explosion in drug therapy, the hazards escalated accordingly, but it is only relatively recently that we began to recognize the severity of adverse drug reactions and gather enough data to assess the consequences. In his excellent reference book, *Hazards of Medication,* Dr. Eric Martin has documented the extent of the problem:

> **During the 1960's, at the zenith of the misuse of medications in this country, the damage to patients was staggering . . . In the United States during that period some 1,500,000 of the 30,000,000 patients hospitalized annually were admitted *with* adverse drug reactions (ADR's) and about 850,000 *because* of such reactions. In one general hospital 25 percent of the deaths on the public medical record resulted from ADR's.**[26]

Fortunately, the reporting of this situation has made patients and doctors more aware that drugs must be handled with care and that the risks must be weighed against the benefits before commencing treatment. Consequently, there has been a significant reduction in adverse drug reactions in recent years and when they do occur people are better prepared to recognize them and act accordingly to reduce the danger.

ODIOUS ADVERTISING

The Federal Trade Commission (FTC) has gotten into the act as well. Its regulatory efforts have given buyers of mouthwash cause for a mini celebration. After years of resistance and appeals all the way up the judicial ladder, the makers of LISTERINE finally threw in the towel and complied with the Federal Trade Commission's ruling: they could no longer push the idea that their yucky-tasting antiseptic was good for sore throats and cold symptoms. Even better than that, the Warner-Lambert Company actually had to use "corrective" advertising to tell people that LISTERINE did not live up to their old inflated claims. This gives us an important precedent which in theory should promote more responsible advertising.

Unfortunately, every silver lining has its cloud. In undoing the damage of past transgressions, the drug company dug deep into its bag of tricks. A commercial was created that touted the superiority of LISTERINE over SCOPE in fighting *odious* onion breath. Two men were seen breathing in the direction of their girlfriends. Both women beat a hasty retreat in order to avoid a visible cloud of halitosis. Our two heros then gargled with their respective mouthwashes (almost as if they were dueling), and presto, the fellow who used LISTERINE was back in business with his girl.

What is so aggravating about this commercial is that while our attention is being directed toward the horrors of onion breath, the announcer introduces in a subtle and gentle manner the message that LISTERINE can't do anything for colds or sore throats. What's the matter with that? Well, if you are going to correct old errors you sure as heck ought to do it straightforwardly, without any flim-flam. Not only does the ad dilute the corrective message, but it's a reasonable bet that we're facing another inflated claim.

If you are going to devour those wonderful raw onions on your hot dogs and hamburgers, face reality. They are going to end up in your stomach where, after a short time, they will be digested and absorbed into your bloodstream. From there the onion essence will circulate through the body and eventually end up in the lungs where with each breath the aromatic extract will be exhaled in the form of onion breath. Holding your breath might solve the problem, but in our estimation that's a rather drastic and potentially permanent solution for a minor dietary indiscretion. The point of all this silliness is that although the FTC finally won a major battle to correct misleading advertising, the results have not been as far-reaching as we might have hoped. One of these days we may get to see the drug companies correcting the so-called corrective commercials.

AND NOW FOR THE BAD NEWS

Now that you've heard the good news, it's time to flip the coin and look at the other side. So hold on tight, there's some rough water ahead. Throughout the book we're going to try to help you avoid some of the rocks and sinkholes. For one thing, although the number of prescriptions filled in pharmacies has been steadily declining over the last few years, we are spending more and enjoying it less. In 1972 Americans shelled out 6.3 billion dollars for prescription drugs in pharmacies.[27] This does not include the almost $4 billion spent for medications in hospitals.[28] By 1975 pharmacy sales of prescription drugs had jumped to over $8 billion and by 1978 they exceeded $12 billion. [29] If you add $4 billion for hospital drugs (a conservative estimate) and another $5 billion for over-the-counter products you reach a mind-crunching total of over 21 billion dollars being spent on drugs of one kind or another.

Big deal. What difference does it make if we spend $5 billion or $50 billion? Well, it *is* a big deal! Ounce for ounce, VALIUM is much more valuable than gold. Americans spend more on medicine and beauty aids than they commit to private education or religious donations and charity. These comparisons should give you some idea of the size of the drug market, the size of the drug problem, the scale of the stakes, and the way it's accelerating. It is a cliché, but we *are* a pill-popping society. People are still falling for the sophisticated hucksterism of the drug companies and their ad-agency hypesters. Doctors are still prescribing an irrational number of drugs and people are still dying from adverse drug reactions.

There are many reasons for our ever-increasing dependence upon drugs. We live in an "instant" society. We have instant food, instant banking, instant copies, instant replay, and of course we demand instant relief—fast, Fast, FAST! The drug companies have promoted this philosophy by encouraging us to treat symptoms rather than seek causes or solutions to our problems. Don't worry about *why* you have anxiety—take a pill. You say you've got problems, Bucky, well then take our "Extra Strength" pain reliever. Perhaps you'd like "Arthritis Strength" pain reliever or would you prefer the "Adult Strength" stuff? If you're really hurting we've got "Maximum Strength" relief and one of these days there will be "Super Strength" pain relievers. Don't be at all surprised if some company doesn't bring out an **"Industrial Strength"** pain reliever for industrial-sized headaches.

While the consumer is partly to blame for swallowing this sophisticated sophistry, doctors must also shoulder a good chunk of the responsibility for overmedicating. They are apparently just as gullible as consumers when it comes to buying the drug companies' advertising pitch, as a recent article in the *Journal of the American Medical Association (JAMA)* corroborates:

> **Although a complete picture of prescribing practices are not at hand, the conclusions of two influential groups of physicians and researchers who have studied the matter are that the average physician is insufficiently educated in clinical pharmacology, often misled by industry advertising and "detail men," and inadequately informed of the alternatives to pharmacologic therapy.[30]**

Another article, this time in the prestigious *New England Journal of Medicine,* comes to a similar conclusion:

> **"Detail men" [salesmen] have been found to constitute the most influential single source of information for physicians during the period when a drug is first prescribed. Physicians frequently rely on advertising in medical jour-**

nals and material in the *Physicians' Desk
Reference* in matters such as dosage and adverse
reactions for drugs.[31]

Now that's heavy! And it is not an indictment leveled by a group of wild-eyed consumer advocates who hate doctors. It was written *by* doctors! These were the conclusions of the highly respected Institute of Medicine of the National Academy of Sciences. You could not find a more "establishment" group of physicians and researchers if you searched the country from one end to the other.

Dr. Richard Burack, a renowned expert in the field of medicine and pharmacology (and author of a marvelous book called *The New Handbook of Prescription Drugs*) offers additional insight into the relationship between physicians and pharmaceutical companies:

> It is time to remind medical students, doctors-in-training, and all of the concerned public that the aims of the drug manufacturers are different from the aims of good doctors. The manufacturers wish to maximize their profits by encouraging doctors to write as many prescriptions as possible for the most expensive drugs. Manifestly, good doctors should minimize writing prescriptions and, as purchasing agents for patients, should do all they can to keep the cost of necessary medications as low as possible.[32]

Dr. Ingrid Waldron, from the University of Pennsylvania adds fuel to Dr. Burack's fire with the following remarks:

> Drugs are often prescribed for clinical conditions in which therapeutic benefits do not outweigh the risk of adverse reactions... This paper has presented evidence that drugs are frequently prescribed when their use is not medically justified. This results in increased rates of illness and death due to adverse effects of prescribed drugs as well as inflated costs to the patient. Excessive and irrational prescribing is due in part to the profit-motivated activities of drug companies, including extensive promotional activities and research efforts devoted to the development of combination drug products and "me-too" drugs [instead of creating new drugs].[33]

Whoa, Nelly! Is there any evidence to support such strong statements? Unfortunately, it looks as if there is. Dr. Waldron's article is well documented. But confirmation comes from other sources too. A group of reporters from the *Milwaukee Journal* were investigating the Medicaid program in their city. In the process they learned a lot more than they cared to about the way some doctors prescribe drugs. Reporter John Stevens had this to say:

> **It took just 47 seconds. When the doctor left the examining room, I had three prescriptions— antibiotic pills and cough syrup for a sore throat I didn't have, plus diet pills for weight I can ill afford to lose. A nurse also gave me a shot of penicillin for the sore throat. I spent a total of 2 minutes, 57 seconds in one of the doctor's examining rooms. That brief period climaxed more than two hours I spent waiting—first for an appointment and then to see the doctor. The 47 second examination cost $10. With the prescription for the antibiotic pills [tet- racycline], cough syrup [phenergan], diet pills [apparently stratobex-D] and the shot of penicillin, I paid a total of $33.[34]**

Ouch! That doesn't just smart—it hurts like hell! Now we grant you, that is not your typical physician or even a close cousin. Most doctors are caring, highly competent professionals who do their very best to heal people who are sick or in distress. But even good doctors may bomb out when it comes to understanding drugs and the need to inform patients about side effects.

THE VALIUM TEST

Take VALIUM. It is still numero uno. Doctors write darn close to sixty million prescriptions for the BIG V each year. (If you add LIBRIUM, the combined total is over seventy million prescriptions.) And if ever there was a drug that doctors should understand inside and out, it should be VALIUM (Diazepam). A recent article published in the *American Journal of Psychiatry* suggests that this assumption may not be as valid as you would hope.

A questionnaire designed to test the basic knowledge of the uses, actions, and side effects of VALIUM was given to a group of medical students, residents in both psychiatry and internal medicine, and supervising psychiatrists at a major teaching hospital in New York

City. The questions were not esoteric or designed to stump the doctors. Rather, "all questions had a direct and immediate bearing on such clinically relevant decisions as when to prescribe or withhold a drug, choice of administration route, establishment of a proper dose, administration schedule, and indications for discontinuation of a drug."[35]

How do you think the doctors did on the test? To say that the results were shocking would be dramatically understating the case. For openers, the psychiatric residents and psychiatrists scored no better than the medical students or the medical house staff, even though the head doctors should have had more practical experience with VALIUM. That they all scored comparably would not be bad if they had all done well, but that was not the case. The authors stated that "all groups performed better than chance alone would predict," but big deal, all that means is that they knew a little more than if they were guessing blind.

These doctors blew the test and blew it badly! On basic questions about how the drug works in the body they answered only a little more than one-third correctly. Even more incredible, *fewer* than one-third of the physicians realized that certain groups of patients, particularly older folks, are especially sensitive to the effects of nervous-system depression associated with VALIUM. Worse yet (if you can believe this), only one-fifth were able to call upon their basic pharmacological knowledge of VALIUM in order to set up a rational dosage schedule that would maintain appropriate levels of the medication in the body all the time. A truly terrible showing!

The results of the test show that many of these doctors did not know whether or not to prescribe VALIUM for certain patients, whether it should be given by mouth or by injection, what the proper dose should be, and perhaps most important of all, when VALIUM use should be discontinued.

We usually assume that young doctors-in-training or those teaching at hospitals are more alert and better informed than the average family physician who may be more easily influenced by the drug-company salesmen and have less time to bone up. But this little test demonstrates that there could be a serious question about the adequacy of medical education when it comes to drugs. If these physicians did so poorly on this test and showed such an inadequate understanding of the most frequently prescribed drug in the world, it makes you wonder how they would have fared with less familiar medications.

A personal touch may better serve to emphasize the point. We recently received a letter from Mrs. O.S. from Virginia in which she told of her own experience with VALIUM:

> Before ever accepting this medication I asked *many* questions and was ever so cautious. Never before had I questioned a doctor's prescription so thoroughly—never before or since have I been so fooled, bewildered and befoozled by anything as this VALIUM. Ten years ago I had an auto accident—someone hit me in the rear. Whiplash was the pain problem, VALIUM was to be the cure. *Well, I'm still on the cure.* Headaches, upset stomach, sore throat, blurred vision, ear ringing, deep depression, sleepiness and unsleepiness ... With 10 years of this drug I could *really* go on and on with its *horrible* effects, that was to be a *harmless nerve relaxer* to start with—now I have cut the dosage on my own—pill by pill...And even gotten off, then in about a week, *help*! I was in real trouble, all hell would break loose (I'm taking the little blue devils—10mg). I even called my doctor and asked him to put me in the hospital since I thought I was going crazy— *Answer*—take your VALIUM. And so I'm still with it and fighting like hell to keep my wits. My question is—is there any way to get off this pill? P.S. I am alone in this fight as I lost my husband 8 years ago. Of *course* it was more VALIUM!

Mrs. O.S., Virginia Beach, Va.

This woman's story is not an isolated event. We have heard from many people who have gotten into trouble with VALIUM because a doctor never explained how to taper off gradually. If someone goes cold turkey "all hell" *can* "break loose." We will deal at length with the whole question of VALIUM withdrawal in Chapter 11.

DRUG-INDUCED TRAGEDY

We have received other letters from people who have suffered tragedies because someone failed to relay some important drug information. One letter in particular stands out and we felt duty bound to share parts of it to try to prevent this kind of thing from happening to others:

If I had read your book a month earlier I would have been able to save my mother from death and from three weeks of agony. She went into the hospital in good health, excellent appetite, etc. for a skin graft. She had bad pain from arthritis at times and her doctor prescribed INDOCIN. Not one word that it had any side effects of any kind and she was 85 years old, so it would have been helpful to have had words of caution . . .

My mother's appetite started to dwindle until the mere thought of food could start the most horrible retching. She did not vomit up any food. She went from 142 to 119 pounds in three weeks and neither the doctor or nurses did anything. The doctor said it was "emotional," but he couldn't have been more mistaken. Day after day she got weaker. I told the doctor I wanted to take my mother home and he agreed—she was so weak from lack of food.

She died one week after getting home from the hospital. The doctor took her off INDOCIN the day before she left the hospital at my insistence. I felt it was something they were giving her for medication that was doing this horrible thing to her, but the doctor said the INDOCIN would not do that, and I believed him. When I read the part of your book "The Dangers of Indocin" my hair stood on end. My mother had so many of the symptoms, nausea, vomiting, loss of appetite, blurring of vision, difficulty in breathing, itching (she thought it was due to the soap they used), skin rash, depression, terrible headaches and the feeling that her head was so light it was empty. Can you imagine what that INDOCIN did on an empty stomach?

I will never forget the agony nor her complete bewilderment of going into the hospital well and coming out so sick she could barely believe it. She kept asking, "Whatever is making me so sick?" She put up one big fight, she wanted to live so badly but her heart finally gave out. Other patients in the same room told me they didn't see how she lasted through the night, never mind a week after getting home . . . I have

**already told members of my family to get your
book so we can try not to let anything like this
happen again. Also by spreading the word we
may save someone else's life.**

Mrs. T.N., Wolfeboro, N.H.

Well, we are spreading the word! INDOCIN is no worse than many
other drugs and used correctly it can be a useful medication. But as
with any drug, prescribed incorrectly or without warning patients and
family about side effects it can produce tragic adverse reactions.
Doctors have a legal and moral responsibility to inform their clients
about the most common or most dangerous effects of any medicine
they prescribe. And patients deserve answers to questions they ask.
This kind of tragedy must never happen again.

THE DES NIGHTMARE GOES ON AND ON . . .

Unfortunately, there are still too many drugs on the market that
should have been eliminated years ago. An amazing number of the
hundreds of thousands of non-prescription agents sitting on
pharmacy shelves are not only ineffective (as advertised), but
possibly injurious to the health of millions of Americans. Doctors,
pharmacists, drug companies, and creaky bureaucracies have been
shockingly complacent and too darn slow to initiate needed changes.
We will discuss over-the-counter medications in detail in Chapter 2.
But even worse, there are prescription drugs that have caused more
than their share of misery that still go on and on and on. DES
(diethylstilbestrol) is one example that refuses to go away. In fact, it
only gets worse with time.

Diethylstilbestrol, a hormonal drug, was given to two million
women during the 1940s and 1950s and even well into the 1960s and
early 1970s. It was prescribed to prevent miscarriages in "high-risk"
pregnancies even though research going back to the 1950s suggested
that it might not have been effective for this purpose.

In 1971 it was announced to the world that some of the daughters
of women who had received DES during their pregnancies were
developing vaginal and cervical cancer. The time bomb had been
ticking and no one even knew it was there. Soon, hundreds of young
women between the ages of seven and twenty-eight were diagnosed
as having abnormal cellular changes because of a drug their mothers
received twenty or thirty years earlier. It was also discovered that sons
of DES mothers were not immune to the effects; there were often
abnormalities within their reproductive tracts (small testicular

growths, and cysts) and the possibility of decreased fertility. Clearly, millions of people were at risk.

No one thought much about the danger to the mothers themselves. Only in 1976 did researchers begin collecting information about DES mothers. An initial report forced investigators to start worrying about a possible cancer risk for them as well, and the recommendation was made to have regular breast and gynecologic examinations to check for precancerous changes.

As if the damage done years ago were not enough, the DES nightmare goes on because it is *still prescribed* to women (in some cases the very ones who received it *in utero*) as a "morning-after pill" contraceptive. "It is given routinely to rape victims to prevent rape-associated pregnancies."[36] Amazing as this is going to sound, research conducted at a large municipal hospital in Atlanta, Georgia indicates the

> **routine prescription of DES to rape victims seen in this hospital was not completely effective in preventing pregnancy ... the results appear to be similar to what one would expect if the drug had not been prescribed ... The implications of the above finding suggest that the use-effectiveness of DES as a postcoital contraceptive has not been adequately demonstrated. The safety of DES as a postcoital contraceptive has not been rigorously studied.[37]**

That, friends, is earth-shattering! It seems we are destined to continue to repeat the DES mistakes over and over and over again. When will we learn? The drug is dangerous—we know it has been associated with cancer. Yet it is still being given to young women although there are doubts that it is even effective as a "morning after pill." It is also used routinely to suppress lactation when women choose not to nurse their new born babies, even though there is no good evidence it is beneficial in preventing breast engorgement. Sheer LUNACY!

We have received letters from people who have been there—who have had personal experience with DES. Once again, we feel impelled to share their feelings and experiences:

> **Being a DES mother I am aware of its dangers. I have tried for the past five years to have it banned, in any form. The use of it being given to cattle is my greatest concern, because no one**

knows how many millions of people are ingesting it into their systems. I have found in my five years of frustrating stuggle to have DES banned, that to the politicians, it is too hot of an issue to handle. Senator Kennedy tried his best in 1975 to have it banned and the drug companies had it set aside stating they did not have an adequate opportunity for a hearing, and since then no more has been heard about banning it. Once again thank you for writing about DES because unless someone keeps it in the news, it will continue to be ignored.

If you're not angry after reading that you damn well should be! If the doctors, politicians, and regulators won't do anything to get rid of this blot on American medicine, it's time that just plain folks do something. Send us your letters and we will pass them on to those people who can make a difference. With hard work we can get DES banned. The Health Research Group (a Nader organization) has urged the following steps and we couldn't agree more:

1. Initiate a nationwide effort to notify the 2 million women who took the drug of their increased risk of cancer.

2. Outlaw the use of DES as a "morning after pill." (Hundreds of thousands of prescriptions for DES and other estrogens continue to be written each year for trivial and inappropriate purposes: acne, drying up breast milk after pregnancy, "mental disorders," and use as the "morning after pill.")

3. Ban DES from the food supply. (It is currently permitted in cattle feed, and residues appear in beef.)[38]

HOW TO PROTECT YOURSELF

Where do we go from here? We have pointed out just a few of the problems that still exist. Nothing has been said about hair dyes, food additives, or any of the potential cancer-causing chemicals that seem to surround us no matter where we try to hide. We will attempt to deal with these and many other safety issues throughout this book as they arise. If all this seems terribly depressing, it is. But there is much room for optimism. Just a few years ago we weren't even aware of the problems. Now at least we know they're out there and can begin to do something.

By now, you may be saying to yourself, "I'll never take another pill again as long as I live." That would not only be foolish, it would be a terrible mistake. And it certainly is *not* the message of this book. We have not discussed the "bad news" in order to frighten people out of taking needed medication. The point is that drugs have benefits *and* risks. While there have been abuses and scandals, never forget that drugs also save lives—lots of lives. They relieve suffering and cure us when we are ill. We may be an overmedicated society but that does not mean you throw away the life raft when the ship is sinking.

Arthritis victims would have great difficulty functioning without aspirin and other anti-inflammatory agents. People with high blood pressure would be more likely to develop serious complications and die at an earlier age without appropriate hypertension treatment. Folks with ulcers would be in terrible shape without antacids and other therapeutic medications. Heart patients would have to throw in the towel if we didn't have such an impressive array of modern pharmacological tools available. If our child had a strep throat or pneumonia we would be the first in line for penicillin. So please don't think we are against drugs. But as we have said before, drugs are double-edged swords and to use them wisely the patient needs the most complete access to information and a few fencing lessons. That is what we hope to provide in *People's Pharmacy-2*.

When you have an ailment, first and foremost try to find out what is really going on. It is crucial to understand what has caused the problem, what the symptoms are, and what they mean. All too often we either ignore the symptoms or treat them exclusively, without paying any attention to the underlying causes. That is rather like sticking a penny in the fusebox when the fuse blows. You may think you are doing yourself a favor, but the next time it blows you could really be in trouble.

Before initiating any drug therapy you should go down a check list (like a pilot preparing for take off). Here are some rules of thumb we would like to share because we think that they are important. Although we mentioned many of these points in *The People's Pharmacy* we feel that they are so crucial they should be repeated here:

1. **Why is the drug being prescribed?**

   All too often people focus exclusively on the side effects of a given medication. While that

is vital, it is equally important to understand the anticipated benefits and what the doctor's expectations are. That way it is possible to evaluate benefits against risks. And keep in mind, sometimes there are alternatives to drug therapy. For example—some people with high blood pressure can reduce or eliminate the need for a prescription if they lose weight, exercise (with supervision), cut out salt, reduce stress, and monitor their progress with their own sphygmomanometer.

2. Know the name of your drug!

It is absolutely crucial to find out exactly what you are supposed to be taking (brand name and generic name). It is important for many reasons. There are many drugs that look a lot alike. While most pharmacists are very careful to double and triple check their work, sometimes accidents do happen. If you want to see exactly how similar some drugs are, check out table 1. If a heart medicine like Digoxin were confused with a close cousin called Digitoxin, a disastrous overdose situation might occur that could put a patient in the emergency room of the nearest hospital. Imagine how easy it would be for a pharmacist to make a mistake, especially if the doctor is in a hurry and makes a spelling error. Make sure your doctor pronounces the name of the drug carefully and slowly and then pronounce it back until you get it right. Many medications have difficult names. If your doctor has an unreadable scrawl you have a right to ask him or her to have the name of the drug (with all generic components listed) typed out or printed neatly on a separate piece of paper. If any adverse reaction occurs you will immediately be able to identify the medicine instead of trying to describe a little white tablet or a black and green capsule.

Drugs with Similar Names

ACETAZOLAMIDE—ACETOHEXAMIDE

BENTYL—BENYLIN—BETALIN

BRISTACYCLINE—BRISTAMYCIN

DALIDYNE—DALIDERM

DEXAMETH—DEXAMYL

DIGITOXIN—DIGOXIN

DIMETANE—DIMETAPP

ELAVIL—ELADRYL

HALDRONE—HALODRIN

KEFLEX—KELEX

LASIX—LAXSIL

ORINASE—ORNADE

PREDNISOLONE—PREDNISONE

QUINIDINE—QUININE—QUINAMM

SULFAMETHOXAZOLE—SULFAMETHIZOLE—SULFISOXAZOLE

VALIUM—VALMID—VALPIN

3. **How do you take the drug?**

Most people take their medicine incorrectly, if they take it at all. Some studies have shown that one quarter to one half of all patients either don't get the doctor's prescription filled, or fail to take the drug once they do buy it. Of the ones who do take their medications, more than half may make serious errors by taking too much, not enough or by taking the drugs at the wrong time. One group of researchers discovered that the reason so many people were making so many mistakes was because doctors were not taking enough time to give them simple, easy-to-understand instructions nor were they taking the time to find out if their prescribed regimen was understood.[39] So make sure you know exactly how to take your medicine. "Before meals" and "three times a day" are too ambiguous—you need specific instructions. Can you take the medicine with milk or is water best? Find out what you need to know!

4. What are the drug's side effects?

No matter what your doctor may say, every drug has the potential to cause some side effects in some people, and you may be that person. Your physician has the legal and moral responsibility to inform you about the most common and the most dangerous adverse reactions associated with any medication he prescribes. It would also be useful to find out if there are any screening tests to detect early signs of side effects—such as an occasional blood check or urine analysis. If you do experience a side effect, even a minor one, get back in touch with your physician. She needs to know exactly how you are making out. And there is another benefit—the next time she prescribes the same drug to another patient she will think to warn of a side effect that might have otherwise gone unmentioned.

5. What about drug interactions?

Glad you asked that question! A great many drugs are totally incompatible with other medicine. One chemical can negate the benefits of a second, or make a side effect worse. Liquor and Valium are a classic dangerous interaction. When different doctors prescribe different drugs to different patients a problem can be created. Always take a list of every remedy you take (including non-prescription medications like laxatives, antacids or cold pills) when you visit a doctor. That way the potential for dangerous interactions can be reduced. And also get a list of any foods or beverages that might not mix well with your prescription.

6. Get it down on paper!

Visiting a doctor's office is usually a traumatic experience for most people. There is a lot of anxiety associated with sickness and often the nature of the doctor-patient relationship can be stressful in itself, especially if you have to wait a long time in the waiting room. By the time you see the doctor, and get through with the examination you may not be in any frame of mind to really understand or remember verbal instructions or warnings. So get your doctor to write down all the important stuff. That way you won't have to go through the trauma of trying to remember all the pieces to the puzzle when you get home and begin recuperating from the visit to the doctor.

Well, there you have it. If you follow these *People's Pharmacy Rules* we don't guarantee something bad won't happen, but the chances are much improved that if it does you will be prepared.

WHERE DO WE GO FROM HERE?

This is a book about direction finding and decision making. No, we're not going on a trip, but we will try to provide you with a map and a compass that should make your passage through the maze of prescription drugs and over-the-counter remedies a little less confusing. We may destroy some myths and illusions along the way. For example, the doctor is not a "pill fairy" who can dispense magic bullets to cure everything that ails you. She or he is a human being who has doubts and insecurities just like you, and who is just as vulnerable and fallible as other mortals.

Health care should be a shared responsibility between the patient and the physician. Instead of the usual lopsided arrangement, you should seek a collaborative relationship with your doctor where knowledge is shared equally. Instead of acting as a passive receptacle for the pills and potions that the doctor prescribes, you can be an active health consumer learning about all the significant consequences of the medications and evaluating the benefits as well as the risks. And then you can monitor the therapeutic response and remain vigilant for side effects.

Our goal is to provide you with the tools to take back some of the power and control that has been taken away from you. You have a lot of good common sense and you make decisions about your health care every day. But you need a little extra input to counteract all the horrible hogwash delivered to you in television and radio commercials. So, dear reader, sit back in a comfortable chair, put your feet up, and prepare to discover a lot of new information about prescription drugs, over-the-counter medications, home remedies, and dangerous drug interactions. We will do our best to enlighten you and entertain you, save you some money, and maybe even save your life.

In the following chapters we will bring you up-to-date on the latest drug developments. You will discover some wonderful wacky do-it-yourself stuff. You will learn about aphrodisiacs and what to do for stomach gas—in fact, you will probably end up knowing more than you ever wanted to about flatulence.

For the adolescents among us there will be plenty on pimples. New research offers some real hope for them thar zits. And parents will be better prepared to treat their youngsters after reading our chapter on drugs and children. There are too many booby traps waiting on pharmacy shelves for you to go shopping unprepared.

Because older people are especially vulnerable to drug effects and are often exposed to more medicines than any other segment of the population, there will be a wealth of information on new arthritis medications. We will also let you know what's happening in the treatment of high blood pressure. You will also receive the most recent update on the value of aspirin for preventing heart attacks and strokes. And for those who care about nutrition and vitamins, there will be some solid material that should help blow away some of the smoke that has been clouding the issues.

If you've ever had trouble getting to sleep, there's good news ahead. We will evaluate most prescription and OTC products. Some new rulings by the FDA have profoundly changed what is available in the drugstores. You will also benefit from some new and impressive home remedies. And if you've been feeling anxious and depressed lately, relax. You will get a guided tour through VALIUM land with some side trips to the candy mountain of antidepressants.

There will be lots of good self-care information including an analysis of diagnostic tools that belong in most people's little black bags. And naturally, we will update your medicine chest, advising you what to throw out and what to add. All this and much, much more. So strap on your seat belt and adjust your crash helmet, *The People's Pharmacy-2* is about to blast off.

REFERENCES

1. "Can You Read These Rxs?" *Pharmacy Times* 43(2):8, 86, 1977.

2. "Can You Read These Rxs?" *Pharmacy Times* 43(3):78, 98, 1977.

3. "Can You Read These Rxs?" *Pharmacy Times* 45(1):19, 86, 1979.

4. "Can You Read These Rxs?" *Pharmacy Times* 45(12):66, 84, 1979.

5. "Can You Read These Rxs?" *Pharmacy Times* 44(4):102, 114, 1978.

6. "Can You Read These Rxs?" *Pharmacy Times* 45(10):85, 118, 1979.

7. Anonymous. "A Study of Physicians' Handwriting as a Time Waster." *JAMA* 242:2429–2430, 1979.

8. Hecht, Annabel. "On Reading Prescriptions." *FDA Consumer* Dec. 1976–Jan. 1977, pp. 17–18.

9. National Prescription Audit in Continuing Education. "1977: Top 200 Drugs: Total Number of Rxs Slumps Again for 4th Year in a Row." *Pharmacy Times* 44(4):41–48, 1978.

10. Schreiber, Donald. "Somebody Do Something...About Rehumanizing the Patient-Physician Relationship." *Mod. Medicine* 47(2):37, 1979.

11. Hecht, Annabel. "Developing Drug Information for Patients." *FDA Consumer* 11(7):17–19, 1977.

12. Smith, R. Jeffrey. "Jere Goyan Brings Innovative Record to FDA." *Science* 206:200–201, 1979.

13. News Highlights. "Zirconium Removed from Antiperspirants." *FDA Consumer* 10(5):29, 1976.

14. Cormia, F. E., and Sheard, C., Jr. "Granuloma of Axilla (Zirconium?) from Deodorant Stick." *Arch. Derm.* 75:903–905, 1957.

15. Epstein, W. L.; Shahen, J. R.; and Krasnobrod, H. "Granulomatous Hypersensitivity to Zirconium: Localization of allergen in tissue and its role in formation of peitheloid cells." *J. Invest. Derm.* 38:223–232, 1962.

16. Lewe, I. A. "Granulomas of the Axillae Caused by Deodorant." *Arch. Derm.* 75:765–767, 1957.

17. Kleinhans, D., and Knoth, W. "Axillare Granulome (Zirkonium?)." *Dermatologica* 152:161–167, 1976.

18. News Highlights. "Zirconium Removed from Antiperspirants." *FDA Consumer* 10(5):29, 1976.

19. News Highlights. "FDA Completes Action on Zirconium Ban." *FDA Consumer* 11(7):29, 1977.

20. Silverberg, S. G., and Makowski, E. L. "Endometrial Carcinoma in Young Women Taking Oral Contraceptive Agents." *J. Obs. Gynecol.* 46:503–506, 1975.

21. Lyon, F. A. "The Development of Adenocarcinoma of the Endometrium in Young Women Receiving Long-Term Sequential Oral Contraception: Report of Four Cases." *Am. J. Obstet. Gynecol.* 123:299–301, 1975.

22. Kelley, H. W.; Miles, P. A.; Buster, J. E.; and Scroggs, W. H. "Adenocarcinoma of the Endometrium in Women Taking Sequential Oral Contraceptives." *Obstet. Gynecol.* 47:200–202, 1976.

23. Kaufman, R. H.; Reeves, K. O.; and Dougherty, C. M. "Severe Atypical Endometrial Changes and Sequential Contraceptive Use." *JAMA* 236:923–926, 1976.

24. News Highlights. "Sequential Birth Control Pills Discontinued." *FDA Consumer* 10(3):25, 1976.

25. Martin, E. S. (ed.) "HEW Secretary Suspends General Marketing of Phenformin." *FDA Bulletin* 7(3):14, 1977.

26. Martin, Eric W. *Hazards of Medication.* 2nd ed. Philadelphia: Lippincott, 1978, p. 1.

27. Marketing Emphasis. " '76 Drug, Cosmetic and Toiletry Expenditures." *Product Marketing* July/August, 1977, pp. 43–51.

28. Silverman, M., and Lee, P. R. *Pills, Profits and Politics.* University of California Press. Berkeley, 1974.

29. "PM's Consumer Expenditure Study Shows HBA Sales at $23.2 Billion." *Product Marketing* 31st Annual ed., July, 1978, pp. A–V.

30. Medical News. "Physician Prescribing Practices Criticized; Solutions in Question." *JAMA* 241:2353–2360, 1979.

31. Solomon, Fredric, et al. "Sleeping Pills, Insomnia and Medical Practice." *N. Engl. J. Med.* 300:803–808, 1979.

32. Burack, R. *The New Handbook of Prescription Drugs.* Ballantine, New York, 1976, p. *xxii.*

33. Waldron, Ingrid. "Increased Prescribing of Valium, Librium, and Other Drugs—an Example of the Influence of Economics and Social Factors on the Practice of Medicine." *Int. J. Health Serv.* 7:37–61, 1977.

34. Stevens, John. "Physicians Took 47 Seconds for Diagnosis, Prescriptions." *Milwaukee Journal* March 8, 1977, p. 1.

35. Gottlieb, R. M.; Nappi, T.; and Strain, J. J. "The Physician's Knowledge of Psychotropic Drugs: Preliminary Results." *Am. J. Psychiatry* 135:29–32, 1978.

36. Jones, V. C. J. "The Routine Prescription of Diethylstilbestrol as a Postcoital Contraceptive in Rape Victims." Speech Presentation on the OB/GYN Advisory Committee of the Food and Drug Administration, January 30–31, 1978.

37. Ibid.

38. Thomas, C. "Mothers are DES Victims." *Public Citizen,* Spring, 1978, p. 3.

39. Hulka, B. S.; Cassel, J. C.; et al. "Communication, Compliance and Concordance Between Physicians and Patients with Prescribed Medications." *Am. J. Pub. Health* 66:847−853, 1976.

Over-the-Counter Medications: Bewitched, Bothered, and Bamboozled

Federal regulators aren't doing their job—ineffective and dangerous drugs abound and misleading advertising is commonplace • DOAN'S PILLS & PREPARATION H • **Phenacetin** in pain killers can hurt • **Saccharin** spells trouble • Diet-Pill Disaster • Sleeping pill nightmares • Hair dyes aren't harmless • How to be an informed consumer: building a reference library and stocking your own black bag • Taking care of your skin: safely stalk that elusive tan; zap the zits once and for all • Dietary indiscretion: surprising use of PEPTO-BISMOL • How to save money over-the-counter.

Once upon a time, not so very long ago, there existed across our land the Traveling Medicine Show. Promoters of such old favorites as Kickapoo Tonic and Barker's Nerve and Bone Liniment would put on a show that dazzled and delighted the curious crowds while hucksters sold the highly touted tonic. Most of the marvelous remedies were supposed to cure practically anything that ailed you— from hemorrhoids and "pain around the chest" to dandruff and constipation. Today sophisticated Americans scoff and smile knowingly at the naiveté, ignorance and gullibility of past generations taken in by those old-timey snake-oil peddlers. Instead, we huddle around the television set while a bunch of loonies sing "Plop Plop, Fizz Fizz" or some announcer authoritatively exhorts us to shrink the swelling of hemorrhoidal tissues with PREPARATION H.

When most people walk into a pharmacy these days they automatically assume that the non-prescription drugs they'll find on the shelves will be both safe and effective. That seems like a perfectly reasonable assumption since in 1962 Congress amended the Food, Drug and Cosmetic Act to guarantee all drugs would have to meet those basic criteria. Unfortunately, that assumption is false. Even though people demanded protection from unscrupulous promoters and Congress mandated change, our "protectors" haven't done their jobs. The federal regulatory agencies like the Food and Drug Administration and the Federal Trade Commission were given the responsibility of making sure that our present-day drugs are both safe and effective and that we are no longer subjected to deceptive or misleading advertising. Despite some progress, there are still a great many non-prescription medications on the market that have not been proven to be either safe or effective. According to the FDA itself, only about 50 percent of the ingredients available in over-the-counter (OTC) drugs have been demonstrated to meet those standards.[1] And much of the advertising ignores the spirit if not the letter of the law. What all this means is that every day we are throwing away good money on products that not only may do us little good but could actually cause us harm.

Americans spend about five billion dollars on over 300,000 OTC products each year.[2, 3] Three hundred thousand sounds like a tremendous number of different drugs. You could almost pity the poor bureaucrats at the FDA who have to monitor that many medications. Before you shed any tears, however, bear in mind that there is unbelievable duplication and repetition in the pharmaceutical marketplace. According to Dr. William E. Gilbertson, Director of the OTC Drug Evaluation Branch of the FDA, "there are only about 500 significant active ingredients used in all of these 300,000 products."[4] Take antacids for example. There are over eight thousand brands available to consumers but only about half a dozen actual acid-buffering ingredients are used in all those different antacids.

By now you would think that the FDA would have figured out which drugs worked and which didn't and which are dangerous to your health, especially since they have had almost twenty years to get cracking. Unfortunately, their track record is atrocious. In 1972 they geared up to start analyzing all major non-prescription products. Panels of experts were established which were supposed to bring together individuals with broad experience in each area of concern — cough/cold, internal analgesics (pain killers), laxative, antacid, contraceptive, hemorrhoidal, sedative, sleep aid, stimulants, and so on. At the time of this writing only the antacid panel has come to any final decisions and had them implemented. We are still waiting for the other groups to finish their investigations. And even when they finally do complete the task it will still be years before their recommendations are actually put into effect. Meanwhile, consumers will continue to be at the mercy of the modern-day "medicine show."

As for the poor Federal Trade Commission, the agency that is supposed to protect us from deceptive commercials on television, radio, and in the newspapers, forget it. The people there are well meaning and really want to reduce the misleading garbage you have to put up with whenever you turn on the TV or radio, but about the best they can do is stick their fingers in the dike while the crapola pours over the top. They have neither the manpower, budget, nor expertise to really monitor the advertising that spews forth in all media. And even when they do take action the advertisers fight back every inch of the way.

A perfect example is the Warner-Lambert Company, maker of LISTERINE. As mentioned in the Introduction to this book, when the FTC challenged the claim that their antiseptic mouthwash was good for sore throats and cold symptoms, this giant of the pharmaceutical industry dragged it into court and tied up the case and the Commission's resources for nearly a decade, wasting untold taxpayer dollars. The company finally agreed to corrective advertising in order to rectify the misleading ads of past years. The LISTERINE case was one of the few victories the FTC can brag about. The majority of the commercials are never even reviewed, let alone corrected.

Take DOAN'S PILLS, for instance. This "bestseller" cornered the backache market years ago. Commercials on television have always implied that there was something special about DOAN'S that made it perfect for relieving the sore muscles and pain of a nagging backache. Until just recently this "marvelous" remedy contained some extraordinary ingredients. Included in the green tablets were extract of Uva Ursi and extract of Buchu. Now, both of these old-fashioned remedies were once utilized as diuretics and as urinary antiseptics. Whether they were successful is anyone's guess, but even if they were it's unlikely such action would be of any benefit for a backache. In fact, about the last thing someone with a sore back needs is to run back and forth to the bathroom to pee.

The old DOAN'S also contained Theobromine, a chemical cousin of caffeine that is commonly found in cocoa and tea. Theobromine also has some weak diuretic effects and can, in large enough doses, stimulate the nervous system and the heart. Once again, such pharmacological action hardly seems beneficial for a nagging backache.

In addition to the diuretics, DOAN'S contained vitamin A, and as far as I can tell, this vitamin has never been shown to be useful for any sort of muscular disorder. Last, but not least, was Sodium Salicylate, an aspirin-like drug that may actually have provided some relief from pain if it was used in a high enough dose. Unfortunately, the amount of salicylate in each DOAN'S pill was equivalent to less than a third of an adult aspirin tablet. And while the instructions on the label were to take four pills four times a day, that was still less than a standard dose of aspirin.

But all that has changed. The old DOAN'S is gone. In 1979 DOAN'S came out with a "NEW FORMULA: America's leading pill for the relief of backache pain is now even better." It's hard to believe that anything could be better than Buchu or extract of Uva Ursi, but according to the television commercial, "New DOAN'S takes the ache out of backache." As we watch some poor woman grasp her lower back in pain we hear the following spiel:

> **Are you an overdoer? Someone who occasionally gets an over-doer's backache? Then you should know about new DOAN'S PILLS. New DOAN'S is stronger and starts to work faster than ever before. With a medically proven pain killing ingredient that relieves backache pain and strained muscles for hours. Remember new stronger DOAN'S. It takes the ache out of backache.**

Okay, what's in this new, stronger formula? Well, they did remove the Theobromine, Vitamin A, Buchu, and Uva Ursi. Instead of sodium salicylate they added magnesium salicylate, a pain reliever approximately equal to sodium salicylate or aspirin in analgesic potency. And for good measure they threw in a little caffeine, about enough to amount to a half a cup of coffee. This "special" analgesic is supposed to provide "temporary relief of backache, headache, muscular aches and pains due to factors such as overexertion, stress and strain." And the price for this new "stronger formula"? Well, I paid $1.29 in a local discount drugstore for twenty-four pills. For the same price I could have purchased almost three hundred aspirin tablets which probably would have been just as good for my theoretical bad back and would have avoided the caffeine which won't do a darn thing for a nagging backache and may make you jumpy. To say that DOAN'S is special for backache would be about the same as saying that aspirin was special for muscular aches due to overexertion. The makers of ANACIN, BUFFERIN, CAMA, COPE, and a host of other pain relievers might just as easily make the same claims. What bothers me most, however, is that many bad backs require professional treatment. Reliance on something simplistic like DOAN'S PILLS might delay appropriate diagnosis and therapy.

So even in our "enlightened" 1980s the consumer cannot believe the ad man's claims and there is no guarantee that all non-prescription medications on drugstore shelves will be safe and effective. One assumption does hold, however: the hucksters we see on television screens care little if at all about our health; their preoccupation is with profits.

You may be thinking that is strong language and wondering where's the evidence. For starters, let's take a look at hemorrhoidal preparations. To give you some idea of the magnitude of the pile problem, over $75 million is spent on more than 200 different brands of hemorrhoidal suppositories and ointments each year. Hemorrhoids are not nice. First, they can be very painful, and second, they are not considered a subject for polite company. Most people are easily embarrassed about "sensitive" body areas and hate to visit a doctor about such a problem, especially since hemorrhoid operations have a painful reputation and a high price tag.

As much as the victims would probably prefer to suffer (or obtain help) in silence, that is practically impossible since the makers of the most popular pile product, PREPARATION H, broadcast and publish their now familiar promise with great regularity: "Helps shrink swelling of hemorrhoidal tissues . . . gives prompt, temporary relief in many cases from pain and itching." If you don't recognize those famous words you have been living in a cave. With the kind of come-on this advertisement offers it's no wonder millions of sufferers use this product regularly.

What makes PREPARATION H so popular? The ingredients are unique, we'll give them that. There's shark liver oil for starters. It's terrific for sharks; they can't live without it, but I'm not convinced the slimy goo is any more effective than petroleum jelly when it comes to soothing inflamed tissues. Next there's live yeast cell derivative. Experts for the FDA did not find evidence to support claims that this ingredient speeds healing of hemorrhoids.[5] Last, but not least, is phenylmercuric nitrate, a mild antiseptic. According to the *Medical Letter on Drugs and Therapeutics,* a highly respected independent medical journal, "There is no acceptable evidence that any of these ingredients, alone or combined in PREPARATION H, can reduce inflammation, cure infection, or shrink hemorrhoids."[6]

When I called Whitehall Labs, makers of PREPARATION H, to get their side, I was told the *Medical Letter* quote was "probably correct." A spokesman confessed that there was "virtually no acceptable evidence," and that they "have not had good clinical studies on PREPARATION H." Needless to say, I was flabbergasted with such candor and I asked him if they had *any* research information at all to substantiate the advertising claims. I was referred to a study done at the University of California in San Francisco and I immediately headed for the library to check it out. The investigators did indeed study PREPARATION H, and interestingly, their results were favorable.[7] The yeast-cell derivative did seem to speed wound healing—in rats and rabbits. Now I don't know if rats and rabbits get hemorrhoids, but even if they do, the relevance of such a study seems questionable. Since the doctors weren't studying hemorrhoids at all, but rather surgically induced wound healing, I think it would be fair to say that any conclusions drawn from this rat research would have little bearing on human hemorrhoids.

Perhaps you're thinking, even if PREPARATION H isn't completely effective and doesn't always live up to advertising promises, at least it is safe. Well, I'm not so sure about that either. Remember I mentioned that the last ingredient was phenylmercuric nitrate. Although there is no evidence it will shrink hemorrhoids it does contain mercury, and as everyone knows, mercury is a highly toxic chemical. All forms are "poisonous if absorbed."[8] And it seems hard to imagine that some wouldn't be absorbed from a suppository since the sensitive tissue within the rectum can absorb almost anything that comes into contact with it. A panel of experts who reviewed OTC contraceptive products banned all mercury-containing compounds because they knew absorption from the vaginal tract could cause serious problems, especially if a woman became pregnant unknowingly. Here are some of the conclusions they came to about the spermicidal compound, phenylmercuric acetate (PMA):

> **Experimental studies on animals indicate that (1) PMA is readily absorbed from the vagina, enters the systemic circulation, and is distributed in various tissues of the body; (2) in the event of pregnancy, PMA and its metabolic product, the inorganic mercuric ion, are distributed in various tissues of the fetal compartment as well; (3) PMA is embryotoxic; (4) mercurial compounds are excreted in milk; and (5) PMA and mercuric ion adversely affect critical biochemical systems in the cells of most**

> tissues, particularly the nervous system. . . . the
> panel concludes that it is evident from the
> animal studies reviewed above that the use of
> PMA in vaginal contraceptive preparations is
> potentially hazardous to the human fetus and to
> the breast-fed infant.[9]

I have little reason to believe that the possible danger of phenylmer-curic acetate (PMA) absorption from the vaginal tract would be any different from the possible danger of phenylmercuric nitrate (PMN) absorption from the rectum, especially if a woman were pregnant.

Signs of chronic mercury poisoning are often hard to diagnose because they are subtle and creep up slowly. Symptoms may include weakness, fatigue, loss of appetite, weight loss, stomach upset, nervousness, irritability, and a metallic taste.[10] Various malformations have been reported after fetal exposure to mercury and there is little doubt in my mind that any woman who becomes pregnant should avoid all contact with mercury-containing products. That is why the PREPARATION H ads upset me. The makers actually go out of their way to pitch the product to pregnant women since hemorrhoids are often a common complaint during pregnancy. Although the level of phenylmercuric nitrate found in PREPARATION H is extremely low and no one knows if it's absorbed from these suppositories, even the possibility makes me shudder.

Since the FDA and the FTC don't seem to be protecting us, we consumers would do well to protect ourselves by preventing hemorrhoids in the first place. Hard stools and constipation that leads to huffing and pushing in the bathroom often aggravate the condition. A diet that is high in roughage and bran will go a long way toward preventing hemorrhoids in the first place. Oatmeal, whole wheat, prunes, raw fruit, vegetables, and bran cereals are often recommended. Lots of liquids can also be helpful. And for the immediate pain and itch a hot tub bath three or four times a day often works wonders. It can reduce irritation and facilitate the retraction of protruding piles. Some folks swear that a little witch hazel will also help eliminate these symptoms if applied to the tender tissues after each visit to the "john."

If you really start to suffer you might want to use something that truly will relieve inflammation. A cortisone cream (now available without a prescription by the name CORTAID) will usually do the job quite nicely. And if all else fails you really don't need to fear the surgeon's scalpel. A new procedure that can be done in the doctor's office has replaced surgery in many instances. It involves tying off the hemorrhoids with special rubber bands and is much less painful and expensive than surgery. Best of all, most people can resume normal activities almost immediately. So before you fall for the advertiser's banana oil remember that you can't count on the Food and Drug Administration or the Federal Trade Commission to protect you from hemorrhoidal preparations that have dubious benefits.

PAIN KILLERS CAN HURT

Even though hemorrhoids are a pain for people who have them, they provide a bonanza for the drug companies. But compared to analgesics, hemorrhoidal products are just a drop in the bucket. Each year over 1,000,000,000 (one billion) dollars is spent on over-the-counter pain relievers. If you add in prescription products like DARVON, DARVOCET, PERCODAN, and EMPIRIN WITH CODEINE the figure is astronomical. And once again, federal regulation has been lackadaisical.

The history of non-prescription pain killers in the United States is fascinating. Opium, morphine, and cocaine were the mainstays of patent medicines during the nineteenth century. Such sweet-sounding products as "Mrs. Winslow's Soothing Syrup" and "Godfrey's Cordial" were loaded with potentially addicting "relief." Billions of jars of these "women's friends" and pain killers were sold at traveling medicine shows, in groceries, general stores, pharmacies, and even through the mail.[11] It's hardly surprising that drug dependency became a problem for many very straightlaced Americans:

> **The ready availability of the opium-containing nostrums combined with misleading advertising and a general consumer ignorance of the drugs' hazards led to virtually thousands of cases of chronic opium intoxication and dependence during the two decades before and after the turn of the twentieth century. In 1900, for example, it was estimated that 3,300,000 doses of opium were sold every month in the state of Vermont alone—enough to provide every man, woman, and child in that state with a continuous daily supply of one and one-half doses. Reports from this period also suggested that the national population of those who had become physically dependent on opium well exceeded 200,000.[12]**

The Pure Food and Drug Act of 1906 slowly began to call a halt to the chaos of this patent-medicine madness of the 1800s. But even in the 1980s there are still abuses and the FDA has some way to go before Americans can rest easy. Are you aware that some of the popular pain remedies on your drugstore shelf or possibly in your medicine chest have been banned or restricted in Canada, Britain, Sweden, Denmark, and Australia? The problem is with phenacetin, an ingredient that has been popular in many prescription and over-the-counter analgesics. Long-term use of this drug can result in hazardous effects to the urinary tract and may ultimately lead to kidney damage.[13-17] We have known about the potential toxicity of phenacetin for over eighty years. What we didn't know was that it might cause cancer. Recent reports in the medical literature have raised a haunting new specter:

> **More than 100 cases of renal pelvic [kidney] tumors in abusers of phenacetin-containing analgesics have been reported in the literature... There are epidemiologic studies in humans and metabolic and experimental data in rats that strongly support the assertion that phenacetin is a carcinogen. We therefore question the justification of keeping such a drug on the market.[18]**

> **Although phenacetin is not as potent a carcinogen as some others to which we are exposed daily, we believe that its use in non-prescription analgesics should be banned. The ever-increasing body of data from animal and human studies concerning the metabolism, mutagenicity, and carcinogenicity of phenacetin is impossible to ignore. Swedish and Australian authorities have long since taken action to minimize exposure to phenacetin. The documented cumulative effects of carcinogens argues strongly for the reduction of exposure to phenacetin. Alternative analgesics are available.[19]**

Despite these strong warnings the FDA still allows both over-the-counter and prescription pain relievers that contain phenacetin to be sold. Fortunately, the manufacturers of ANACIN, EXCEDRIN, BROMO-SELTZER, GOODY'S HEADACHE POWDER, and EMPIRIN COMPOUND had the good sense to remove it from their products voluntarily, but many other drug companies still continue to market analgesics and cold remedies that contain this potentially dangerous ingredient. According to the 1979 edition of the *Handbook of Nonprescription*

Drugs, published by the American Pharmaceutical Association, the following products still contain phenacetin: A.P.C., A.S.A. COMPOUND, ASPHAL-G, CAPRON CAPSULES, PAC, SAL-FAYNE CAPSULES, S.P.C., CENAGESIC, HISTA-COMPOUND NO. 5, PYRROXATE, and RHINIDRIN. Prescription products that contain phenacetin include DARVON COMPOUND, EMPRAZIL, FIORINAL, NORGESIC, SOMA COMPOUND, and SYNALGOS.[20]

Although none of these pain relievers will cause kidney damage if used in low doses for short periods of time, they could cause problems if used in excess. And the FDA has concluded that phenacetin has a considerable abuse potential because it provides a slight euphoria and mild stimulation. In other words, people can get high. Factory workers in the southern part of the United States used to be able to purchase phenacetin-containing pain killers from dispensing machines right on the job. It has been suggested that the companies abetted drug abuse in order to increase work output. The result of this practice, however, is apparently showing up in a greater incidence of kidney disease.

An FDA panel of experts concluded as far back as 1977 that phenacetin "is not safe for OTC use because of the high potential for abuse, the high potential for harm to the kidney . . . and the lack of compensating benefits of the drug." They also suggested that it "should be removed from analgesic preparations."[21] But as usual, the recommendations are slow to be implemented and many drug companies will be slower yet in their willingness to comply. And doctors seem totally unaware of the problems they can create when they casually write prescriptions for potent pain killers. A letter that I received from one of our column readers tells a tragic story:

> I am an intense abuser of the drug "SOMA COMPOUND." Six months ago a doctor gave me a "standing order" (any amount I want anytime) after I complained to him of a tense neck due to nerves. Since then I've taken 500-600 of these pills (just bought another 100 today). SOMA COMPOUND makes me feel relaxed, confident and "high" after a certain point. At first 3 or 4 did the job . . . then 6 at a time—then 8. Twice I've taken 12 within two hours. Time flies on this drug. Errands and such that I despise fly by with ease. By now I feel I can't face a somewhat difficult day without a bunch. I am very psychologically addicted—feel as though I

> couldn't live without SOMA COMPOUND, nor do I
> want to. God . . . I pray I can get myself off this.

Anonymous, Seattle, Wash.

SOMA COMPOUND is no more addictive or dangerous than many similar medications. Some people are just more susceptible to drug dependence than others. Doctors should never give out open-ended prescriptions for potent, abusable drugs, especially when they can do such damage to the kidney. Until the FDA gets its house in order and eliminates phenacetin from both over-the-counter and prescription drugs consumers will have to take it upon themselves to use good judgment and restraint when using any combination product that contains this ingredient. Better yet, why not avoid phenacetin-containing drugs altogether?

Plain old aspirin will do the job quite nicely, thank you, and don't get snookered with claims of extra strength. Two 325-mg tablets (5 grains each) of aspirin are all you need for most minor pains. If you took ten pills they wouldn't take your headache away any faster or better and they could do a nasty job on your stomach. So when Whitehall Laboratories advertises that ANACIN has "more pain reliever (400 mg) plus a special combination of medical ingredients," don't fall for their line. All they've done is add an extra 75 mg of aspirin per tablet and 32.5 mg of caffeine, about as much as you would get from an average cup of tea. As far as I'm concerned, the only thing that's really "extra" is the high price.

SACCHARIN SPELLS TROUBLE

Sometimes when the Food and Drug Administration does act to protect the public their efforts may be blocked by politicians who know little or nothing about pharmacology or toxicology and who care more about corporate profits than people's health. On March 9, 1977, the FDA proposed the elimination of saccharin from foods and diet drinks because of scientific evidence that it caused cancer in laboratory animals. Public reaction was immediate and emotional; jokes flew fast and furious badmouthing the research findings. "Warning: saccharin may be hazardous to your rat's health" was one popular wisecrack. The politicians immediately realized that they had a great campaign issue and so they stood up for motherhood, apple pie, and the right to saccharin. A little lobbying from the soft-drink industry just put the icing on the cake and in a highly charged atmosphere Congress acted quickly to impose an eighteen-month moratorium on the FDA saccharin ban.

And so saccharin remained on supermarket shelves. It was everywhere—in soda pop, chewing gum, candy, toothpaste, and even medicine. And children were the prime targets since many consume huge quantities of sweets and sodas. They also take most of their drugs in liquid form and saccharin often replaces sugar to help make the medicine go down. Because they are smaller than adults, they receive a higher concentration relative to body weight. The effects of the artificial sweetener are probably cumulative, so prolonged exposure could cause damage that may take years to assess. Although saccharin is reported to be only a "mild" carcinogen in comparison to other agents, it may make people more susceptible to cancer from other hazardous substances. It's as if saccharin "primes the pump" by making the cells less capable of resisting other carcinogens. This is a process scientists have dubbed "tumor promotion." For example, smokers might be at greater risk of cancer than they normally would be if they were also heavy saccharin users.

Even though Congress acted to prevent a ban on saccharin it did ask the National Academy of Sciences (NAS) to evaluate all the research available and report back as soon as possible. The conclusions of the NAS weren't what the legislators wanted to hear: saccharin "must be viewed as a potential cause of cancer in humans." The Congressmen didn't like the findings of the National Cancer Institute (NCI) either. In the largest and most costly epidemiology research project of its kind ever undertaken, NCI scientists interviewed nine thousand people between 1978 and 1979. They wanted to find out if there was any link between heavy use of artificial sweeteners and bladder cancer. What they found just added more fuel to the fire. Those people who used six or more servings daily or who consumed two or more diet drinks each day had a 60 percent greater risk of bladder cancer than people who didn't use sugar substitutes.[22]

Cancer is not an act of God. Despite the fact that we are all tired of hearing about yet another carcinogen loose in the environment, most people are terrified of cancer. It's a disease that justifiably inspires fear:

> **One of every four Americans now living will eventually have cancer. During the 1970's there will be an estimated 3.5 million deaths from cancer, 6.5 million new cases, and more than 10 million persons under medical care for cancer. Every day 1,000 Americans die of cancer—that is, one person every one and a half minutes.[23]**

And most scientists now believe that "the majority of cancers, perhaps as many as 80 or 90 percent, are caused by substances in our environment—substances in the food we eat, the air we breathe, the water we drink, and the products we make and use."[24]

So even though it was easy to joke and laugh about rat studies and diet soda when the first reports came out, no one should be laughing now. Dr. Richard Bates, Assistant to the Director for Risk Assessment at the National Institute of Environmental Health Sciences, had this to say about saccharin: "FDA scientists calculate that even moderate use of saccharin over a lifetime by every American might lead to the possibility of up to 1,200 additional cases of bladder cancer a year. With thousands of Americans dying from cancer every day, this additional risk is one we can do without."[25]

It's about time legislators in this country forgot about economic interests and political expediency and allowed the FDA to do its job. They should follow the lead of the Canadian government in eliminating saccharin from food, diet drinks and most drug products. Until they do, parents should take it on themselves to regulate their children's intake of sweets, at least until some safer sugar substitute is marketed.

DIET-PILL DISASTER

Have you taken a look in the mirror lately? If you're like me, the tummy roll is a little embarrassing. Some folks may call it love handles, but me, I call it fat. According to the folks who should know (the makers of diet pills), "In the United States 80 million adults are overweight, 70 million want to lose weight, and 40 million dieted within the last year."[26] With such an alluring market you could guess the drug companies would do their best to satisfy our urge to eliminate those extra pounds. Walk into any pharmacy and in a corner somewhere you will find the "Weight Control Center." The ads appeal to the lazy streak in most of us, promising results with little or no effort: "LOSE FAT FAST—TAKE WEIGHT OFF—BE SLIM—NO DIETING, NO STRENUOUS EXERCISING, LOSE POUNDS IN DAYS." Sounds great. But what's in those diet pills and how safe are they?

The most common ingredient in non-prescription diet aids like DEXATRIM, PROLAMINE, APPEDRINE, ANOREXIN, GRAPEFRUIT DIET PLAN WITH DIADOX, and SPANTROL is a tongue twister called phenyl-propanolamine or PPA for short. It is a decongestant that is also found in many cold and allergy products such as ALKA-SELTZER PLUS,

ALLEREST, CONTAC, CORICIDIN "D," SINE-AID, and TRIAMINICIN. Because PPA is chemically related to amphetamine it does seem to have some ability to suppress appetite. But how much and for how long is controversial. Even the "high-powered" prescription diet drugs like BENZEDRINE, DEXEDRINE, PRELUDIN, FASTIN, and TENU-ATE are not terribly effective. The FDA-required package insert that accompanies these restricted diet pills tells the story best:

> **The magnitude of increased weight loss of drug-treated patients over placebo-treated patients is only a fraction of a pound a week. The rate of weight loss is greatest in the first weeks of therapy for both drug and placebo subjects and tends to decrease in succeeding weeks ... The amount of weight loss associated with the use of an "anorectic" [appetite suppressant] drug varies from trial to trial, and the increased weight loss appears to be related in part to variables other than the drug prescribed, such as the physician-investigator, the population treated, and the diet prescribed.**

It is hard to believe that an over-the-counter diet aid would be any more effective or long-lasting in its action than these prescription products. And since they lose their ability to suppress appetite within a few weeks it seems only natural that the non-prescription drugs would too. The respected journal *Medical Letter on Drugs and Therapeutics* unequivocally concluded that "There is no good evidence that phenylpropanolamine, oral benzocaine or any other drug can help obese patients achieve long-term weight reduction. The only satisfactory treatment for obesity is a life-long change in patterns of food intake and physical activity."[27]

Just because these drugs are of dubious value does not mean that they are not without risks. It has been known for a long time that PPA can cause nervousness, insomnia, restlessness, nausea, and headache. More recently the British medical journals have reported serious elevations in blood pressure. In a study of 140 healthy medical students there was a dramatic increase in blood pressure after only one dose of a non-prescription diet pill.[28] Approximately one-third of those receiving the active medication had their diastolic blood pressure go from 70 mm to over 100 mm and one person's pressure reached the dangerous level of 190/142. The students who had the greatest elevations in pressure also noted symptoms such as dizziness, palpitations, headache, chest tightness, rash, tremor, nausea, and lassitude. Remember that these were healthy medical students. I shudder to think what could happen in an overweight, middle-aged person with hypertension, especially if he were taking some other drug simultaneously.

Many medications can interact with PPA in a dangerous way. A hypertensive crisis (blood pressure of 200/110) occurred when one woman combined her arthritis drug (INDOCIN) with her OTC diet pill.[29] Doctors are also concerned that there may be problems when PPA is taken simultaneously with a blood-pressure medication like ALDOMET, antidepressants such as MARPLAN, NARDIL, and PARNATE, and possibly oral contraceptives. So, as far as I'm concerned, phenylpropanolamine is a dangerous drug and not a very effective way to lose weight. Let's face it, the answer to the spare tire is not in a pill—it's in ourselves. The most successful weight-reduction programs are those that utilize group support and insist on behavorial changes in eating patterns.

SLEEPING PILLS

Sometimes the Food and Drug Administration actually does protect the public by out and out banning of a dangerous drug. In 1979 the FDA eliminated the ingredient methapyrilene from OTC sleeping pills, daytime sedatives, and allergy remedies because it was shown to cause cancer in animals. (Most sleep researchers doubted that the non-prescription sleep aids provided much benefit anyway.) Over eight hundred products were pulled off pharmacy shelves, including ALLEREST TIME CAPSULES, ALVA TRANQUIL, COPE, COMPOZ, EXCEDRIN P.M., NYTOL, SOMINEX, and TRANQUIL CAPS. Drug companies were hopping mad about the loss of business and the threat to years of carefully nurtured advertising images. Many manufacturers rushed to salvage the reputation of their highly promoted products. The makers of such well-known sleeping pills as SOMINEX and NYTOL quickly moved to reformulate. Advertisements soon boasted of a "New Formula."

NYTOL promised to make you drowsy to help you "get the sleep you need," while SOMINEX billed itself as "The effective night-time sleep aid." While the ads may have been different, both sleeping pills contained the same identical ingredient—pyrilamine, an antihistamine that is chemically very similar to the banned drug methapyrilene. While there is nothing yet to indicate that the new ingredient is dangerous, there isn't very much data to support its value either. The head of the FDA has required additional testing to establish the effectiveness and safety of pyrilamine. In the interim, of course, the drug companies exhort us to buy the "new formula for safe, restful sleep." I sincerely hope that they're right.

Why can't people be protected from potentially dangerous products *before* they're marketed? Why should millions of Americans be guinea pigs for untested remedies, especially if the benefits are questionable at best? The law is quite specific. Drugs must be safe and effective—now! Not tomorrow, or next year, but today. It's incredible that we are exposed to so many medications that have neither proved their worth nor their long-term safety.

HAIR DYES AREN'T HARMLESS

Sometimes the FDA can't do anything about hazardous products even though it wants to. Despite a sizable amount of evidence that many coal-tar dyes found in permanent hair colors are carcinogens, the FDA is powerless to protect the public from their inclusion in hair dyes because of a law that was passed in 1938 which forever exempts these dyes from regulation. All the bureaucrats can do is warn people of danger. And many hair dyes may be more dangerous than you suspect.

During the early 1970s a pioneering biochemistry professor from the University of California at Berkeley discovered a quick-and-easy screening procedure to detect potential cancer-causing chemicals. Until Dr. Bruce Ames came along with his test-tube method of checking up on environmental agents, researchers had to perform long and expensive animal experiments or wait until so many people died that it was obvious the material in question was a hazard. Because it often takes cancers twenty or thirty years after exposure to a carcinogen before they become apparent the wait-and-see technique is outrageous. The Ames test quickly told researchers which chemicals caused changes in the genetic material of bacterial cells and sent up a red warning flag that the compound in question required further testing.

Because Dr. Ames was an innovative teacher as well as a superb researcher he sent his biochemistry students out to perform a fascinating experiment. Their task was to buy up hundreds of common household products and test them to see if any caused mutations in the Ames test. Fortunately, there were only two substances that turned up positive. No one was surprised to discover that cigarette tar caused changes in the genetic material of bacterial cells. But they were dismayed to discover that hair dyes produced mutations. In a follow-up investigation it was found that 150 out of 169 different hair colors were mutagenic.

As a result of Dr. Ames's initial work researchers at the National Cancer Institute undertook a large-scale study in order to verify or reject his suspicions. They also tried to pinpoint exactly which chemicals in hair dyes might be the culprits. After extensive animal tests investigators came up with some bad news for the cosmetic industry—Dr. Ames was right. Many of the dyes found in popular products were carcinogens. Their list contained names which were real jaw-breakers to pronounce: 4-methoxy-m-phenylenediamine (abbreviated 4-MMPD or 2,4-DAA); 4-amino-2-nitrophenol; 2-nitro-1,4-phenylenediamine; 2,4-toluene-diamine; Direct Blue No. 6; and lead acetate.

It should come as no surprise to learn that the hair-dye manufacturers raised a ruckus once they learned of the NCI report. They tried to belittle the significance of the research by claiming that it was ridiculous to test these chemicals by feeding them to animals since obviously humans never eat hair colors. That argument was quickly put to rest when the investigators proved that the dyes are easily absorbed through the surface of skin and scalp.

But the real proof of the pudding came when researchers began calculating cancer incidence in people who came into contact with hair dyes—beauticians and women who frequently colored their hair. Two studies uncovered a higher rate of lung cancer among female hairdressers than among other women.[30, 31] And investigators at New York University found that women over fifty who had used hair dyes for at least ten years had a higher incidence of breast cancer than non-users.[32] This study was particularly significant because it took into account both the amount of exposure the women had to hair dyes and the long lag time between use and the actual development of the disease.

In 1977 the Controller General of the United States offered the following report to Congress:

> **About 33 million women use hair dyes to temporarily or permanently change their hair color. There is increasing evidence that some colors used in coal tar hair dyes—the dyes most widely used—may carry a significant risk of cancer to users. Cosmetics, including hair dyes, are regulated under the Federal Food, Drug and Cosmetic Act. Exemptions in the act do not permit the Food and Drug Administration to regulate coal-tar hair-dye products effectively; they bar the agency from banning or restricting the use of cancer-causing coal-tar hair dyes.[33]**

Even though there is a clear-cut reason to ban suspect coloring agents, the FDA must resort to the only weapon it has—warning labels. In 1980, five years after Dr. Ames let the cat out of the bag, the FDA finally required the following caution on products that contained 4-MMPD (4-methoxy-m-phenylenediamine): *"Warning: contains an ingredient that can penetrate your skin and has been determined to cause cancer in laboratory animals."* [my italics]

So what? Warning labels have about as much effect as a *pffft* in the wind, you're thinking. Well, you'd be surprised. In the competitive world of cosmetics about the last thing anyone wants is a frightening label on their appealing package. Just the threat of such a caution caused most major companies to throw out 4-MMPD. That's the good news. But what about the reformulated products, are they any safer? Ah, there's the rub. According to *Consumer Reports* some of the manufacturers have perfected a molecular shell game that has the FDA and the National Cancer Institute discombobulated:

> **To avoid the warning label, Revlon took out 4-methoxy-m-phenylenediamine sulfate. In its place the company put 4-ethoxy-m-phenylenediamine sulfate (4-EMPD). You don't have to be an organic chemist to suspect that 4-MMPD and 4-EMPD may be very similar. To find out if the new chemical posed the same danger as the old one we consulted Dr. Benjamin Van Duuren . . . "There's not one iota of difference between their potential for causing cancer," said Van Duuren. Revlon, he said, had merely added three atoms to the 4-MMPD molecule to make 4-EMPD . . . When NCI testing shows that a chemical is carcinogenic, manufacturers using that chemical may replace it with an "analog"—a closely related chemical with properties similar to the original, but one not yet tested by the NCI. By juggling atoms this way, manufacturers can stay a step ahead of government regulators almost indefinitely.[34]**

Does all this mean that men and women are stuck with their yucky natural hair color forever—no dashing brunette, daring red, or bouncy blond? Does it mean dark roots or streaks of gray? Not necessarily. While it would probably be safer to opt for the natural look there are ways to minimize your risk. First, select a hair dye that has as few suspect chemicals as possible. Here is the list again:

**4-METHOXY-M-PHENYLENEDIAMINE (4-MMPD
OR 2,4-DAA)
2-NITRO-1,4-PHENYLENEDIAMINE
4-AMINO-2-NITROPHENOL
2,4-TOLUENE-DIAMINE
DIRECT BLUE No. 6
LEAD ACETATE**

We definitely do not recommend Revlon's SALON FORMULA COLORSILK. The expert consulted by Consumers Union found that besides making a mockery of reformulation the product contained 10 chemicals that were "potentially hazardous." Semi-permanent dyes, tints and rinses may be safer than the longer-lasting permanents and Clairol's LOVING CARE did not contain any ingredients that were considered human carcinogens. So our first choice would be LOVING CARE. It would also be wise to wait as long in life as possible before hopping on the hair-dye bandwagon. Once you get started the process can be almost addicting. You hate to see those ugly roots start to show so you go for the dye one more time. Limit the frequency of your indulgence. And don't spare the water during rinsing. If you like the frosted look it will probably be safer since there is significantly less contact between the dye and your scalp. And if you are pregnant let vanity take a backseat to safety. Wait till the baby is born and weaned before resuming your former look.

AND NOW A WORD FROM OUR SPONSOR

By now you may be thinking there isn't anything that's good for you. Perhaps you're one of those people who just throws your hands up in despair with the comment "Everything causes cancer, so what's the use of worrying! Bring on the cigarettes, saccharin, hair dyes, bacon, and damn the torpedoes." Or maybe you are at the opposite end of the spectrum and are paranoid about all chemicals. In that case your battle cry could be "I don't take anything!" If someone offered you an aspirin for a headache it would probably provoke a look of disdain. However, chances are you are none of the above, but rather a person caught in the middle, with only a lead balloon for escape. You read the frightening stories in the newspapers and magazines and tend to believe them but you don't know quite what to do. "To dye or not to dye, that is the question." Should you drink that diet soda and use SWEET'N LOW? Is everything you buy over-the-counter either ineffective or dangerous?

The answer is an emphatic NO: not everything is bad for you. In fact there are only a relative handful of problem drugs and chemicals compared to the number that are safe. Remember that of all the hundreds of household products that Dr. Ames's students studied only two (cigarettes and hair dyes) caused problems. Very few chemicals lead to cancer, but the ones that do deserve the headlines they receive and prudent caution always makes good sense. That does not mean you have to empty your medicine chest or throw the baby out with the Tris-treated pajamas. There are many safe and effective non-prescription drugs on pharmacy shelves. I am an advocate of informed self-care and I sincerely believe that most folks are capable of taking an active role in their own health care if only they are given the knowledge and tools to do so.

Before you start building up your own little black bag you should develop a resource library so you can become a knowledgeable consumer. You don't have to buy lots of expensive medical books; your local library should be well stocked with some of the treasures we are about to present to you. But *DO* subscribe to *Medical Self-Care* magazine. It is the finest publication you can purchase in order to find out about the latest self-care techniques and what resources (both written and human) are available. It can be obtained by sending $15.00 for a year's subscription to:

Medical Self-Care
Post Office Box 717
Inverness, Calif. 94937

Next, because you will need allies within the health-care community you should order the *Client Brochure & Self-Help Manual* from Dr. Walt Stoll. This doctor is incredible. He knows what is meant by physician/patient communication and more than anything he wants to keep his patients well by *preventing* illness rather than treating it. Here are just a few of the gems you will find in Dr. Stoll's brochure:

OBJECTIVES

To return the client to his rightful place as the most important member of the health care team.

A. To involve the client in decisions regarding delivery of health care.

B. To utilize client education so as to reduce costs and need for utilization of professional skills.

C. To forge communication into a clinical tool.

Your primary care facility is responsible for coordinating your total health program. This includes:

A. Giving you the opportunity to learn to: (1) prevent all preventable problems, (2) eventually manage all minor problems without professional input;

The object of a client/physician encounter is to transfer, from the client to the doctor, as clear a picture as possible of what the problem is; followed by a transfer back of, hopefully, appropriate knowledge and experience to *assist the client to solve his problem*. The patient is ultimately the one who does all the suffering, expends all the effort, suffers the consequences, or reaps the benefits of this encounter.[35]

It would be wonderful if we could all have Dr. Stoll for our personal physician, but since that isn't possible the next best thing would be to order his publication. Send $2.00 to:

Client Brochure & Self-Help Manual
Holistic Health Center
Walt Stoll, M.D., A.B.F.P.
1412 North Broadway
Lexington, Ky. 40505

Equipped with this extraordinary resource you will be in a powerful position to maximize your interactions with health-care providers and turn these people into your allies. Next, I recommend the Bible of the self-care movement—Dr. Keith Sehnert's *How to Be Your Own Doctor (Sometimes)* (Grosset & Dunlap). It became an instant classic. Not only will this wonderful book help you learn how to "listen when your body talks" but it provides some excellent tips on how to deal with minor ailments.

If you have children in your house then there are two books that I think are winners. First, *Healing at Home: A Guide to Health Care for Children,* written by Dr. Mary Howell, a truly excellent pediatrician, and second, *Child Health Encyclopedia: A Comprehensive Guide for Parents,* prepared by the Boston Children's Medical Center and Dr.

Richard I. Feinbloom. It can be obtained from Consumers Union for $7.50 by writing to: Consumer Reports Books, Dept. AA89, Orangeburg, New York 10962. And of course no home should be without Dr. Benjamin Spock's *Baby and Child Care*. Well I could go on and on about such favorites as *Take Care of Yourself* by Drs. Donald Vickery and James F. Fries or *Our Bodies Ourselves* by the Boston Women's Health Collective, *A Guide to Physical Examination* by Dr. Barbara Bates or so many more. Instead, order all the back issues of *Medical Self-Care* magazine and discover for yourself the vast number of excellent publications on the market.

Now you are almost ready to start shopping for a little black bag, but first you need some specific drug resources. Our number-one recommendation is a fabulous book compiled by the American Pharmaceutical Association called *The Handbook of Nonprescription Drugs*. It is surprisingly objective. This one is the self-medicator's Bible. Not only does it list the ingredients in most products, but it also gives an overview of the various families of medicines, such as asthma products, laxatives, menstrual products, antacids, and so on. There is no axe to grind and no effort to distort. The language is straightforward, though since it is directed toward the pharmacist you may find a few words you will have to look up in a medical dictionary. The book is a mite expensive but I think well worth every penny. It can be obtained by sending $20.00 to:

Handbook of Nonprescription Drugs
The American Pharmaceutical Association
2215 Constitution Avenue, N.W.
Washington, D.C. 20037

There is another book that is a good buy: *A Doctor's Guide to Non-Prescription Drugs* (Signet) by Morton K. Rubinstein, available at the time of this printing in bookstores for $1.95. Also high on our list of "*must haves*" is *The Medicine Show* by the Editors of Consumer Reports. A 1979 revised edition of this old friend will cost $5.50 including postage and handling. You can order it by writing to:

The Medicine Show
Consumer Reports Books
Dept. AA10, P.O. Box 350
Orangeburg, N.Y. 10962

If you just want an all-purpose dictionary-type reference for prescription drugs I highly recommend *The Pill Book* by Drs. Harold M. Silverman and Gilbert I. Simon (Bantam). This is the poor man's version of the *Physician's Desk Reference (PDR)*, which, by the way, is an unsatisfactory reference book. Very few people (and that includes doctors) realize that it is mainly advertising—drug companies have to pay to get their products into this behemoth. It is a sad commentary on the medical profession that it is most doctors' primary prescribing reference. The *Pill Book,* on the other hand, is easy to use and cheap—at the time of this writing the price is $2.95, one-fifth the cost of the *PDR,* and it even comes equipped with a color-photograph section that will enable you to identify commonly prescribed pills by color code. The drugs (over 950) are listed alphabetically by generic name. For checking out the nuts and bolts of the most common prescription drugs, this is one of the best—and certainly the lowest-priced—references on the market. It is widely available in bookstores. But you don't have to buy *The Pill Book* or any of the other books we have mentioned. Just have your local librarian order them for your reading pleasure.

Okay, *now* you are ready. Would you like a ready-made black bag? The "Black Bag of Medical Tools" can be purchased ready-stocked from the Health Activation Network, P.O. Box 923, Vienna, Virginia 22180. "It comes with a stethoscope, blood-pressure cuff, otoscope (for looking into ears), high-intensity penlight, oral and rectal thermometers, tongue depressor, dental mirror, a self-help medical guide by Keith Sehnert, M.D., and a sturdy vinyl bag in which to carry everything. Family health record forms and directions for using the black bag tools are also included."[36]

STOCKING THE MEDICINE CHEST

The first thing that you should not do is store drugs in the medicine cabinet. While that may seem like the most logical location, in reality the bathroom cabinet is the last place you should store medications. You don't believe me, right? Well, all you have to do to prove that the medicine chest is the worst place in the house to store medicine is look at yourself in the mirror after your next shower. You won't be able to see a darn thing and the reason is steam. Nothing can damage drugs faster than heat and humidity. But wait a minute, you might reply—if the lid to your medicine is on tight how can steam cause any problems? That's just the trouble, the lid to your medicine is not on as tight as you might think. Most prescription drugs and many over-the-counter medications come with child-proof tops and these safety closures are not always airtight. In addition, a lot of people who have trouble getting the lids off their medicine often leave the tops open to avoid the hassle.

So where should you store drugs, if not in the bathroom? Well, just about any place else is fine, as long as it's away from sunlight and heat. Perhaps a kitchen closet that is out of children's reach, or a high shelf in a bedroom. By the way, have you ever noticed how many drugs come with the caution to "store in a cool dry place?" What does it mean? According to the United States Pharmacopeia, cool is "any temperature between 46 and 59 degrees. If storage in a cool place is directed, the drug may be stored in a refrigerator unless otherwise specified on the label."[37] But not every medication should be stored in the fridge, since cold can damage some prescriptions almost as fast as heat. If room temperature is the order of the day then that means between 59 and 86 degrees. You might not think that temperature makes much difference. You'd be wrong. Oxacillin (BACTOCILL, PROSTAPHILIN) capsules should be stored at room temperature. But if your doctor prescribed the antibiotic in liquid form it would only last three days if stored between 59 and 86 degrees, whereas if you kept it in the refrigerator it would be good for two weeks. Always check with your pharmacist about proper storage conditions.

Wouldn't all this trouble be eliminated if we just got rid of those annoying child-proof tops? Nothing can drive a relatively sane person crazy faster than safety lids. True, but they save lives, lots and LOTS of children's lives, and as far as I am concerned any inconvenience is worth a young person's life any day! And if you don't have children you could always request the pharmacist to put your prescription in one of the old-fashioned pop-top containers. Better yet, request the new reversible caps. On one side they have a safety closure, but flip them over and they become a simple screw-off lid. If the grandchildren come to visit or a neighbor's child stops by you can rely on the protection of the child-proof side and when you are by yourself the easy-off side can be used. If your man with the mortar and pestle never heard of such a thing he is a pretty punk pharmacist. Just tell him to order these new containers for you from M&M Plastics, Inc.; P.O. Box 6134; Chattanooga, Tenn. 37401. And if there are toddlers or young children in the house, I highly recommend a drug "safe." One brand that I have only praise for is called MEDICO SAFE available from the Horchow Collection; P.O. Box 34257; Dallas, Texas 75234.

TAKING CARE OF YOUR SKIN

Almost everyone has problems with their skin at one time or another. Maybe a little rash or some itching or perhaps even a nasty case of eczema. If you went to the dermatologist the last time your skin acted up chances are very good that she or he gave you some sort of cream or lotion, and darned if it didn't work. What was that magical stuff? Well, almost inevitably it would have been a cortisone ointment. I don't know what dermatologists would do if we took away their "miracle" drug. Cortisone demands respect. It's a powerful drug, especially when used orally to treat difficult ailments like arthritis, lupus, or ulcerative colitis. When used in large doses for too long a period of time people experience all sorts of unpleasant side effects including greater susceptibility to infection, thinning of bones (osteoporosis), bleeding stomach ulcers, fluid retention, unattractive acne, muscle weakness, cataracts, nervousness, and mood changes. Despite these serious side effects and the fact that many doctors used to overprescribe it, it may surprise you to learn that the Food and Drug Administration recently approved the sale of mild hydrocortisone creams (CORTAID etc.) over-the-counter. How safe are such steroid drugs when they are applied to the skin? Can consumers really use such powerful medications without risk? To get an answer to that question I discussed these issues with our dermatological consultant, Dr. Stanley B. Levy. He pointed out that "topical" or local application of a cortisone or steroid-based preparation to the skin doesn't cause nearly the troublesome side effects people have experienced when they take these drugs internally. For the most part they can be used safely without fear of immediate or even long-term adverse effects.

Dr. Levy says that he can select from more than one hundred brands of cortisone in order to clear up skin problems that may range from a case of diaper rash and eczema to the much more impressive-sounding seborrheic dermatitis. Many of these medications are quite similar, but as a group they vary widely in strength when applied to the skin. Generally the potency of a given preparation depends upon the chemical structure. Fluorination of steroids greatly increases their ability to penetrate the skin and reduce inflammation. But like a double-edged sword, greater strength brings with it a higher risk of adverse effects. Prolonged use of the more potent fluorinated preparations can weaken and thin the skin, which makes it fragile and may bring on what seem to be stretch marks.

Now before you get nervous, keep in mind that many months of repeated use in the same area is needed before this problem is noticed. Some areas of the body are more sensitive than others, so be extra careful around armpits or in the groin where the folds of skin can trap the medication. This prolonged contact is what increases absorption. And if you use the more potent fluorine-containing medications too often on your face you may develop an acne-like condition that is very hard to treat. Initially, the drug appears to improve things, but in the long run it may be worsening the situation. A few extremely sensitive persons may develop burning, itching, dryness, and irritation in response to the lotion—the same symptoms they are probably trying to clear up, so some caution is necessary.

But all in all, cortisone creams have established an admirable track record over the last twenty years. They have brought excellent relief to millions of people by blasting minor inflammation and mild itching almost like magic. The FDA should be saluted for making **HYDROCORTISONE** available over-the-counter. I wouldn't be without some in my black bag. And I wouldn't go anywhere without my favorite skin book: *Manual of Dermatologic Therapeutics* by Kenneth A. Arndt, M.D. (available for $12.95 at the time of this writing from Little Brown, 34 Beacon St., Boston, Massachusetts 02106, or a local bookstore). However, this should not be interpreted as an "open sesame" to self-diagnose and treat every skin ailment that occurs. Many problems require professional attention.

STALKING THE ELUSIVE TAN

The sun is terrible for your skin. The dermatologists are absolutely right when they tell you that following Zonker's quest for the perfect tan will only lead to premature spotting, aging, wrinkling, and drying, not to mention a significantly greater sensitivity to cancer. Youth fades fast enough, you don't have to help it along. But how can you resist those glorious rays even with all of that? The answer to your dilemma is to compromise. There are now so many excellent sunscreen products on the market that no one need get a sunburn ever again. But there are also a lot of turkeys out there so you better shop carefully.

When shopping for a good sunscreen forget the sex appeal. Products with names like **SAVAGE TAN TROPICAL BLEND, SWEDISH TANNING SECRET LOTION, NATURAL WOMAN SUNTAN LOTION** and **HAWAIIAN TROPIC PROFESSIONAL TANNING OIL** rarely live up to the promise. Usually they contain only oils—mink oil, avocado oil, coconut oil, olive oil, baby oil—and oil won't do a thing to protect your skin from the sun. With all that grease on your body you will simply fry instead of broil. What you do want to look for is the "SPF" number you will find on most lotions these days. The FDA now requires manufacturers of tanning lotions to include on the label a Skin Protection Factor number so that consumers will be better able to match the correct kind of sunscreen with their particular skin. People who are especially sensitive should use a brand with an SPF number of 8 or higher. (The numbers range from 2 to 15, with the highest numbers offering the most protection).

My favorite brands are SUPER SHADE 15; ELIZABETH ARDEN SUN CARE 15 (which, by the way, is extremely water- resistant and won't come off so easily after a dip in the ocean); PIZ BUIN EXCLUSIV CREME; PABANOL; PRE-SUN; PABAGEL; and SUNGUARD. If you want a tan and don't want to burn, start exposure to the sun slowly—pamper that delicate epidermis. Start out with just a few minutes of unprotected basking (fifteen minutes max) and then smear on one of the really effective screening agents that will block out the nasty rays. That way your skin will react to the limited assault by darkening gradually over the course of a few weeks and there will be less damage overall. There is no reason why you have to look like a boiled lobster ever again.

TAKING THE ACHE OUT OF ACNE

Zits, pimples, papules, pustules, comedones, blemishes, white-heads—no matter what you call them, they're a bummer. We usually think of acne as the penalty you pay for passing through adolescence, but kids aren't the only ones who suffer. Adults are also susceptible and in recent years dermatologists have seen a rash of "post- pill" pimples in some women when they stop taking oral contraceptives. The acne may rear its ugly face a few months after the Pill has been discontinued and can affect women who never had a blemish while they were teenagers.

The reason that pimples often occur during adolescence is that this is the time when glands in the skin begin making a fatty substance that collects around tiny, invisible hairs. Going on and off birth-control pills may also stimulate an overproduction of oil. As dead cells and oil start to build up they can clog the pores of the hair follicles and it is this process that brings on the blemishes. Since it is all going on beneath the surface of the skin no amount of face washing will help pimples. In fact, excessive scrubbing can only add to the problem. Our dermatological consultants recommend ordinary hygiene: washing two, or at most, three times a day with a mild soap. (DOVE is a reasonable choice).

You can forget all those special diets too. There is no good evidence that avoiding milk, nuts, butter, or chocolate will make a darn bit of difference. And as for sex, that old devil will neither increase nor decrease the prevalence of pimples. You can make matters worse by gunking your face up with greasy makeup, however, so never use anything that would prevent your skin from "breathing."

What should the acne victim do? If he were to listen to the disc jockeys the answer would appear simple. All that is necessary is to buy the brand they're hawking and all skin worries will be over. Unfortunately, most popular brands are pure promotion. Many highly advertised remedies are of no proven value or contain ingredients in such low concentrations it is unlikely they will do much good. Pat Boone, for example, got caught in a nutcracker for advertising a brand that couldn't live up to the claims. Pat and his four daughters appeared on the tube claiming that the high-priced ACNE STATIN ($10 a bottle) was better than other pimple products. The Federal Trade Commission said baloney! Since neither the drug company (Karr Medical Products) nor Boone could verify the claims for ACNE STATIN they were forced to cough up "restitution" money to recompense product purchasers who might have been misled by the overzealous advertising. Karr paid $175,000, the advertising agency paid $60,000, and Pat Boone paid $5,000 for a grand total of $240,000.[38]

That ruling may have made other companies a little more cautious, but not much. If you can't trust the commercials where do you go? Well, by logic the treatment of acne should be directed at unplugging the oil glands which are at the root of the problem. Since it takes almost three months for an oil gland to plug up and rupture it takes persistence to clear up the skin again. In order to succeed you need plenty of patience.

Most successful programs rely on three different medications: benzoyl peroxide, retinoic acid (or Tretinoin), and antibiotics like tetracycline. A mild case of zits can usually be handled with just benzoyl peroxide which is available over-the-counter under various brand names including LOROXIDE, OXY-5, PERSADOX, TOPEX, and VANOXIDE. It does the job by drying and peeling the skin. Since it can be irritating when used in excess or after washing with harsh soaps or astringents you should be cautious. When starting, use the lower, 5-percent concentration and apply a thin film once a day or once every other day. If too much dryness or irritation occurs cool it for a few days. Usually the redness and scaling will disappear after continued use.

A more serious case of acne will probably require a dermatologist's use of retinoic acid (RETIN-A). This medication will actually loosen existing plugs and prevent the formation of new ones. It is a powerful tool and the backbone of most effective treatment programs. Unfortunately, many doctors don't take full advantage of this drug. Here is what Dr. Sidney Hurwitz, professor of dermatology at Yale, had to say about his colleagues' use of retinoic acid:

> **It is unfortunate that Tretinoin, perhaps the single most effective topical remedy for acne, is potentially irritating and is improperly used by so many physicians. Because of its known capacity to cause severe irritation and peeling, topical Tretinoin therapy should be started conservatively, on an alternate-day or, occasionally, an every-third-day regimen, preferably with the less irritating cream. If tolerated, this may then be gradually worked up to the more penetrating and slightly more drying and potentially irritating gel formulation. Patients should be instructed to wash with a mild soap, no more than two or three times a day, and to wait at least 30 minutes after washing (to ensure that the skin is completely dry) before the application of Tretinoin. If prolonged sun exposure is anticipated patients must be cautioned to use a sun-protective lotion.[39]**

Surprisingly, if you use both benzoyl peroxide and RETIN-A together (for example one in the morning and the other at night before bed) there may be less irritation than if you use just RETIN-A alone. And success is faster.

People who have a really bad case of acne or who have extensive pimples on their backs can benefit from antibiotics. It used to be that doctors immediately prescribed oral tetracycline and forgot about the problem. While it works quite well, prolonged treatment is not without side effects. Women may come down with vaginal yeast infections and this broad-spectrum antibiotic can cause stomach upset. Fortunately, a new development in therapy enables patients to apply the antibiotics directly to the skin and avoid all unpleasant side effects. Dermatologists report excellent results with topical clindamycin (CLEOCIN) and erythromycin. Topical tetracycline (TOPICYCLINE) works but it seems to be a little less effective than the other two.

The really big news in dermatology, however, is an experimental synthetic vitamin-A drug called ISOTRETINOIN (13-cis-retinoic acid). Reserved for very severe, resistant cases, this new oral medication can really clean up the skin. According to Dr. Gary L. Peck, a researcher in the Dermatology Branch of the National Cancer Institute:

> The antibiotic-resistant acne conditions of the first group of 14 patients now have been in remission for an average of 30 months. In the second group, 22 of 33 patients have been free of acne lesions for 12 to 18 months; the other patients have about 95% clearing of lessions... The first group of 14 acne patients had an average of 26 nodules or cysts before therapy in this study. After four months' treatment with an average dosage of 2 mg/kg/ day of isotretinoin in capsule form, 13 patients had complete clearing of their acne lesions and the 14th person had 75% clearing when last observed... Centers at which the retinoid is now being used experimentally for acne in this country are the University of Iowa, Iowa City, Boston University, and the Down State Medical Center, State University of New York, Brooklyn.[40]

ISOTRETINOIN is still in the experimental stages of development and won't be available for another year and a half. Before it is released for widespread use researchers must determine if there are any long-term side effects. Until then, be patient, and DO NOT take larger doses of vitamin A as a substitute. That vitamin can cause dangerous toxicity when used in excess and has not been proved effective for severe acne.

Even without this new therapy there is no reason for most acne victims to suffer anymore. Old-wives tales and high-pressure hip talk from record jocks won't make those nasty little red blips disappear. A well-informed doctor who is willing to take the time to work together with his client and create an individualized treatment program can help keep those zits at bay.

SAVING THE STOMACH

Indigestion is as American as apple pie, or pizza or sauerkraut or chili. Every year we fork over 500 million dollars on antacids in order to relieve our massive dietary indiscretions. It's hardly a mystery why we belch our way through life—Americans don't take enough time eating. Like everything else we do we gobble at a gallop. Every day one-third of the adult population eats out, and a big chunk of that is done at plastic fast-food joints. No wonder the burgers bite back.

The typically American solution to solving our dietary excesses is with antacids. And considering the way Americans casually consume these neutralizers you'd think they were perfectly safe and totally effective. For the most part you would be right. They do tame our troubled tummies without much in the way of problems.

Sodium bicarbonate, or baking soda, is a cheap and effective old standby. It wipes out excess stomach acid and is found in products like BISODOL POWDER, SODA MINT, and ROLAIDS (as sodium carbonate). ALKA-SELTZER also contains sodium bicarbonate coupled with aspirin which makes about as much sense as driving with your foot on the brake and the gas pedal at the same time. While the bicarbonate soothes the irritation the aspirin makes it worse.

Baking soda can bring relief from overindulgence, but it can also be a real problem for millions of people with hypertension or heart failure. Most people with high blood pressure are told to cut back their salt intake. Even a moderate reduction in salt can lead to a normalization of pressure for some people. This sort of regimen usually means limiting the diet to 1,000 milligrams (mg) of sodium each day. Good-bye Big Macs and fries, adiós anchovies, say so long to sauerkraut. One big handful of pretzel sticks or 3½ handfuls of potato chips contain around 1,000 mg of sodium. And a regular dose of "Plop Plop, Fizz Fizz" contains about as much—1,042 mg. If you were foolish enough to follow the suggestions on the label and consume the maximum dose recommended you would take in a whopping 4,168 mg in a day, which, as far as I am concerned is excessive even for a healthy person. The body requires no more than 200 mg of sodium a day in order to function normally. Although most people consume six to forty times that amount through their normal diets it is foolish to add to this sodium overload with a drug. Although there is a warning on the label that tells people "Do not use this product except under the advice and supervision of a physician if you are on a sodium restricted diet," I wonder how many people take the time to glance at that fine print. And even if they did, how many really would bother their doctors about something that seems as benign as plopping and fizzing? But long-term use of this sort of antacid could make high blood pressure worse or even precipitate heart failure in some very sensitive individuals. Even if you are in good shape I recommend that you only rely on the baking soda once in a while and leave the plopping and fizzing to the characters on television.

Calcium carbonate is another common ingredient in heartburn remedies. This antacid is found in ALKA 2, ALKETS, DICARBOSIL, TITRALAC, and TUMS. While it is fast-acting and safe in small doses, regular use can lead to constipation. There is also concern that large amounts of calcium carbonate may actually cause increased gastric acid secretion after three or four hours, thereby setting up a vicious cycle of antacid—acid secretion—antacid—acid, etc., etc., etc.

Aluminum hydroxide is one of the most popular constituents in antacids. It is available in AMPHOJEL, DIGEL, GELUSIL, MAALOX, and MYLANTA. Like calcium carbonate, aluminum could cause constipation in large doses. Most aluminum-containing remedies don't, however, because they usually contain magnesium as well, which has a counteracting laxative effect. Any combination of aluminum and magnesium is a pretty safe bet unless you are getting on in years and may be susceptible to weakening of bones. Aluminum antacids can make osteoporosis worse by depleting the body of phosphate, which in turn messes up the calcium balance and ultimately may weaken bones. Moderation should prevent problems.

TRAVELER'S DIARRHEA

PEPTO-BISMOL is the sleeper in the stack. It contains bismuth subsalicylate, an ingredient that the FDA has not been overly impressed with as an antacid. But for traveler's diarrhea this remedy is dynamite! Dr. Herbert Dupont, a gastroenterologist at the University of Texas Medical School at Houston, has been studying the effects of bismuth subsalicylate on American students attending summer classes in Guadalajara, Mexico. What he found was that a prophylactic course with this drug could significantly reduce the incidence and the severity of "turista":

> Diarrhea developed in 14 (23%) of 62 students receiving subsalicylate bismuth compared with 40 (61%) of 66 students taking a placebo. The protective effect of subsalicylate bismuth was apparent within a day or two of the study onset and became more obvious as the number of days at risk increased. The students treated with subsalicylate bismuth experienced fewer intestinal complaints and were less likely to pass soft or watery stools of any number. Once diarrhea occurred, enteropathogens were less

> commonly identified in stools of students
> receiving subsalicylate bismuth (33%) com-
> pared with placebo (71%). Subsalicylate
> bismuth was well tolerated by students during
> the 21-day trial ... We believe that since the
> current data indicate no overt side effects of
> subsalicylate bismuth administered for three
> weeks, daily subsalicylate bismuth is a reasona-
> ble means of preventing diarrhea for adults
> traveling briefly to high risk areas including
> Latin America, Asia, Africa, Eastern Europe,
> and certain Mediterranean countries.[41]

It seems very much as if there is finally some degree of protection
from traveler's diarrhea, otherwise known to travelers as "Mon-
tezuma's Revenge" in Mexico, "Delhi Belly" in India, and "the
Trotskys" in the Soviet Union. It is not entirely clear what the ideal
dose would be to prevent the cruds. The students in Dr. Dupont's
study took 60 milliliters (4 tablespoons or 2 ounces) four times a day
but less might work just as well. An editorial written by Dr. Sherwood
L. Gorbach in the *Journal of the American Medical Association
(JAMA)* recently offered this comment on Dr. Dupont's research:

> Sophisticated tourists know about unpeeled
> fruits, leafy vegetables, unsanitary drinking
> water, and—the most deceitful vehicle—ice
> prepared from unclean water floating in their
> mixed drinks ... Despite the possible limita-
> tions of subsalicylate bismuth, the study by
> Dupont et al. is, in my opinion, a most
> important contribution to this difficult problem
> of prophylaxis in traveler's diarrhea. It shows
> that a pharmacologic agent with low toxicity can
> prevent this disease. As the authors point out,
> this approach avoids the unpleasant side effects
> of antibiotics. Certainly, there will be other
> advances in this field, but the subsalicylate
> bismuth regimen is the first to offer safe
> prophylaxis to the beleaguered wayfarer who
> suffers the intestinal agonies of foreign travel.[42]

So my friend, if an occasional overdose of pizza and pickles doesn't
agree with you, go ahead and smother that smoldering volcano with
an antacid. And if you travel abroad, remember to check out the local
pharmacies for a good stock of PEPTO-BISMOL.

BRINGING HOME THE BACON

Most folks take non-prescription drugs for granted. They assume, incorrectly, that if a remedy doesn't require a prescription it must be innocuous. As I have already pointed out, that is not the case at all. Many of these drugs can be hazardous, especially if used incorrectly or by someone who is sensitive. For example, people with high blood pressure or glaucoma must be extremely cautious when it comes to using over-the-counter cough and cold remedies. Decongestants and drying agents may stop the sniffles but they can raise pressure within the eye as well as within the arteries and complicate successful treatment of these ailments.

What this means is that reading labels should become a matter of habit. And if the warning on the bottle says not to drive or operate machinery, take it seriously. You'll be inviting an accident if you think you can handle an antihistamine and still function effectively. Which is why I would never "give my cold to CONTAC." The ads tell you that six hundred tiny time pills will provide you with relief "all day while you work, all night while you sleep." But the warning on the label states unequivocally—"Do not drive or operate machinery." How, I wonder, do the makers of CONTAC expect people to get to their jobs if they aren't supposed to drive? Public transportation is not always convenient or available, and even if someone does make it in one piece, how are they supposed to work efficiently if the medicine causes drowsiness? Maybe if you are an advertising executive no one would notice that you were spaced out, but a telephone lineman, a construction worker, or a welder could get into serious trouble. As far as I'm concerned, the commercials don't match the cautions on the label. So stick with the warning and skip the claptrap.

For most people, shopping for over-the-counter medications is a little like playing blind man's bluff. Most products contain a slew of active ingredients with names that are virtually impossible to pronounce, let alone understand. Who but a pharmacist or a pharmacologist could pronounce *XYLOMETAZOLINE* (a nasal decongestant), *CETYLPYRIDINIUM* (an antibacterial found in throat lozenges), or *OCTYLDIMETHYLAMINOBENZOIC ACID* (a sunscreen) without stumbling. Just attempting to say these drugs could dislocate a virgin tongue. So most folks just skip trying to read the label, or shop comparatively and pick the brand they see advertised most often on television. Which is how come DOAN'S PILLS, COMTREX, EX-LAX, TYLENOL, TUMS, and ANACIN have become such big winners.

People know that they can save money by asking their doctor to write generic prescriptions instead of brand names or by getting the pharmacist to substitute equivalent generic medications. But few people realize that they can save a whole lot more by buying generic equivalents in over-the-counter medications. DOAN'S PILLS can cost one hundred times more than the house brand of aspirin and as far as I can tell, won't be any more effective in "taking the ache out of backache."

You don't have to be able to pronounce the names of the ingredients to shop wisely and save money. Just grab a handful of similar products and compare labels. Chances are that they will all have pretty much the same stuff anyway. Remember, there are over 300,000 different products available over-the-counter but only about 500 actual active ingredients in most remedies. So in most cases there is incredible duplication. For example, the following OTC contraceptives all contain the spermicide nonoxynol 9: BECAUSE, CONCEPTROL, CONTRA-FOAM, DALKON, DELFEN, EMKO, ENCARE OVAL, KOROMEX, SEMICID, and S'POSITIVE. If I were shopping for a spermicidal contraceptive I would look for the foam with the highest concentration of nonoxynol 9 at the lowest price.

The same thing would hold true if I wanted an acne treatment. I would look for all the products with benzoyl peroxide (BENOXYL, CLEARASIL ANTIBACTERIAL ACNE LOTION, DRY AND CLEAR ACNE CREAM, LOROXIDE, OXY-5, OXY-10, PERSADOX, PERSADOX-HP, TOPEX, and VANOXIDE) and then I would compare prices. It is ludicrous to pay through the nose for a high-priced ad-agency's blitz. And the best way to defend yourself from their razzmatazz is to go to the pharmacy armed with a list of the ingredients you want. Copy down the names or take along a reference book if need be so you can shop intelligently. Not only will you get safer, more effective medications but you will save gobs of money as well.

What about the pharmacists? Can't they supply useful information? Yes and no. It pretty much depends upon the individual you are dealing with. Pharmacists are caught in a classic double bind. They are highly trained professionals who are more than capable of supplying accurate and useful information about prescription and over-the-counter medications. Better yet, they can tell you when to skip a pill and allow the body to heal itself. But there is the little matter of money. Pharmacists are also business people who rely on the sale of these products to survive. If they tell you to avoid a laxative and eat a proper diet instead, there go the profits. Or if they recommend the cheaper house aspirin over the most expensive brand-name pain reliever, they lose dollars. So on the one hand there is the ethical responsibility to provide safe and effective medications at the lowest price to the consumer, while on the other there is the need to survive economically.

In my opinion it's possible to do both and that's why you should shop for a pharmacist you can trust just the way you would shop for a doctor or a lawyer. You want someone who can talk to you in plain language you can understand and who will watch out for your welfare. A good pharmacist won't stock garbage and will tell you when to avoid a drug entirely even if it means a lost sale. And if the pharmacist is really on the ball she or he will keep a "patient profile" that will keep track of every medicine you are taking, both prescription and OTC. She will never allow a clerk to hand you the prescription after it has been filled but will give it to you personally and tell you how to take it and what side effects to be alert for. And a good pharmacist will never be too busy to answer your questions with a smile. When you find someone like this, treasure him or her and be willing to pay a little bit more for the valuable service you receive.

Finally, and most important of all, remember that before you treat any "minor" ailment with a drug, very few non-prescription medications can cure anything. They generally tend to mask symptoms. Sometimes that's fine. If you are suffering from a headache or menstrual cramps there is no reason to tough it out if two aspirins will make you feel well again. And if you occasionally pig out at meal time and suffer a case of indigestion, there is no reason in the world not to seek relief with an antacid. However, some symptoms are alerting you to take action. If you have serious bad breath it would be foolish to continue to gargle with LISTERINE or SCOPE instead of trying to track down the reason for the problem. It would be equally reckless to treat a persistent hack with a cough remedy and ignore the cause of the discomfort.

Informed self-care requires solid information, common sense and the smarts to know when to discontinue treatment and seek professional attention. Let's hope you are now a little better prepared to resist the commercials and take a giant step down the road to becoming a knowledgeable consumer.

REFERENCES

1. Lessing, Melvin. "Influences Affecting Self-Medication: The Government's Viewpoint." Presentation to the 23rd Annual Ohio Pharmaceutical Seminar, April 24–26, 1978, Ohio State University.

2. "Annual Consumer Expenditures." *Drug Topics* June 1, 1979, pp. 26–29.

3. Hecht, Annabel. "Progress Report: The OTC Drug Review: (An Interview with Dr. William E. Gilbertson, Director of OTC Drug Evaluation). *FDA Consumer* 13(1):18—22, 1979.

4. Ibid.

5. "Tentative Findings of the FDA OTC Panel on Hemorrhoidal Drug Products," Information Copy, 1977.

6. "Preparation H." *Med. Letter* 18:108, 1976.

7. Goodson, William; Hohn, David; Hunt, Thomas K.; and Leung, Daniel Y. K. "Augmentation of Some Aspects of Wound Healing by a Skin Respiratory Factor." *J. Surg. Res.* 21:125—129, 1976.

8. Gosselin, Robert E.; Hodge, Harold C.; Smith, Roger P.; and Gleason, Marion N. *Clinical Toxicology of Commercial Products* 4th ed., Baltimore: Williams and Wilkins, 1978.

9. "OTC Contraceptives and Other Vaginal Drug Products," Information Copy, November, 1978.

10. Koos, Brian J., and Longo, Lawrence D. "Mercury Toxicity in the Pregnant Woman, Fetus, and Newborn Infant." *Am. J. Obstet. Gynecol.* 126:390—409, 1976.

11. Inciardi, James A. "Over-the-Counter Drugs: Epidemiology, Adverse Reactions, Overdose Deaths, and Mass Media Promotion." *Addictive Diseases: An Internal. J.* 3(2):253—272, 1977.

12. Ibid., p. 255.

13. Ferguson, Ian, et al. "Aspirin, Phenacetin, and the Kidney: A Rheumatism Clinic Study." *Med. J. Austral.* 1:950—954, 1977.

14. Wilson, D. R., and Gault, M. H. "Analgesic Nephropathy." *Can. Med. Assoc. J.* 117:16 (July 9), 1977.

15. Kincaid-Smith, Priscilla. "Analgesic Nephropathy." *Kidney International.* 13:1—4, 1978.

16. Molland, Elizabeth Ann. "Experimental Renal Papillary Necrosis." *Kidney International.* 13:5—14, 1978.

17. Carro-Ciampi, Giovanna. "Phenacetin Abuse: A Review." *Toxicology* 10:311—339, 1978.

18. Johansson, Sonny, and Angervall, Lennart. "Carcinogenicity of Phenacetin." *Science* 204:130, 1979.

19. Vaught, J. B., and King, C. M. "Phenacetin Studies." *Science* 206:637—639, 1979.

20. Corrigan, L. Luan, ed. *Handbook of Nonprescription Drugs.* Washington, D. C.: American Pharmaceutical Association, 1979.

21. "OTC Drugs, Establishment of a Monograph for OTC Internal

Analgesic, Antipyretic and Antirheumatic Products." *Federal Register* 42(131):35346—35494, 1977.

22. Associated Press. "Saccharin Danger Reported Real." *Durham Sun* December 21, 1979, p. 6C.

23. Culliton, Barbara J., and Waterfall, Wallace K. *Cancer,* Washington, D.C.: American Association for the Advancement of Science, p. 4.

24. "Saccharin: Where Do We Go From Here." *FDA Consumer* 12(3):16—21, 1978.

25. Interview between Timothy Larkin, Special Assistant to the Commissioner of Food and Drugs, and Dr. Richard Bates. "Animal Tests and Human Health." *FDA Consumer,* September, 1977, pp. 12—15.

26. Martin, Frances. "Diet Aids: New Reason For Close Counseling." *Drug Topics* January 18, 1980, pp. 45—50.

27. "A Nasal Decongestant and a Local Anesthetic for Weight Control?" *Medical Letter* 21(16):65—66, 1979.

28. Horowitz, J. D., et al. "Hypertensive Responses Induced by Phenylpropanolamine in Anorectic and Decongestant Preparations." *Lancet* 1:60—61, 1980.

29. Lee, K. Y.; Beilin, L. J.; and Vandongen, R. "Severe Hypertension After Ingestion of an Appetite Suppressant (Phenylpropanolamine) with Indomethacin." *Lancet* 1:1110—1111, 1979.

30. Garfinkel, J.; Selvin, S.; and Brown, S. M. "Possible Increased Risk of Lung Cancer Among Beauticians." *J. Natl. Cancer Inst.* 58:141—143, 1977.

31. Menck, H. R., et al. "Lung Cancer Risk Among Beauticians and Other Female Workers." *J. Natl. Cancer Inst.* 59:1423—1425, 1977.

32. Shore, Roy E., et al. "A Case-Control Study of Hair Dye Use and Breast Cancer." *J. Natl. Cancer Inst.* 62:277—283, 1979.

33. Report of the Controller General of the United States. "Cancer and Coal Tar Hair Dyes: An Unregulated Hazard to Consumers." December 6, 1977.

34. "Are Hair Dyes Safe?" *Consumer Reports* 44(8):458—460, 1978.

35. Stoll, Walt. "Patient Brochure & Self-Help Manual." Lexington, Kentucky, 1979.

36. "Black Bag Changes." *Med. Self-Care* No. 5, p. 46.

37. Lipman, Arthur G. "Temperature Requirements for Drugs Storage." *Mod. Med.* 45(14):103, 1977.

38. "Acne-Statin Mfr.'s Consent Agreement with FTC Establishes Trust Fund." *FDC Reports—The Pink Sheets* 41(28):T&G-9—T&G-10, 1979.

39. Hurwitz, Sidney. "Acne Vulgaris." *Am. J. Dis. Child.* 133:536—544, 1979.

40. Gunby, Phil. "Experimental Retinoid Effective in Treatment of Severe Acne." *JAMA* 243:11, 1980.

41. Dupont, Herbert L. "Prevention of Traveler's Diarrhea (Emporiatric Enteritis) Prophylactic Administration of Subsalicylate Bismuth." *JAMA* 243:237—241, 1980.

42. Gorbach, Sherwood L. "How to Avoid Running With Escherichia Coli." *JAMA* 243:260—261, 1980.

DRUG INTERACTIONS
Eat, Drink and Be Wary!

Drug incompatibility with foods and beverages: **Ampicillin, Amoxicillin, Aminophylline, Aspirin,** COUMADIN, **Digoxin, Erythromycin,** INDERAL, LANOXIN, **Theophylline**, laxatives, antacids, blood pressure medicines and so many more ... ● Smokers metabolize drugs differently ● Heartbreaking case histories ● Drugs that mess up laboratory test results ● Drug Interaction Tables, for easy reference: Food/drug, Alcohol, Antacids, Aspirin, Cold Remedies, Asthma Drugs, Diarrhea Medication, Digitalis, Hypertension Medicine, Pain Relievers, Thyroid Hormones.

Drug interactions are complicated, confusing, and the complexities can be downright mind-boggling. There are so many combinations and permutations that it practically takes a computer to sort out the whole thing. It's no wonder that doctors sometimes throw their hands up in despair. One drug may cancel out the benefits of another. For example, some tuberculosis medications can reduce the effectiveness of birth-control pills and lead to an unwanted pregnancy. On the other hand, one drug may amplify the side effects of a second drug. Antihistamines may magnify the incoordination and drowsiness often caused by sedatives. For example, the combination of CONTAC for a cold and VALIUM for nerves could be lethal if you got in your car and tried to drive. In some instances the combination of two or more drugs could create a totally unexpected reaction. If a woman who was taking a drug called FLAGYL for a vaginal infection also had a few drinks, she might discover some very unpleasant side effects: headache, flushing, nausea, and vomiting. Vitamins can alter the effectiveness of certain drugs and some medicines really mess up nutritional levels. Even food can dramatically alter the fate of your medicine.

Doctors have a terrible time with drug incompatibilities. For one thing, there is just too much information to memorize. A physician who is rushed may not take the extra effort to check for possible interactions. Another problem is that doctors rarely know what non-prescription drugs their patients are taking. Laxatives, pain killers, and cold remedies are just a few of the over-the-counter medications that can have a profound effect upon prescription drugs. If the doctor doesn't ask about these "unofficial" products, a dangerous interaction could occur. And since physicians generally look down their noses at patients' interest in vitamins, most folks are reluctant to mention that they take a B complex, vitamin C, or vitamin D. But this kind of incomplete communication is guaranteed to cause problems.

FOOD AND DRINK

Now you would think that something as basic as how to take your medicine would be obvious, straightforward, and at your doctor's fingertips. Guess again. In researching this chapter we were absolutely amazed to discover that there is an appalling scarcity of information about drug-food relationships. That doesn't mean they don't exist; just that people don't know about them. The doctor's "Bible" for prescribing advice, the *Physician's Desk Reference (PDR)*, is a poor resource. It's no wonder that doctors resort to ambiguous and amorphous instructions like: "Take four times a day." Is that every six hours, and if so does that mean you are supposed to get up in the middle of the night? Or how about: "Take before meals"? What does that mean anyway? It could be five minutes, half an hour, or two hours before meal time. And how many times has your doctor told you whether to take the medicine with water, juice, or milk? If you can't answer these questions, then you haven't been getting enough specific information.

If all this seems confusing, it is. But don't despair. Our goal is to try to bring some clarity to this chaos. Let's take a magical mystery tour through the incredibly complicated world of food and drug interactions. With a little luck we may even slay the Jabberwock and come galumphing back.

In order to get those tablets and capsules into your stomach in the first place you have to swallow them with something. (There are a few people out there who can pop a pill without any liquid, but because pills can easily get stuck in the esophagus and cause problems there, that is just plain silly. So let's forget it and deal with the more common practice.) Most folks choose a beverage pretty much at random, unless they have a super doc who gives specific instructions. They need something to help the medicine go down, so they reach for whatever is handy. In the morning it might be a glass of orange or grapefruit juice with breakfast; at lunch a glass of milk or a soft drink. We even heard about one old codger who took his blood-pressure pill and his vitamins with a shot of whiskey. Well, watch out! The liquid you use to chug-a-lug your medications can make a big difference in how well they do their job once they hit your stomach.

Fruit and vegetable juice, soda pop, and wine are all acid drinks. They reduce the effectiveness of some important antibiotics including ampicillin, erythromycin, and penicillin.[1] On the other hand, juice that is high in vitamin C is an excellent choice if you have to take an iron supplement. Ascorbic acid improves the absorption of iron. But watch out for milk. It doesn't mix with iron and quite a few other drugs.

We thought the whole world knew that cow's milk fouls up the proper absorption of tetracycline antibiotics so that the drugs don't get into the bloodstream adequately and are ultimately less effective. Well, we were wrong. Periodically we hear from someone who was never told by a doctor or a pharmacist to avoid this combination.

Milk is also a poor choice if you use bisacodyl laxatives. BISACODYL, DULCOLAX, or FLEET Bisacodyl should not be taken within one hour of milk or antacids since these drugs may not dissolve correctly in your stomach if you create an alkaline environment. The presence of the laxative in the stomach without its protective enteric coating may cause gastritis.

As bad as milk is for some drugs, it can be very good for medications that are irritating to your gut. Aspirin will do less damage when taken with a full glass of milk. We have said it before and we'll say it again: take a mouthful of milk, pop in two aspirin tablets, and chew them up with the milk. Then wash the whole mess down with the rest of the glass. Seems terrible, but it will make your tummy happier. Potent arthritis remedies are also less likely to injure your innards when you take them with milk.

Whoops! We promised clarity and here we are getting things tangled up already. Fruit juice is good for some drugs but bad for others. Milk may interfere with antibiotic absorption but if you are taking a potent arthritis medication milk can be helpful because it may reduce some of the irritation. All right, before your brain gets fuzzy, relax: there is a table at the end of this chapter that summarizes all this drinking and drugging stuff and will help bring the picture into focus.

TRUSTY H$_2$0

As a general rule, it is always safe to take a drug with a glass of water (especially if it's an antibiotic). Now many people are concerned with conservation these days and instead of drinking the whole glassful they may glug the medicine down with one frugal swallow. That can be a real mistake. Take a drug like erythromycin (BRISTAMYCIN, E-MYCIN, ERYTHROCIN, ETHRIL, ILOTYCIN, PEDIAMYCIN, ROBIMYCIN) for example. Skimping on liquid can reduce the amount of drug that gets into your bloodstream by as much as one-half. [2] Another antibiotic called amoxicillin (AMOXIL, LAROTID, POLYMOX, TRIMOX) can also be affected by how much you drink when you swallow the capsule. Even aspirin is sensitive to your fluid intake. If you want the drug to go to work as fast as possible don't economize on water and never chew or swallow your aspirin dry (it can irritate gums). Since it is sometimes hard to convince children to "drink it all down," take a little extra time and try some gentle persuasion.

While all of this may not seem monumental, it really is terribly important. What it means is that unless you take in enough water the proper doses of medicine may never reach your bloodstream in high enough concentrations and may never do its job effectively. If you had an infection, that could prolong the illness. The doctor could be left shaking her head in bewilderment because her prescription hadn't done the job. So, if you want to be on the safe side, guzzle those pills with an eight-ounce glass of water.

WHEN DRUG MEETS FOOD, WATCH OUT!

Well, what about food? There is shockingly little known about effects of diet upon medications. Information supplied by pharmaceutical companies is often woefully inadequate and doctors may not be able to provide patients with specific instructions on how to take a particular drug. There are many foods that can practically wipe out the benefits of certain prescriptions. Neither the patient nor the physician would be able to explain a therapeutic failure that might result from this sort of interaction. The time you take your medicine in relation to when you eat can also influence the treatment outcome as can the type of food you eat. For example, a high carbohydrate meal may slow down the absorption of a pain killer like TYLENOL and delay headache relief. Even the way in which food is prepared can have an effect on drugs. A fried-chicken dinner increases the effectiveness of an antifungal agent like FULVICIN (griseofulvin) while if the same chicken were broiled it would be of no benefit. (This is because fatty food significantly facilitates absorption.) If you would like to get an overall bird's-eye view of which drugs are best with food take a look at the handy-dandy guide found at the end of this chapter, pages 77–81.

Some drugs are very irritating to the digestive tract. Taken on an empty stomach they can cause pain, nausea, vomiting, diarrhea, and ulcers. Arthritis medications are particularly notorious for this problem. Drugs like BUTAZOLIDIN, CORTISONE, DECADRON, DELTASONE, INDOCIN, MOTRIN, OXALID, STERAZOLIDIN, and TANDEARIL are just a few that cause less irritation when buffered by food. Asthma medicines like AMINOPHYLLINE, BRONDECON, BRONKOTABS, MARAX, QUADRINAL, TEDRAL, and THEOPHYLLINE are irritating to the stomach and should generally be taken during or after meals or with a snack. Even iron supplements are better when taken with a meal.

Many medications will be incompletely absorbed (and therefore less effective) if you swallow them within a few hours of a meal. Antibiotics are particularly susceptible. Tetracycline, penicillin, ampicillin, amoxicillin, and erythromycin are some broad categories that should almost always be taken on an empty stomach. The anti-Parkinson drug, LEVODOPA, and the tuberculosis medicine, ISONIAZID (INH) may be less effective when swallowed close to meal time. *By the way, the instructions "Take on an empty stomach" usually mean at least one hour before meals or at least two hours after eating.* If a drug isn't irritating, most doctors tend to recommend this approach in order to guarantee therapeutic blood levels and a successful treatment program. But lately we are discovering a growing list of drugs that are actually absorbed more completely if they are taken with food. This is shaking up traditional practices and forcing everyone to re-examine the whole foundation of their prescribing instructions. A few drugs that may be absorbed more effectively with food include ALDACTAZIDE, ALDACTONE, ALDORIL, APRESOLINE, DILANTIN, DYAZIDE, ELIXOPHYLLIN, FULVICIN, GRIFULVIN, GRISACTIN, HYDRALAZINE, HYDRODIURIL, INDERAL, LOPRESSOR, MACRODANTIN, MARAX, QUIBRON, SER-AP-ES, and TEDRAL.[3]

As the eminently respectable *British Medical Journal* stated the problem in a recent editorial:

Despite recent improvements in the information provided about drugs, comparatively few data sheets say whether the product should be taken with food or on an empty stomach—though food

> may have any one of several effects on the
> processes which determine bioavailability. Most
> studies have been based on single doses of
> drugs, and we need more work on patients
> taking regular medication. [4]

One of the leading authorities on food and drug interactions is Dr.
Peter Welling at the University of Wisconsin School of Pharmacy. He
has made some extremely important observations on the subject and
concluded:

> Food may have varied influences on drug
> absorption, from a significant increase—as with
> griseofulvin, nitrofurantoin, and lithium ion—
> to a marked decrease—as with ampicillin pro-
> pantheline [PRO-BANTHINE], and some tetracyc-
> line. It is also apparent—as observed with
> penicillin V and alcohol—that the time interval
> between eating and dosing can change the
> intensity of drug-food interaction. The reports
> on acetaminophen [TYLENOL, DATRIL, DAR-
> VOCET, etc.], also show that specific dietary
> components may influence drug absorption in
> different ways . . . Evidence has been presented
> that drug-food interactions may vary with the
> type and size of meal, the time interval between
> eating and dosing, the volume of fluid ingested
> with a drug, and the . . . forms in which the drug
> is dosed . . . For drugs like some tetracyclines,
> propantheline, levodopa, and some penicillin
> and erythromycin products, drug-food interac-
> tions could cause depressed circulating drug
> levels and may result in therapeutic failure.[5]

To bring some order to this chaos we dug deep into the
pharmacological literature in order to find out which medications
should be taken with meals and which should be swallowed on an
empty stomach. You should confirm these recommendations with
your doctor.

DRUGS THAT MAY BE ADVERSELY AFFECTED BY FOOD

Food can interfere with the proper absorption of many drugs. Unless otherwise directed, it is usually a good idea to take medicine on an empty stomach with a full eight-ounce glass of water. The following medications are particularly susceptible to the effects of food. Absorption may be impaired and the effectiveness of the drug reduced. Check with your doctor or pharmacist for specific instructions. If you are supposed to take a drug on an "empty stomach" it usually means at least one hour before meals or two hours after eating.

AMPICILLIN
- Alpen
- Amcill
- Omnipen
- Pen A
- Penbriten
- Pensyn
- Polycillin
- Principen
- SK-Ampicillin
- Totacillin

AMOXICILLIN*
- Amoxil
- Larotid
- Polymox
- Robamax
- Trimox
- Wymox

DECLOMYCIN

ERYTHROMYCIN*
- Ilotycin
- Pediamycin Tabs
- Robimycin

ERYTHROMYCIN STEARATE
- Bristamycin
- Erythrocin
- Ethril
- Pfizer-E

ISONIAZID
- INH
- Laniazid
- Niconyl
- Nydrazid
- Triniad

LEVODOPA
- Bendopa
- Dopar
- Laradopa
- Sinemet

LINCOCIN

OXYTETRACYCLINE
- Abbocin
- Dalimycin
- Oxlopar
- Oxy-Kesso-Tetra
- Oxymycin
- Terramycin
- Urobiotic

*When taking **Amoxicillin** and **Erythromycin**, the more water you drink the better. If you skimp, there will be significantly less drug absorbed. Chug-a-lug with at least 8 ounces of water.

DRUGS THAT MAY BE ADVERSELY AFFECTED BY FOOD (continued)

If you are supposed to take a drug on an "empty stomach" it usually means at least one hour before meals or two hours after eating.

PENICILLAMINE*

Cuprimine*

PENICILLIN G

Omnipen
Pathocil
Pensorb
Pentids
Principen
SK-Penicillin

PENICILLIN V

Betapen
Compocillin-VK
Lanacillin V
Ledercillin VK
Pen-Vee K
Pfizerpen
Robicillin VK
Uticillin
V-Cillin K
Veetids

PENTAERYTHRITOL
TETRANITRATE

Cartrax
Duotrate
Miltrate
Pentritol
Pentryate
Peritrate

PROPANTHELINE**

Pro-Banthine**
Robantaline**
Ropanth**
Spastil**

PROSTAPHLIN

RIFAMPIN

Rifadin
Rifamate
Rimactin

TAO

TEGOPEN

TETRACYCLINE

Achromycin
Amtet
Bicycline
Bristacycline
Centet
Cyclopar
Mysteclin-F
Panmycin
Retet
Robitet
SK-Tetracycline
Sumycin
Tet-Cy
Tetrachel
Tetracyn
Tetrex

UNIPEN

*Drink, drink, drink! When taking CUPRIMINE the more water the better. Short of drowning yourself, keep the liquids coming since the greater the fluid intake the less drug necessary to do the job. You may have to get up in the middle of the night to drink some more.

**Brand new information—hot off the press! Doctors used to tell ulcer patients to take PRO-BANTHINE at meal time. New research indicates that just the opposite might be true: that is, it may be better on an empty stomach. Check with your doctor.

DRUGS BEST TAKEN WITH FOOD

Many medications can really mess up your stomach because they are so irritating. Food may reduce the damage, diminish the yucky feeling and prevent nausea or vomiting. Some drugs may actually be absorbed better when they are taken at meal time. Drugs that appear below (in large, bold print) are those that may be more effective when accompanied by food.

We recommend that you check with your doctor to confirm these recommendations. If the instructions you were given differ from our suggestions, find out why. There may be a good reason for your doctor's recommendations.

"With meals" generally means just before, during or immediately after eating—and it doesn't mean a morsel. Eat well! If you have to take a drug between meals make sure you take it with milk or a snack.

ALDACTAZIDE
ALDACTONE
ALDORIL
Amesec
Aminodur
Aminophylline
APC
APRESAZIDE
APRESOLINE
APRESOLINE-ESIDRIX
Aristocort
Artane
Aspirin*
Ascriptin
Azolid
Brondecon
Bronkotabs
Butagesic
Butazolidin
Butazolidin Alka

Celestone
Chlorothiazide
Codeine**
Colace
Cortisone
Cortef
DARVON COMPOUND
Decadron
Decagesic
Delta Cortef
Deltasone
Dialose (plenty of water)
Dilantin
Di-Phen
Diupres
Diuril
Diphenyl
Diphenylan

*Food may slightly reduce the effectiveness of **Aspirin**, but if you are sensitive to stomach irritation take it with a full eight-ounce glass of water or milk and have a snack.

Some people are sensitive to **Codeine. Taking it with food should reduce the upset stomach somewhat.

DRUGS BEST TAKEN WITH FOOD (continued)

"*With meals*" generally means just before, during or immediately after eating. Drugs that appear below (in large, bold print) are those that may be more effective when accompanied by food.

DOXYCYCLINE
DRALSERP
DRALZINE
DYAZIDE
Edecrin
E.E.S.
Ekko
Elixophyllin
Empirin Compound/
   Codeine
Emprazil
Enduron
Enduronyl
ERYTHROMYCIN
  ETHYL SUCCINATE
ESIDRIX
ESIMIL
Flagyl
Ferrous Sulfate†
Feosol†
Fer-In-Sol†
FURADANTIN
FURALAN
FURALOID
FURANTOIN
GRIFULVIN**
GRISACTIN**
GRISEOFULVIN**
GRIS-PEG
Hexadrol
HYDRALAZINE

HYDROCHLOROTHIAZIDE
HYDRODIURIL
HYDROPRES
HYDROTENSIN
HYDRO-Z-25/50
Hygroton
Indocin
Indomethacin
Iron Supplements†
INDERAL*
LEXOR
LITHIUM CITRATE
LITHONATE-S
LOPRESSOR*
MACRODANTIN
Malcogesic
Marax
Medrol
Mefenamic Acid
METOPROLOL
Metronidazole
Mol-Iron†
Motrin
Neggram
NITREX
NITROFOR
NITROFURANTOIN
ORETIC
Oxalid
Oxyphenbutazone
PARFURAN

†Use fruit juice instead of milk.

**For a list of foods that are particularly beneficial for absorption of these drugs turn to pages 102—103.

*INDERAL (**Propranolol**) and LOPRESSOR (**Metoprolol**) can be affected by food and while it is not necessary to take them at meal time, consistency is important. Don't take them with food one day and between meals the next, but pick one time that suits you and stick with it.

DRUGS BEST TAKEN WITH FOOD (continued)

"With meals" generally means just before, during or immediately after eating. Drugs that appear below (in large, bold print) are those that may be more effective when accompanied by food.

PEDIAMYCIN
Percodan
Phenbutazone
Phenylbutazone
Ponstel
Potassium (not with milk)
PROPOXYPHENE
PROPRANOLOL
Pyridium
Prednisolone
Prednisone
Quadrinal
Quibron
Quinamm
Quinidine
Quinine
Rau-Sed
Rauzide
Regroton
Renese-R
Reserpine

RIBOFLAVIN
Salutensin
Sandril
SER-AP-ES
Serpasil
SERPASIL-APRESOLINE
SERPASIL-ESIDRIX
Spironolactone
Sterazolidin
Tandearil
Tedral
TRANTOIN
Triamterene
UNIPRES
UROTOIN
VIBRAMYCIN
WYAMYCIN

HEARTBREAKING CASE HISTORIES

So far all this sounds pretty theoretical. Let's bring it closer to home with a few examples. Molly Mallone was delighted when her doctor diagnosed her as having a sluggish thyroid gland. She used to say she was born tired and her symptoms of dry skin, constipation, puffy eyelids, low body temperature, and tendency to gain weight had been distressing for years. Once her doctor prescribed thyroid medication for her hypothyroid condition, however, she felt better than she could have ever imagined. But every once in a while Molly's old symptoms returned. Her doctor forgot to mention that vegetables such as Brussels sprouts, cauliflower, kale, kohlrabi, rutabagas, and soybeans have an anti-thyroid effect. Since she loves vegetables and is an avid gardener she often indulges heavily in some of these low-calorie goodies and unknowingly reduces the benefits of her medication.

Bill Bailey had a serious stroke last year. His doctor prescribed an anticoagulant called COUMADIN to "thin his blood" and prevent more clots. The drug works by blocking Vitamin K. Vitamin who?

Well, we grant you, it's not a name everyone will recognize from a high school health class, but this vitamin is crucial to the normal blood clotting process. You produce this vitamin in your intestinal tract, or rather we should say the billions of bacteria that normally live in your gut produce it. These friendly parasites are responsible for manufacturing about half the normal levels of Vitamin K your body requires. The other half comes from the food you eat, especially green leafy vegetables.

Bill Bailey has a middle-aged paunch and his doctor wanted him to cut back on the high cholesterol foods he loved. He was encouraged to eat lots of fruits and vegetables. Unfortunately, no mention was made about foods that are high in Vitamin K such as broccoli, beef liver, cabbage, lettuce, spinach, turnip greens, asparagus, and watercress. Bill's wife included generous portions of these foods in his low-calorie, low-fat diet. Although Bill was successfully losing weight and was taking his COUMADIN conscientiously he suffered another stroke. The doctor checked his blood to see why the medicine hadn't prevented the new clots and was surprised to discover that the drug was not having the expected effect. All those vegetables Bill had been eating had increased the level of Vitamin K in his body beyond the point where the medicine could counteract it. So the extra Vitamin K was doing its usual thing—making the blood clot.

Margery Daw has asthma. Sometimes her breathing gets so bad that she has to rush to the hospital emergency room. Her doctor has tried a lot of different medicines and always comes back to a brand of theophylline (ELIXOPHYLLIN, MARAX, or QUIBRON) as a mainstay in her treatment. Margery usually controls her asthma pretty well with this medication but in the summertime she gets into trouble, especially on weekends and when the family goes on their annual vacation. That is when her husband Bob is declared official cook, and you will usually find him tending a batch of hamburgers or a steak on the charcoal grill. Margery doesn't know why her asthma always seems to get worse after Bob barbeques, but her medicine just doesn't seem quite as effective at those times. Who in a million years would ever think that a charcoal-broiled steak or hamburger could have any effect on a drug?

Well, according to a team of investigators from Columbia University, Rockefeller University, and the Hoffmann-LaRoche Drug Company the charcoal process can exert a profound influence on the metabolism of some drugs. They carried out some elegant research that demonstrated charcoal-broiled hamburgers and steaks (normal-sized portions) could dramatically increase the speed with which drugs like phenacetin and theophylline are metabolized. [6,7] Phenacetin is a pain reliever found in A.P.C. TABLETS, DARVON COMPOUND, EMPRAZIL, FIORINAL, NORGESIC, and SOMA COMPOUND. After only a few days on a charcoal-broiled diet (lunch and supper) the subjects had from 59 to 82 percent less phenacetin in their bloodstreams.

In their study of theophylline these same investigators discovered that charcoal broiling sped up the elimination of this asthma medicine from the body by as much as 42 percent. Their conclusions, although written in medicalese, are significant:

> **The data ... on the effects of food composition and food preparation on drug metabolism, make it clear that dietary factors, in the general sense, can be major influences on drug and chemical disposition in man. These influences, which result in altered biological actions of drugs and in altered impact of environmental chemicals, must be taken into account when evaluating host responses to such agents. In view of the wide disparity in dietary intakes of various populations, it is not unreasonable to suppose that nutritional-pharmacological interactions of the types described ... may be significant in ... adverse reactions to various drugs in man.[8]**

So poor Margery Daw is probably having trouble controlling her asthma in the summer because of all the charcoal-broiled beef her husband keeps serving her. The medicine is not having its usual effect because it is being metabolized faster than usual. The answer to her dilemma is simple. All she has to do is ask her husband to wrap her portion in aluminum foil before sticking it on the grill. The food may not be as tasty, but she will be better able to stay healthy and avoid taking a higher dose of the medicine, which is probably what her doctor would recommend.

Tom Dooley is a swinger. He's hot at the disco and can really put some moves on the honeys. Last week the doctor gave him the bad news—he was hot all right, too hot! He had the clap and it was complicated by prostatitis. Despite the fact that Tom got around, this was the first time he had ever had a venereal disease. The diagnosis of gonorrhea really shook him up and Tom vowed to swear off those casual relationships—at least until he was completely cured.

The doctor prescribed a broad-spectrum antibiotic called ampicillin (brand names include AMCILL, OMNIPEN, PENSYN, POLYCILLIN and PRINCIPEN). It was supposed to cure gonorrhea quickly. Unfortunately, no one bothered to give Tom specific information on how to take the drug. There were no instructions to take it with a tall glass of water and no warning to avoid food. Tom unwittingly took the medicine just before sitting down to a big dinner and instead of swallowing it with water he popped it down with his wine.

Three weeks later Tom still noticed symptoms. If anything, the prostatitis was worse. When he visited his doctor he was given a tongue-lashing for continuing his naughty ways and possibly spreading the bug around. His physician was convinced that the presence of the infection must have been due to a new sexual contact because it was inconceivable to him that the original prescription hadn't worked. Well, the doctor was wrong. Because he hadn't warned Tom to take the medicine on an empty stomach with a full glass of water, the antibiotic never reached an adequate level in his bloodstream to cure the clap.

Barbara Allen was depressed most of the time. She was only twenty-nine but life had stopped having any meaning for her. Some days she wondered if even getting up out of bed was worth the effort. Her doctor tried her on VALIUM and if anything it made her feel worse. He tried another medication called ELAVIL but it hadn't done much good either. Finally he gave her a different kind of antidepressant called MARPLAN, classified as an MAO inhibitor.

When she received this drug Barbara was feeling so low that she barely listened to what her doctor was saying. She vaguely remembered hearing something about avoiding beer and wine and some foods like cheese and chicken livers but it wasn't clear what the danger was and it all sounded pretty flaky at the time. About two weeks after she started taking the drug Barbara began to feel better for the first time in a long while. Slowly, life didn't seem quite so bleak. But around the fourth week she began to notice the occurrence of severe headaches. They were more painful than any she had ever had before but they went away after a day or so and she never thought to call her doctor about something as ordinary as a headache. Around the second month it seemed as if the headaches were occurring with increasing frequency, and sometimes she could feel her heart pounding in her chest. The attacks, as she was beginning to call them, usually occurred a few hours after supper and were very distressing because sometimes they made her nauseous and she would sweat profusely. But she still didn't think they were important enough to call her doctor, and anyway the medicine was really working. She felt optimistic for the first time in years and was feeling so well she decided to throw a party.

Barbara invited all her friends and really went all out to make the affair a success. She made some fantastic onion and guacamole dips and set out gobs of caviar and camembert cheese. There was a wonderful chicken liver pâté and some extraordinary little sausages. She really splurged on wine and bought a special brand of chianti that was usually out of her price range.

The party was everything she wanted it to be and more. Her friends were delighted to see her happy for a change. But midway through the evening the headache came back and this time the pain was excruciating. Her neck became stiff, she was nauseated, and she even threw up. Her skin felt cold and clammy and her heart was beating so fast her chest felt as if it were going to explode. Her friends called an ambulance, but by the time it arrived she was dead!

Barbara Allen died because of an interaction between her drug and the foods she ate that night. Her doctor never told her how dangerous the reaction could be if she ate certain kinds of food—he didn't want to scare her unnecessarily. And he didn't realize that when he prescribed MARPLAN she was in no frame of mind to remember a casual warning. Everything she had served at the party contained a substance called TYRAMINE—the avocados, the sour cream in the dip, the caviar, the camembert cheese, the pâté, the sausages, and the chianti wine. For anyone taking an MAO-inhibitor type of drug (EUTRON, EUTONYL, FUROXONE, MARPLAN, MATULANE, NARDIL, PARNATE), tyramine-containing foods could be lethal. Blood pressure can go so high that a person can experience a stroke. Severe headaches are just one of the early-warning signals of a hypertensive crisis. If Barbara Allen had only known how dangerous those foods were and if she had been told what side effects to be alert for she probably would not have died from a stroke. Other foods and beverages that should be avoided by anyone taking an MAO-inhibitor medication include chicken liver, pickled herring, cheddar cheese, yogurt, beer, sherry, fava beans, chocolate, ripe bananas, canned figs, coffee, soy sauce and yeast.

If you haven't begun to appreciate the significance of food and drug interactions by now, you never will. The "case histories" we have related are imaginary. Any similarity with persons living or dead is purely coincidental. But the interactions are all too real. They could happen to anyone and no doubt have at one time or another. If you want to avoid a food and drug interaction or find out whether to take your medication with meals or on an empty stomach ask your doctor or pharmacist for specific information. And check the tables at the end of this chapter. Our difficulties in compiling them have only further convinced us of how crucial and little known and appreciated this information is.

DRUGS, HABITS, AND OTHER DRUGS

Drug interactions can be subtle or they can hit you over the head with a sledgehammer. Instead of diving into the swamp of confusing incompatibility reactions, let's first dabble our big toe into the muddy waters in order to get a feel for things. Most people don't think of cigarettes or coffee as drugs and they would never imagine that these two "vices" might interact. Well, friends, the name of the tune is "Think Again." Nicotine and caffeine have a profound pharmacology and cigarette smoking appears to have a pronounced influence upon caffeine metabolism.

An unusually inventive investigation was recently carried out by the Department of Pharmacology and Therapeutics of McGill University in Canada.[9] The researchers wanted to know whether smokers who puffed more than twenty cigarettes a day differed from non-smokers in the way their bodies metabolized caffeine. The results were astonishing. The smokers eliminated caffeine in about three hours, more than twice as fast as the six it took non-smokers. Quite clearly the effect of cigarettes on drug metabolism is formidable.

Wait a minute. So smoking increases metabolism, so what? Well, it's important for a couple of reasons. Just as an aside, smokers tend to drink more coffee than non-smokers. The authors of the research article hypothesized that "It is intriguing to speculate that the smoker consumes more coffee than the non-smoker in part to compensate for increased caffeine clearance."[10] While interesting, that is hardly shattering information. What is really exciting in all this is that cigarette smoking may have an important impact upon the metabolism of other, more therapeutic drugs than caffeine.

Smokers are different. There is definite evidence that smoking increases the metabolism of pain killers like TALWIN (pentazocine) and DARVON (propoxyphene, phenacetin, etc.) and the asthma medication theophylline (found in BRONKAID, BRONKOTABS, ELIXOPHYLLIN, MARAX, TEDRAL, QUADRINAL, etc.)[11-13] among other drugs. The result is that smokers probably don't get the same therapeutic benefits and a doctor should take this into account when prescribing certain kinds of medicine.

THE LONG HAUL
Well, so much for subtlety. There are a vast number of interactions that are much more obvious and dangerous. A great many people take more than one drug, and a lot of the time they have no idea that the pill they so casually pop into their mouth may be incompatible with something else. A woman who swallows a birth-control pill every day for years often starts to take it for granted. She never even thinks that the laxative she occasionally uses or the antihistamine she takes for her allergies could interact to reduce the effectiveness of the oral contraceptive. If she smokes, the combination of the cigarettes and the Pill could dramatically increase the likelihood of a stroke or heart attack.

A person who must regularly take an anticoagulant medication is almost always warned to avoid aspirin-containing pain relievers because the two drugs could be lethal together. The blood-thinning effect is magnified and a life-threatening hemorrhage could result. The problem is that a great many pain relievers and cold remedies sold on pharmacy shelves contain aspirin but there is often no mention made of that fact unless you look at the very fine print on the back of the package. Products like ALKA-SELTZER, ANACIN, ARTHRITIS PAIN FORMULA, COPE, CORICIDIN, EMPIRIN COMPOUND, EXCEDRIN, SINE-OFF, TRIAMINICIN, and VANQUISH all contain aspirin. If someone didn't check carefully they might use one of these products and in combination with their anticoagulant end up in the hospital, or worse yet, dead.

A person who is taking a digitalis heart drug like LANOXIN or DIGOXIN must be extremely alert for side effects if the doctor adds another medication called INDERAL (used for irregular heart beats, angina, migraine headaches, and hypertension). Such a combination could be very hazardous unless a doctor were carefully monitoring the patient's progress. But even with careful supervision the patient might get into serious trouble if he independently added a laxative to the already touchy combination. Digitalis toxicity might be increased and the heart could stop.

In order to bring this critical issue into finer focus let's look at another case history. Patrick Finkelstein is a middle-aged businessman. He worked his way up to vice-president of marketing in a high-powered ad agency. Pat is a pretty tense individual. He smokes about a pack a day and in the evening it takes at least two drinks before he starts to unwind. If his boss is on his case he might even indulge in a martini at lunchtime.

It's hardly surprising to learn that Pat has high blood pressure and a cholesterol level that makes his doctor unhappy. And you should hardly be amazed to learn that Pat lives with a chronic state of indigestion and an ulcer that comes and goes. When the pressure really starts to mount it is not unusual for Pat to come down with a nasty headache that drives him right up the wall. Pat is not very different from many other American businessmen.

Here is a list of the various drugs that Patrick Finkelstein consumes: (1) His cardiologist recently prescribed a medication called SER-AP-ES (a combination of reserpine, hydralazine, and hydrochlorothiazide) for the high blood pressure. (2) In order to get the cholesterol levels down the doctor also put Pat on ATROMID (clofibrate). (3) Pat has a bottle of VALIUM (diazepam) handy just in case the pressure cooker at work gets to be too much to handle. (4) For indigestion he relies on a combination of antacids including the "Plop, Plop, Fizz, Fizz Relief" ALKA-SELTZER. He also uses the "How Do You Spell Relief" ROLAIDS. And TUMS is never far from reach. (5) When the ulcer acts up Pat can grab for a prescription drug called TAGAMET (cimetidine) that his gastroenterologist prescribed last year. (6) Since Pat has hay fever he usually takes some sort of non-prescription remedy like ALLEREST or CONTAC or SINE-OFF when his nose feels stuffy. Well, that's about it. When the headaches get really bad he might reach for (7) BUFFERIN or EXCEDRIN.

Patrick Finkelstein is walking a dangerous tightrope. He is taking a lot of drugs that are capable of interacting in some very unpleasant ways. Let's follow Pat for a few months after he started taking the new high blood pressure medicine called SER-AP-ES and see what happened with all the various combinations. We should also point out that the doctor did not ask about any of the other drugs he was taking, and it didn't occur to Pat to mention many of these OTC products since he didn't think of them as "drugs," so when he asked about side effects he was told there weren't any to be concerned about.

The first thing that he noticed after about a week with the new drug was that his old ulcer pain started acting up again. Pat didn't associate the upset with the drug though, because the pressure at work was particularly high (a new account) and he just chalked it up to the rat race. (The heart doctor was unaware of Pat's ulcer problem. One of the ingredients in the high blood pressure pill was reserpine, a drug that often leads to irritation of the digestive tract and is contraindicated in ulcer patients). Pat also noticed that his nose was much stuffier than usual (also as a result of the reserpine) and he began to feel very depressed. In fact as the weeks passed Pat sank so low that he began to wonder if the ball game was worth playing anymore. He actually started contemplating suicide. This too was a side effect of reserpine. Pat started taking his ALKA-SELTZER with great regularity to try to relieve the constant pain and indigestion. Even the ulcer medicine TAGAMET didn't help much. For the stuffy nose he took the ALLEREST almost constantly. The headaches were becoming unbearable and the EXCEDRIN didn't even touch the pain. One night the pain of his ulcer and the pain in his head got so bad that he couldn't stand it. He headed for the emergency room at the local hospital. That probably saved his life. A young resident took a careful medical history and upon hearing about the various drug combinations poor Pat was taking told him to stop everything. Would you like to know why the resident shook his head in disbelief when he realized what was going on?

For one thing the drug called SER-AP-ES was a terrible mistake. It would interact with the ASPIRIN in the ALKA-SELTZER and the EXCEDRIN to severely irritate his stomach. In fact, it's a wonder he didn't perforate his gut with that combination. What's more, the ASPIRIN wasn't helping his headaches (exacerbated by the SER-AP-ES) because the reserpine eliminates the analgesic action of ASPIRIN. The decongestants in the allergy medicine actually were working against the blood pressure medicine and undoing what benefit was to have been achieved. (Remember, the stuffy nose was caused by the hypertension drug—it caused him to treat the congestion with a drug that should not have been used). The sodium level in ALKA-SELTZER and ROLAIDS also acted to defeat the purpose of the SER-AP-ES. The drug that he was taking for the cholesterol problem, ATROMID S, also added to his stomach upset and made him feel tired. The combination of VALIUM and booze, antihistamines (in the sinus medicine) and RESERPINE were making Pat feel depressed and tired most of the time. It's a wonder he *didn't* jump out a window. Well, we could go on and on, but you get the point. All Pat's drugs are commonly prescribed and the over-the-counter products are in practically everyone's medicine chest. But taken in the wrong combinations these relatively safe drugs become dangerous weapons. At the end of this chapter you will find a table that will assist you in avoiding some of the traps that poor Pat Finkelstein fell into.

DRUGS AND LABORATORY TESTS

Drugs don't just interact with other drugs. Something that is often overlooked is that many medications can raise havoc with the results of lab tests. Say you go in for your annual check-up. The doctor tells you that she wants to do a routine laboratory work-up. Chances are pretty good that you will have to donate some blood to a lab tech with a good-natured gleam in his eye and more likely than not you will be encouraged to produce a urine specimen. So far, so good. But in all probability no one will ask you what vitamins, prescription, or OTC drugs you are taking and if they don't ask this crucial question it is quite possible that the results of the test will be completely mucked up. According to Dr. Eric Martin, a renowned expert in the field of drug interactions, "The most frequently encountered sources of error in clinical laboratory testing are interfering chemicals, including drugs and food constituents."[14] Drugs can cause abnormally high or low test results and can lead to false interpretations and ultimately an incorrect diagnosis. The consequences can be very serious. For one thing your doctor might prescribe an unnecessary drug to treat a nonexistent malady. You might be hassled by a life insurance company over a test that showed you had diabetes even though your blood sugar is perfectly normal. Even worse, you might be scheduled for needless surgery based on false data. According to Dr. Martin, two researchers saved a patient from this fate when they "reported that a high value for catecholamines [a urine test] in one of their specimens was actually due to the presence of previously administered methyldopa [ALDOMET, a drug used to treat high blood pressure] rather than to adrenal pathology. They thereby prevented a patient from undergoing unnecessary surgery and the pathologist and his staff from receiving unjustified criticism."[15,16]

In order to appreciate the significance of this problem let's take a look at some examples. Many drugs can make it look as if there is sugar in the urine when there is none. ASPIRIN can produce this "false positive" glucose test as can a sleeping pill called NOCTEC (chloral hydrate).[17] Vitamin C, PYRIDIUM (a drug for urinary tract infections) and LEVODOPA (a drug used by Parkinson patients) may do just the opposite—that is they may cause false confidence in a diabetic by creating normal results when a person actually *is* spilling sugar into the urine.

ASPIRIN and ESTROGEN hormones can interfere with thyroid function tests. Both drugs can create utter confusion by simultaneously producing high levels on one test and abnormally low levels on another. A doctor who tries to make sense out of the lab results could end up scratching his head in dismay. TETRACYCLINE antibiotics can interfere with laboratory values for gallbladder, liver, and kidney tests. Sodium bicarbonate (ALKA-SELTZER, baking soda) could mistakenly produce evidence of protein in the urine and make a doctor think there was kidney disease where none existed. Major tranquilizers like **THORAZINE** may cause untold anguish for a woman who goes in to have a pregnancy test. These drugs can produce false positive results. In other words, a woman who is not pregnant might be told that she is going to have a baby because her head drug threw a monkey wrench into the laboratory machinery.

The moral of this tale is that whenever you have a lab test done make darn sure your doctor and the laboratory technician know every drug and vitamin you are taking. Make a list and check it twice so as to include the over-the-counter medications as well. And if by chance you end up in the hospital where they will run about every conceivable test in the world, make sure someone is familiar with the drugs that could interfere with the laboratory values. The last thing you need is to "develop" a new illness that you don't really have.

PINNING THE TAIL ON THE DONKEY

By now, you should have begun to appreciate the complexity and confusion that surround the whole world of drug interactions. We clearly did not promise you a rose garden when we started this chapter but we hope that the new awareness you have gained will prevent you from getting pricked the next time you receive a new prescription. As you have seen, drugs can interact with beverages, with foods, with other prescription drugs or over-the-counter remedies. They can influence nutrition (see Chapter 5 on vitamins) and they can interfere with laboratory test results.

The significance of drug interactions is hotly debated. Some doctors claim that "One patient in 10 is admitted to the hospital because of adverse interactions."[18] Other experts insist that the problem is actually insignificant. Researchers can't even agree on how frequently interactions occur. In one study of people in North Carolina a group of investigators "found that one-third of all Medicaid patients who habitually use anticoagulants were exposed to potentially harmful interactions with another drug."[19]

> **What's more, these potential interactions could not be attributed to the use by patients of more than one physician or pharmacy. In 79 percent of the patients exposed to drug interactions, both drugs were prescribed by the same physician, and in 94 per cent, the prescriptions were filled by a single pharmacy.**[20]

Most dangerous drug interactions are preventable, or at least they should be. It takes careful cooperation and communication between every doctor you visit and your pharmacist as well to prevent incompatibility reactions from occurring. Insist that these health care providers take a little extra time to check their reference books to make sure there is no danger when a change is made in your drug regimen. You also have an important responsibility to keep precise records of every medicine you take, including that occasional laxative, antacid, or sleeping pill. A team effort can practically eliminate the problems of adverse drug interactions.

At the end of this chapter you will find many different tables that summarize the points we have tried to make. You will discover which specific foods and drinks can foul up the effectiveness of your drugs and which non-prescription products may interact to cause serious adverse reactions. Although we did our best, there is no way in the world that we could have included every possible food and drug interaction or every dangerous drug-drug combination. We have tried not to duplicate information that can be found in *The People's Pharmacy*, so if you do not find your particular drug in these tables you may want to check in that book. (It is available in most libraries.) And of course, you should always consult your physician.

Not every interaction you will find in the tables will lead to problems. Some of these potential situations are controversial and experts often disagree about their significance. Nevertheless, we feel that forewarned is forearmed. It's your body and with a little knowledge you are the one who is best able to prevent an adverse interaction from occurring. If you allow yourself to be blindfolded, ultimately you have only yourself to blame.

REFERENCES

1. Lambert, Martin L. "Drug and Diet Interactions." *American J. of Nurs.* 75(3):402–406, 1975.

2. Welling, Peter G. "How Food and Fluid Affect Drug Absorption." *Postgrad. Med.* 62(1):73–82, 1977.

3. Melander, Arne. "Influence of Food on Bioavailability of Drugs." *Clin. Pharmacokin.* 3:337–351, 1978.

4. Editorial. "Drug Administration and Food." *Br. Med. J.* 1:289, 1979.

5. Welling, Peter G. "Influence of Food and Drug on Gastrointestinal Drug Absorption: A Review." *J. of Pharmacokin. and Biopharm.* 5(4):291–335, 1977.

6. Pantuck, E. J., et al. "Effect of Charcoal-Broiled Beef on Phenacetin Metabolism in Man." *Science* 194: 1055–1056, 1976.

7. Kappas, et al. "Effect of Charcoal-Broiled Beef on Antipyrine and Theophylline Metabolism." *Clin. Pharmacol. Ther.* 23:445−449, 1978.

8. Ibid.

9. Parsons, William D. and Neims, Allen H. "Atmospheric Pollution on Caffeine Clearance." *Clin Pharmacol. Ther* 24:40−44, 1978

10. Ibid.

11. Kerri-Szanto, M. and Pomery, J. R. "Atmospheric Pollution and Pentazocine Metabolism." *Lancet* 1:947−949, 1971.

12. Boston Collaborative Drug Surveillance Program. "Decreased Clinical Efficacy of Propoxyphene in Cigarette Smokers." *Clin. Pharmacol. Ther.* 14:259−263, 1973.

13. Hunt, S. N.; Jusko, W. J.; and Yurchak, A. M. "Effect of Smoking on Theophylline Absorption." *Clin. Pharmacol. Ther.* 19:546−551, 1976.

14. Martin, Eric W. *Hazards of Medication: A Manual of Drug Interactions, Contraindications and Adverse Reactions, with Other Prescribing and Drug Information.* Second Edition. Philadelphia: Lippincott, 1978.

15. Wirth, W. A., and Thomson, R. L. "The Effect of Various Conditions and Substances on the Results of Laboratory Procedures." *Am. J. Clin. Path.* 43:579−590, 1965.

16. Martin, op. cit. p. 129.

17. Wallach, Jacques. *Interpretation of Diagnostic Tests.* Third Edition. Boston: Little Brown, 1978.

18. What's New in Drugs. "Clinically Speaking." *Drug Topics* 22(3):39, 1978.

19. Chi, Judy, Ed. "A Look at Drug Interaction." *The State of The Art.* (A publication of the Health Services Research Center, The University of North Carolina), pp. 3−5, December 1977.

20. Ibid.

> *The following references were not cited in this chapter but were crucial in the research and preparation of much of the material. They are included here so that you may track down the original research.*

21. Lehmann, Phyllis. "Food and Drug Interactions." *FDA Consumer* 12(2):20−23, 1978.

22. Hansten, Philip D. "Clinically Significant Interactions." *In Current Prescribing* 5(3):69−71, 1979.

23. Stanaszek, Walter F. "These 8 Tables Will Help You Prevent Drug Interactions in the Elderly Patient." *Pharmacy Times* 45(1):54−58, 1979.

24. Friedman, et al. "Automated Monitoring of Drug-Test Interactions." *Clin. Pharmacol. Ther.* 24(1):16−21, 1978.

25. Pantuck, E. J., et al. "Stimulatory Effect of Brussels Sprouts and Cabbage on Human Drug Metabolism." *Clin. Pharmacol. Ther.* 25(1):88−95, 1979.

26. Prue, Hart G. C., et al. "Enhanced Drug Metabolism in Cigarette Smokers." *Br. Med. J.* 2:147−149, 1976.

27. Melander, A., et al. "Enhancement of the Bioavailability of Propranolol and Metoprolol by Food." *Clin. Pharmacol. Ther.* 22(1):108−112, 1977.

28. Rosenberg, H. A., and Bates, T. R. "The Influences of Food on Nitrofurantoin Bioavailability." *Clin. Pharmacol. Ther.* 20:227−232, 1976.

29. Musa, M. N., and Lyons, L. L. "Effect of Food and Liquid on the Pharmacokinetics of Propoxyphene." *Cur. Ther. Res.* 19(6):669−674, 1976.

30. Melander, A., et al. "Reduction of Isoniazid Bioavailability in Normal Men by Concomitant Intake of Food." *Acta Med. Scand.* 200:93−97, 1976.

31. Tembro, A. V., et al. "Effect of Food on the Bioavailability of Prednisone." *J. Clin. Pharmacol.* 16:620−624, 1976.

32. Melander, A., et al. "Enhancement of Hydralazine Bioavailability by Food." *Clin. Pharmacol. Ther.* 22(1):104−107, 1977.

33. Melander, A., et al. "Bioavailability of D-Propoxyphene, Acetyl Salicylic Acid, and Phenazone in a Combination Tablet (Doleron): Interindividual Variation and Influence of Food Intake." *Acta Med. Scand.* 202:119−124, 1977.

34. Beerman, Bjorn, and Groschinsky-Grind, M. "Gastrointestinal Absorption of Hydrochlorothiazide Enhanced by Concomitant Intake of Food." *Europ. J. Clin. Pharmacol.* 13:125−128, 1978.

35. Welling, P.G.; Huang, P.F.; and Lyons, L.L. "Bioavailability of Erythromycin Stearate: Influence of Food and Fluid Volume." *J. Pharmaceut. Sci.* 67:764−766, 1978.

36. Greenblatt, D. J., et al. "Diazepam Absorption: Effect of Antacids and Food." *Clin. Pharmacol. Ther.* 24:600−609, 1978.

37. Rosenberg, J. M. "Hormones: How They Complicate Things." *Current Prescribing* 4:78−83, 1978.

38. Marzke, G. R., et al. "Quinidine-Digoxin Interaction." *JAMA* 241:881, 1979.

39. Rosenberg, Jack M. *Prescriber's Guide to Drug Interactions.* Oradell, N. J.: Medical Economics Co., 1978.

40. American Pharmaceutical Association. *Evaluations of Drug Interactions.* Washington, D. C.: APHA Second edition, 1976.

41. "Adverse Interactions of Drugs." *The Medical Letter on Drugs and Therapeutics* 21(2):5−12, 1979.

GUIDE TO DRUG INTERACTION TABLE

DRINK AND DRUG INTERACTIONS

If a person drinks:

THESE BEVERAGES:	WITH THESE DRUGS:	THIS COULD RESULT:
FRUIT JUICE Cherry Cider Cranberry Grapefruit Lemon Lime Orange Pineapple	*Ampicillin* Amcill Omnipen Pen A Penbriten Pensyn Polycillin Principen Totacillin	Fruit juice, soda pop and wine are all acid beverages and can cause problems with some of the antibiotics that are listed here. A large glass of juice may reduce antibiotic activity or interfere with proper absorption of the drug. Unless advised otherwise, it is a good rule of thumb to take antibiotics with a glass of water.
SODA POP Cherry Cola Ginger Ale Grape Grapefruit Lemon/Lime Orange Quinine ALCOHOL Wine	*Erythromycin* Bristamycin E-Mycin Erythrocin Ethril Erypar Ilosone Ilotycin Pediamycin Pfizer-E Robimycin *Penicillin* Pentids Pfizerpen SK-Penicillin *Tegopen*	*Please note that all the drinks interact with all the drugs—that is to say, fruit juice affects ampicillin, erythromycin, penicillin, and tegopen; soda affects ampicillin, erythromycin, penicillin, and tegopen; and wine affects ampicillin, erythromycin, penicillin, and tegopen.*
MILK Non-fat Whole Cream Etc.	*Bisacodyl* Bicol Biscolax Dulcolax SK-Bisacodyl Theralax Ulcolax Vactrol	These laxatives should not be taken with milk (or within one hour of taking antacids or milk). An alkaline environment may cause the drugs to dissolve prematurely. The presence of the laxative in the stomach without its protective enteric coating may cause gastritis.
TEA Hot or iced MILK Non-fat Whole	*Iron Supplements* Feosol Fergon Fer-In-Sol Ferrobid Ferro-Grad-500	Teas, milk, eggs and phytic acid can all interfere with iron absorption. This could, in extreme instances, lead to anemia in sensitive individuals. Pregnant women might be well

DRINK AND DRUG INTERACTIONS (continued)

If a person drinks:

THESE BEVERAGES:	WITH THESE DRUGS:	THIS COULD RESULT:

Cream
Etc.
 	
EGGS
 	
PHYTIC ACID
 	
Whole grains
Breads
Cereals
 	
FRUIT JUICE
	Ferro-Sequels
	Ferrous fumarate
	Ferrous
	  gluconate
	Ferrous sulfate
	Geritol
	Iberet
	Mol-Iron
	Optilets-M-500
	Stresstabs
	  600/Iron
	Tri-Vi-Sol
	Zentrol
		advised to take iron supplements without milk.
		
		Phyhtic acid can also obstruct calcium and zinc absorption. If you are taking mineral supplements, don't take them at breakfast with whole grain cereals or muffins.
		
		Vitamin C can improve the absorption of iron. It is a good idea to take your iron supplement with juice or a little extra ascorbic acid.

MILK Non-fat Whole Cream Etc.	Sodium Bicarbonate Alka-Seltzer Antacid powder (Dewitt) Baking soda Bell-Ans Bisodol Citrocarbonate Diatrol Eno Fizrin Soda Mint	You'd really have to work at this one to get yourself into trouble. Nevertheless, if you are really into packing away these antacids and also drinking milk you could end up with something weird called the "MILK-ALKALI SYNDROME." Symptoms include nausea, headache and weakness and you could ultimately end up with unrecognized kidney damage.
MILK Non-fat Whole Cream Etc.	Tetracycline Antibiotics Abbocin Achromycin Aureomycin Azotrex Bicycline Bristacycline Centet Cyclopar Dalimycin Mysteclin-F Oxymycin Panmycin Retet Robitet	By now it is common knowledge that the calcium in milk products will dramatically interfere with the absorption and effectiveness of **Tetracycline** antibiotics. Nevertheless, you would be absolutely amazed how many folks have told us that they were never warned about this interaction by either their doctor or their pharmacist. If you want your medicine to work, skip the white stuff that comes from cows!

DRINK AND DRUG INTERACTIONS (continued)

If a person drinks:

THESE BEVERAGES:	WITH THESE DRUGS:	THIS COULD RESULT:
	Sumycin Terramycin Tet-Cy Tetrachel Tetracyn Tetrex	

FOOD AND DRUG INTERACTIONS

If a person were to eat:

THESE FOODS:	WITH THESE DRUGS:	THIS COULD RESULT:
VITAMIN-K-CONTAINING FOODS Asparagus Bacon Beef liver Broccoli Cabbage Kale Lettuce Spinach Turnip greens Watercress	Anticoagulants Coumadin Dicumarol Liquamar Panwarfin Sintrom Miradon	Look out! All the foods that are listed are high in **Vitamin K.** If you're not careful you might have real difficulty keeping your blood thinner under control. **Vitamin K** may reverse the effectiveness of your medication. It is not so much what you eat as maintaining a consistent vitamin intake. Once you are stabilized you should maintain the pattern or else you could end up with a clot. Periodic blood tests will tell the story.
ONIONS GARLIC	Anticoagulants Coumadin Dicumarol Liquamar Panwarfin Sintrom Miradon	This may sound bizarre, but there is some evidence that both **onions** (2 ounces or more, fried or boiled) and **garlic** have some anticoagulant activity. So combined with blood-thinning drugs like **COUMADIN** either might increase the anticoagulant effect and in extreme situations lead to bleeding. If in doubt check with your doctor.

FOOD AND DRUG INTERACTIONS (continued)
If a person were to eat:

THESE FOODS:	WITH THESE DRUGS:	THIS COULD RESULT:
GOITROGENS Brussels sprouts Cabbage Cauliflower Kale Kohlrabi Rutabagas Soybean products Turnips	*Thyroid Hormones* Choloxin Cytomel Euthroid Letter Proloid Synthroid Thyrolar	These foods have "goitrogenic" action. Goitrogenic who? You heard right. It means they have an anti-thyroid effect and in rare situations (inadequate iodine in the diet) they might cause goiter. For folks with a weak thyroid gland to begin with, pigging out on these kinds of food could reduce the effectiveness of your medication.
LICORICE (Natural)	Aldoril Anhydron Aquatag Aquatensen Butizide Digoxin Digitoxin Diupres Diuril Diutensin Enduron Esidrix Exna Hydrochloro-thiazide Hydropres Hydrodiuril Hygroton Lanoxin Lasix	This little pig went to market and came home sick as a dog. A lot of us gorp down the licorice, but if you are on any of these drugs, beware, it could spell disaster! More than three-quarters of an ounce (not much for a licorice lover) eaten regularly can really mess up body chemistry and can lead to fluid build-up and high blood pressure. Licorice can reduce the effectiveness of your medication and if you are also taking a diuretic licorice can deplete your body of potassium. This can be *lethal* if you are also on a digitalis heart medicine. So curb your appetite for natural licorice or switch to the stuff with artificial flavor.
FATTY FOODS Avocados Beef Butter Cake Cream Chicken salad French fries Fried chicken	*Griseofulvin* Fulvicin Grifulvin Grisactin Grisowen Grisovin-FP Gris-Peg	Surprise, surprise, surprise! Here's one time when you can indulge your fat tooth and not feel guilty. These antifungal drugs are absorbed better when you eat fatty foods. They should be taken at meal time and you should be encouraged to eat some of the sinful stuff

FOOD AND DRUG INTERACTIONS (continued)

If a person were to eat:

THESE FOODS:	WITH THESE DRUGS:	THIS COULD RESULT:
Gravy Lamb Margarine Mayonnaise Peanut butter Pie Salad dressing Sardines Sour cream Tuna salad Whipped cream		most folks are told to avoid (all things being equal). Incredible as it may sound, this is one time your doctor will probably approve of your little indulgences. So enjoy! These foods will make your medicine more effective. But please don't blame us if you gain some weight — that's your responsibility.
TYRAMINE-CONTAINING FOODS Avocados Bananas Bologna Brie Camembert Canned figs Caviar Cheddar Chicken liver Emmenthaler Fava beans Gruyere Meat tenderizer Pepperoni Pickled herring Salami Sour cream Soy sauce Summer sausage	*MAO-Inhibitors* Eutron Eutonyl Furoxone Marplan Matulane Nardil Parnate	ZAP! This is the infamous and potentially lethal interaction between foods that contain the substance **Tyramine** and a class of drugs called **MAO-Inhibitors**. These drugs are used to treat high blood pressure, psychological depression, infections and cancer. Blood pressure could go so high that you could have a stroke. Early warning signs of this reaction include: terrible headaches, chest pain, sweating, palpitations, rapid pulse, changes in vision, and coma. If your doctor prescribes one of these drugs, please make sure that you watch your diet!
BRUSSELS SPROUTS CABBAGE	*Phenacetin* A.P.C. A.S.A. Compound Darvon Compound	Incredible, mindboggling, bizarre. We wouldn't blame you if you found this one hard to swallow. Nevertheless, reputable researchers recently discovered that a diet high in

FOOD AND DRUG INTERACTIONS (continued)

If a person were to eat:

THESE FOODS:	WITH THESE DRUGS:	THIS COULD RESULT:
	Emprazil Fiorinal Norgesic Pac Soma Compound	**Brussels sprouts** and **cabbage** reduced the levels of **Phenacetin** in the bloodstream between 34 and a whopping 67 percent, thereby reducing its therapeutic effect. The moral of the story is that some pretty common foods can have a significant impact on drug metabolism and can lead to variable drug responses.

CHARCOAL-BROILED BEEF	*Phenacetin*
	A.P.C.
	A.S.A.
	   Compound
	Darvon
	   Compound
	Emprazil
	Fiorinal
	Norgesic
	Pac
	Soma Compound
	
	Theophylline
	Anti-Asthma
	Bronkkaid
	Bronkodyl
	Bronkotabs
	Elixophyllin
	Isuprel
	   Compound
	Marax
	Mudrane Elixir
	Quadrinal
	Quibron
	Slo-Phyllin
	Somophyllin
	Tedral
	Theophyl
	Theospan
		Hold on to your hat. This food-drug interaction is guaranteed to astonish even the skeptical. Research published in *Science* magazine showed that charcoal-broiled beef could have a profound effect on the metabolism of these drugs. The charcoal cooking process is the key. As little as four days on this diet (hamburgers for lunch, steak for supper) can reduce **Phenacetin** levels in the blood an incredible 59 to 82 percent. A similar diet decreased the blood levels of the asthma medicine, **Theophylline**, an average of 22 percent. For someone with asthma, that could reduce the effectiveness of the medication significantly.

FOOD AND DRUG INTERACTIONS (continued)

If a person were to eat:

THESE FOODS:	WITH THESE DRUGS:	THIS COULD RESULT:
Use this Food	**to Counteract These Drugs**	
HIGH-POTASSIUM FOODS	*Potassium-Wasting Drugs*	When it comes to providing patients with solid nutrition information about potassium many doctors have their needle stuck in the same old groove— **oranges** or **bananas**. While these fruits do have potassium, they are certainly not the only ones. If a person is on a diuretic or high-blood-pressure medicine that depletes the body of potassium it is crucial that the diet provide enough to replace that which is lost. The foods listed in this table represent good sources of potassium.
Almonds	Aldoril	
Apricots	Anhydron	
Avocados	Aquatag	
Bananas	Aquatensen	
Beef	Butizide	
(hamburger)	Digoxin*	
Blackstrap	Diupres	
Molasses	Diuril	
Brazil nuts	Diutensin	
Cocoa powder	Enduron	
(not alkali-	Esidrix	
processed)	Exna	
Cress (garden)	Hydrochloro-	
Dates	thiazide	
Flounder	Hydropres	
Green peas	Hydrodiuril	
Halibut	Hygroton	
Lima beans	Lanoxin*	
Oatmeal	Lasix	
Oranges		
Peaches	*Lanoxin or Digoxin require adequate potassium to be safe	
Peanuts		
Pecans		
Potato		
(baked with		
skin)		
Prunes/Raisins		
Wheat germ		
Winter squash		
Yeast		

ALCOHOL

(Beer, Wine, Liquor, Cold Remedies,* Cough Medicine*)

If a person who imbibes alcohol:

ALSO USES:	THIS COULD RESULT:
ANTABUSE Disulfiram	This interaction could be deadly! Even the little alcohol in cough medicine could cause toxicity. The side effects of this interaction are used to persuade alcoholics not to drink.

ASPIRIN (Salicylates)
   Alka-Seltzer
   Arthritis Pain Formula
   A.S.A.
   Ascriptin
   Bufferin
   Cope
   Empirin Compound
   Excedrin
   Fiorinal
   Midol
   Vanquish
	Lots of folks take aspirin to head off a hangover before it hits. Sorry, if you've been drinking you better avoid any product that contains aspirin. The alcohol makes the stomach lining super-sensitive to irritation and aspirin may cause some serious bleeding. Stick with an aspirin substitute if you've had one too many—your tummy will thank you.

ACETAMINOPHEN
   Datril
   Bromo-Seltzer
   Nebs
   Tempra
   Tylenol
   Etc.
	While aspirin substitutes are probably better than aspirin after an occasional bash, watch out if you hit the sauce regularly. A daily drinker may be more susceptible to liver damage from acetaminophen, especially if the headache remedy is used too often.

ANTICOAGULANTS (Blood thinners)
   Coumadin
   Dicumarol
   Panwarfin
   Sintrom
	Stay away from this combination— it's a bag of worms. The effect of the interaction is unpredictable and very dangerous.

*Many cold remedies contain a good slug of booze. For example, NYQUIL runs around 50 proof and COMTREX weighs in at 40 proof. TERPIN HYDRATE cough medicine may run as high as 80 proof, which makes it equivalent to gin, vodka, or whiskey.

ALCOHOL (continued)

If a person who imbibes alcohol:

ALSO USES:	THIS COULD RESULT:
ANTI-DEPRESSANTS Aventyl Elavil Marplan Nardil Norpramin Parnate Pertofrane Sinequan Tofranil Vivactil Etc.	Pop goes the weasel! This interaction can be lethal. Depending upon the type of anti-depressant and the kind of drink all sorts of bad things could happen. For example, **NARDIL** and chianti wine are so incompatible that blood pressure could rise so high a stroke could occur. Other combinations could lead to excessive sedation, incoordination, and stomach upset. To play it safe, avoid booze.
ANTIHISTAMINES Actifed Allerest Benadryl Chlor-Trimeton Contac Coricidin Dimetapp Dramamine Dristan Phenergan Triaminic Etc.	Antihistamines slow you down and often produce sedation. If you have a drink or two on top of your cold medicine or allergy regimen make sure you don't plan on doing anything important—like working or driving. Because many of these drugs are available over-the-counter people take them for granted. Don't! The interaction is dangerous and often ignored.
BARBITURATES Butabarbital Donnatal Nembutal Pentobarbital Phenobarbital Seconal	You might as well point a gun to your head if you start mixing liquor and barbiturates. If you try driving after this combination it's like pulling the trigger. This interaction is suicide city: drunk, drunker, drunkest!
CHLORAL HYDRATE Noctec Somnos	This combination is the infamous "Mickey Finn" or knockout drops. Increased sedation can occur accompanied by flushing, rapid pulse, palpitations, and headache. Don't do it!

ALCOHOL (continued)

If a person who imbibes alcohol:

ALSO USES:	THIS COULD RESULT:
DIABETES MEDICINE (Oral) Diabinese Dymelor Orinase Tolinase	People with diabetes have enough problems without adding to them by drinking. Alcohol really raises havoc with blood sugar and messes up the effectiveness of the medications. Flushing, rapid pulse, nausea, and vomiting may occur as well.
FLAGYL	**FLAGYL** is commonly used to treat vaginitis. It can make you sick as a dog if you also have a drink. Be prepared for nausea, vomiting, stomach cramps, and headaches.
NITROGLYCERIN Nitro-Bid Nitroglyn Nitrong Nitrospan Nitrostat	These heart drugs can lower blood pressure and temporarily make people dizzy. Combined with alcohol the effect is exaggerated and could lead to collapse. Be a wise old owl and stay off the sauce.
SEDATIVES TRANQUILIZERS SLEEPING PILLS Ativan Librium Clonopin Miltown Dalmane Serax Doriden Tranxene Equanil Valium Haldol Quaalude	You're asking for big trouble if you drink and take any of these drugs. There is an increased sedative effect that will interfere with coordination and make concentration difficult. Driving or working could be extremely dangerous. The interaction is potentially lethal and should be considered similar to booze and barbiturates.
PAIN KILLERS Codeine Darvocet Darvon Dolene Narcotics	Analgesics increase nervous-system depression when combined with alcohol. As usual, driving can be very dangerous even after only a couple of beers.

ALCOHOL (continued)

If a person who imbibes alcohol:

ALSO USES:	THIS COULD RESULT:
TIME CAPSULES (SPANSULES) *Long-Acting/Slow Release:* Amphetamines Antihistamines Barbiturates Cold Remedies Compazine Spansule Contac Dexedrine Spansule Diet Aids Eskatrol Spansule Nicobid Nitroglycerin Spansule Ornade Spansule Teldrin Spansule Thorazine Spansule Tuss-Ornade Spansule Etc.	Oh Mama, This Could Really Be The End! Here we have an interaction that very few people would ever even think of because it is so unique. The "Tiny Time Pills" found in spansules are slow to release their active ingredients and are meant to be absorbed gradually over many hours. The outer covering of these pills is often quite soluble in alcohol. If you were to drink something alcoholic while this kind of medicine was in your stomach normal absorption could be dramatically changed. The result may be that instead of receiving the drug over 8 or 12 hours you may get a whopping dose all at once and experience toxic effects. For some drugs, like amphetamines or antihistamines, this could be dangerous.

*Please note that alcohol can interact with over 100 different drugs. We have listed only those combinations that seem particularly dangerous. When in doubt avoid alcohol or check with a reliable professional.

NON-PRESCRIPTION DRUGS
ANTACIDS

Like the eggplant that ate Chicago, antacids are taking over. They're everywhere—gas stations, newsstands, bowling alleys, and even restaurants. We spend over $450 million on over 8,000 different brands. People often take these indigestion aids for granted. They don't even think twice as they casually put away a pack of **ROLAIDS** or **TUMS**. But antacids can interact with many prescription medications. By decreasing the acidity of the stomach contents some drugs will be absorbed more rapidly while others may never reach therapeutic levels because of antacid interference. Some drugs that may be influenced by simultaneous antacid ingestion include **Aspirin, Digoxin, Dilantin, Ephedrine, Indocin, Iron Supplements, LANOXIN, LIBRIUM, Macrodantin, Penicillin, Quinidine, Tetracycline, THORAZINE,** and **TRANXENE**. Unless specifically advised otherwise it would probably be a good rule of thumb not to take an antacid within two hours of the time you take any other medication. The following list of interactions only touches on some of the most important problems. If you're an antacid junkie and have to take any prescription drug, always check with an expert to see if the combination is compatible.

IF A PERSON WHO IS CONSUMING ANTACIDS:

(Alka-Seltzer, Aluminum Hydroxide, Amphojel, Calcium Carbonate, Di-Gel, Gelusil, Maalox, Magnesium Hydroxide, Magnesium Trisilicate, Mylanta, Rolaids, Sodium Bicarbonate, Tums, etc.)

ALSO USES:	THIS COULD RESULT:

ASPIRIN PAIN REMEDIES
 	
  Anacin
  Empirin Compound
  Excedrin
  Salicylates
  Etc.
	No big deal. In fact many pain relievers contain an aspirin/antacid combination to reduce stomach irritation. But the problem is that antacids reduce absorption of aspirin and often speed its elimination from the body. The result is that you get less power from your punch. Aspirin levels may be reduced as much as 50 percent.

NON-PRESCRIPTION DRUGS
ANTACIDS (continued)

IF A PERSON WHO IS CONSUMING ANTACIDS:

ALSO USES:	THIS COULD RESULT:

DIGITALIS HEART MEDICINE
 	
Digitoxin
    Crystodigin
    Etc.
 	
Digoxin
    Lanoxin
    Masoxin
	Antacids that contain aluminum or magnesium (**DI-GEL, MAALOX, MYLANTA,** etc.) can reduce the absorption of **Digitalis** drugs and decrease therapeutic effectiveness. Very serious! Separate antacid use by at least six hours in order to avoid interaction problems with **Digitalis.**

INDOCIN	Less absorption=less effect. Unfortunately, **Indocin** can be terribly irritating to the digestive tract. Doctors often recommend antacids to reduce stomach upset but this may diminish effectiveness. Always take the drug with food.

IRON SUPPLEMENTS
 	
    Feosol
    Fergon
    Fer-In-Sol
    Ferrous compounds
    Geritol
    Etc.
	Watch out for antacids that contain carbonate or magnesium trisilicate (**ALKA-2, A.M.T., CAMALOX, CHOOZ, GELUSIL, TUMS,** etc.). If you have iron-deficiency anemia watch out—these antacids can interfere with proper iron absorption. Give yourself a few hours' separation to prevent this interaction.

ISONIAZID
 	
    INH
    Laniazid
    Niconyl
    Nydrazid
    Rifamate
	These tuberculosis drugs may become less effective if preceded by certain antacids (**Aluminum, AMPHOJEL, MAALOX,** or **RIOPAN,** etc.) If you want **Isoniazid** to really work, take it at least one hour before using any aluminum antacids.

MAJOR TRANQUILIZERS
 	
Phenothiazines
 	
    Compazine
    Mellaril
    Thorazine
    Etc.
	Antacids that contain aluminum hydroxide or magnesium trisilicate can impede absorption of these head drugs. The result could be a return of hallucinations and delusions. In order to maintain an adequate dose make sure that antacid administration is at least two hours before or after tranquilizer use.

NON-PRESCRIPTION DRUGS
ANTACIDS (continued)

IF A PERSON WHO IS CONSUMING ANTACIDS:

ALSO USES:	THIS COULD RESULT:
PROPRANOLOL Inderal	For **INDERAL-Antacid** interaction information turn to **INDERAL** heading.
QUINIDINE Cardioquin Cin-Quin Quinidex Quinora	Antacids such as sodium bicarbonate (**ALKA-SELTZER**, **ROLAIDS**), milk of magnesia, and calcium carbonate (**TUMS**) can make the system alkaline and increase the effectiveness of **Quinidine**. This could produce a toxic reaction. Aluminum-hydroxide antacids (**AMPHOJEL**) may interfere with proper absorption and reduce effectiveness. Play it safe and steer clear of antacids.
TETRACYCLINE ANTIBIOTICS Achromycin Aureomycin Bicycline Bristacycline Declomycin Panmycin Retet Sumycin Terramycin Tetracyn Tetrex Vibramycin Etc.	Ouch! You're caught between a rock and a lead balloon on this one. **Tetracycline** antibiotics tend to cause indigestion and stomach upset. The urge to reach for the **MAALOX** or **TUMS** can be great. But don't! Antacids can dramatically reduce antibiotic absorption and lead to a therapeutic failure. Your doctor would be shaking her head in despair, and not understand why the drug wasn't working. Prolonged treatment might result or a change to a more toxic medication—all because a simple antacid prevented proper absorption. Fifty to 80 percent of the antibiotic may never reach the bloodstream because of this interaction.

ASPIRIN

Aspirin is everyone's favorite drug. Every year over 19 billion doses are sold. OUCH! That's an awful lot of pain *and* profit! Because we pop so many billions of these pills it is not surprising that familiarity breeds contempt. Since aspirin is taken so lightly many advertisers of OTC pain relievers are reluctant to reveal that their "powerful pain killer" is nothing more esoteric than acetylsalicylic acid (aspirin). The advertising makes each product sound unique and they know if they insert the words "extra strength" on the label many people will assume that the product is something special. Now please don't misunderstand us, we are all for aspirin. It's an effective anti-inflammatory agent and pain reliever and is relatively safe—by itself. But combined with other drugs, aspirin can become a hidden enemy. It is incompatible with many other medications and unless you get out your magnifying glass and check out all the ingredients on the label of your cold remedy, allergy medicine, indigestion aid, menstrual product, arthritis formula, decongestant, and sleeping pill you may not even realize that you are taking aspirin. The following interactions only represent the tail of the whale.

If a person who is consuming salicylates:

(Alka-Seltzer, Anacin, Arthritis Pain Formula, A.S.A. Compound, Ascriptin, BC Powder, Bufferin, Cope, Coricidin, Darvon Compound, Dristan, Empirin Compound, Excedrin, Fiorinal, Goody's Headache Powder, Midol, Percodan, Sine-Aid, Sine-Off, Triaminicin, Vanquish, etc.)

ALSO USES:	THIS COULD RESULT:

ALCOHOL
  Beer
  Liquor
  Wine
  You name it
	This interaction really is blood and guts. We've said it before and we'll say it again, don't "Plop, Plop—Fizz, Fizz" if you've been drinking. High doses of alcohol make the stomach lining much more sensitive to the irritating effects of aspirin. The result—gastric bleeding.

ASPIRIN (continued)

If a person who is consuming salicylates:

ALSO USES:	THIS COULD RESULT:
ANTACIDS	For **aspirin-antacid** interaction information turn to **Antacid** heading.
ANTICOAGULANTS (Blood thinners) Coumadin Dicumarol Panwarfin Sintrom	Play this combination and you hit the Big Casino! If you mix aspirin and blood thinners you may get to cash in your chips much sooner than expected. The two drugs may be lethal together because of severe hemorrhaging.
ANTI-CANCER MEDICATION Methotrexate	This is another potential killer. Aspirin increases the toxic effects of **METHOTREXATE** which are bad enough as it is. Watch out for blood disease.
ASCORBIC ACID Vitamin C	Aspirin prevents **Vitamin C** from getting into cells and doing much good. It also speeds the elimination of the vitamin. **Vitamin C**, on the other hand, prolongs and intensifies the effects of aspirin and in large doses may cause salicylate toxicity. The first signs are ringing in the ears—otherwise known as tinnitus.
ARTHRITIS MEDICATIONS Butazolidin Alka Cortisone Indocin Nalfon Naprosyn Steroids Sterazolidin Tandearil	This interaction sounds crazy because aspirin is an arthritis medication, so how could it interact with other arthritis drugs? Well it can! In some cases aspirin reduces the effectiveness of more potent arthritis drugs (**BUTAZOLIDIN, INDOCIN, NALFON, NAPROSYN**, etc.). In other cases aspirin may increase the likelihood of stomach irritation or serious side effects.
DIABETES DRUGS (ORAL) Diabinese Dymelor Orinase Tolinase	Aspirin may make these diabetes drugs work "too" well. That is, blood-sugar levels may drop too low and cause something called hypoglycemia (the opposite of diabetes).

ASPIRIN (continued)

If a person who is consuming salicylates:

ALSO USES:	THIS COULD RESULT:
	The result is that a diabetic could end up bouncing like a yo-yo from too much to too little sugar.
GOUT MEDICINE Anturane Benemid ColBENEMID	These drugs for gout work by lowering uric acid levels in the blood. Aspirin reverses this therapeutic effect and makes them much less efficient. If you don't want your big toe to hurt, avoid the aspirin.

HIGH BLOOD PRESSURE MEDICATION
Propranolol
  Inderal
Reserpine
  Diupres
  Hydropres
  Regroton
  Salutensin
  Ser-Ap-Es
  Serpasil
  Etc.
	Sit back and relax. This is not an earth-shattering drug interaction, but if you've got arthritis, it could pose a dilemma. **INDERAL** may reduce the anti-inflammatory action of aspirin and the result is that you won't get the same relief for those aching joints. **RESERPINE** knocks out the pain relief you normally expect from aspirin so that headache may not disappear. These are not dangerous interactions but may lead to therapeutic disappointments.

COLD REMEDIES, ALLERGY PRODUCTS, ASTHMA DRUGS, DECONGESTANTS, DIET AIDS

Sniffle, sneeze, cough, wheeze—no matter what your symptoms the drug companies have something ready to zap your complaints. Unfortunately, in combination with some prescription medications many of these over-the-counter products may zap YOU! These interactions can be extremely hazardous, and sad to say, are all too often ignored. Few doctors remember to warn their patients about not taking something so mundane as a cough medicine or an appetite suppressant together with a high blood pressure drug or an antidepressant. The result of this oversight could be fatal for the patient. And consumers often do not read the label on their non-prescription cold remedies that usually says: "Individuals with high blood pressure, heart disease, diabetes, thyroid disease, glaucoma, and elderly persons should use only as directed by a physician."

If a person who is taking one of the following drugs:

(ADRENALINE, Alka-Seltzer Plus, Allerest, AMPHETAMINE, Breacol, Bronkaid, Bronkotabs, Contac, Coricidin "D," CoTylenol, Dexatrim, Dimetapp, Dristan, EPHEDRINE, EPINEPHRINE, Isuprel, Neo-Synephrine, Novahistine DMX, NyQuil, Ornade, PHENYLEPHRINE, PHENYLPROPANOLAMINE, Primatene, Prolamine, PSEUDOEPHEDRINE, Ritalin, Robitussin PE, Romilar III, Sine-Off, Sudafed, Tedral, Triaminic, etc.)

ALSO TAKES:	THIS COULD RESULT:
ANTIDEPRESSANTS Aventyl Elavil Endep Limbitrol Marplan Nardil Norpramin	Going, Going, GONE! Watch out for increased blood pressure if you combine your head medicine with your nose medicine. In some cases blood pressure could go so high (hypertensive crisis) that you might end up in the emergency room or the funeral parlor. The interaction

COLD REMEDIES, ALLERGY PRODUCTS, ASTHMA DRUGS, DECONGESTANTS, DIET AIDS
(continued)

If a person who is taking a cold remedy, diet aid, decongestant, or asthma drug:

ALSO TAKES:	THIS COULD RESULT:
Parnate Pertofrane Sinequan Tofranil Triavil Vivactil	between MAO Inhibitor drugs like **MARPLAN, NARDIL**, and **PARNATE** and appetite suppressants, decongestants, and asthma drugs can be particularly dangerous. The moral: if you feed your head with antidepressants be very careful what you feed your nose and lungs. Early signs of hypertensive crisis include: severe headache, neck stiffness, sweating, nausea, vomiting, palpitations, chest pains, and rapid pulse. Call a doctor fast if they occur.
BLOOD PRESSURE MEDICATIONS Aldomet Guanethidine Aldoril Hydralazine Apresoline Ismelin Esimil Reserpine Eutonyl Ser-Ap-Es Eutron Serpasil	Cold remedies, etc., can reduce the effectiveness of blood-pressure-lowering drugs. In some cases there may even be a paradoxical increase in pressure. This is a particular problem with drugs like **ISMELIN, ALDOMET, ALDORIL, EUTONYL**, and **EUTRON**. If you've got hypertension be extremely careful what other drugs you take with your high blood pressure pills.
☠ CORTISONE-TYPE STEROIDS Aristocort Celestone Cortef Cortisone Decadron Deltasone Hydrocortone Medrol Prednisone Etc.	This is a strange and potentially life-threatening interaction. It primarily concerns the use of **ISUPREL**-type asthma inhalers with long term, high dose **CORTISONE**-type medication. Since both are used for asthma treatment this interaction may occur more frequently than it should. The fear is that fatal heart rhythms may occur.
DIGITALIS HEART MEDICINE *Digitoxin* Crystodigin	Decongestants and asthma medications can interact with **Digitalis** heart drugs to cause irregular beats.

COLD REMEDIES, ALLERGY PRODUCTS,
ASTHMA DRUGS, DECONGESTANTS, DIET AIDS
(continued)

If a person who is taking a cold remedy, diet aid, decongestant, or asthma drug:

ALSO TAKES:	THIS COULD RESULT:

Digoxin
   Lanoxin
   Masoxin
	Needless to say, that is about the last thing that a heart patient needs. To be on the safe side, shun all the medications on the cold remedy list unless your doctor gives specific approval.

☠ MAJOR TRANQUILIZERS
   Mellaril
   Novoridazine
   Serentil
   Thioril
	The Canadians have reported a case of a fatal heart rhythm apparently caused by the interaction of a cold remedy (**CONTAC-C**) and **MELLARIL**. They warn that decongestants may sensitize the heart to produce strange irregular beats that could be life-threatening.

☠ MAO INHIBITORS
   Eutonyl   (High blood
   Eutron   pressure)
   Furoxone   (Infections)
   Marplan
   Nardil   (Depression)
   Parnate
   Matulane   (Cancer treatment)
	MAO Inhibitor drugs are used for many different medical problems—from psychological depression to cancer treatment. They are extraordinarily dangerous with certain kinds of foods (see page 103) and with many non-prescription drugs. Decongestants, diet aids, and many asthma medications may increase blood pressure in combination with the MAO Inhibitors. This is a potentially lethal drug interaction!

MIGRAINE MEDICATIONS
Ergotamine
   Cafergot
   Ergomar
   Ergostat
   Gynergen
   Migral
   Oxoids
	Once again, the problem is increased blood pressure. According to Dr. Eric Martin, an authority on drug interactions, the combination could cause "extremely high elevations of blood pressure." Before using an allergy medicine, cold remedy, decongestant, diet aid, or asthma drug, check in with your doctor to get his approval.

DIARRHEA MEDICATION

Anything that affects digestive function can interfere with normal drug absorption. By the way, diarrhea itself can do a nasty number on your medicine by speeding the pills along so quickly that they never have a chance to make it past your GI tract and into your bloodstream. Overuse of laxatives may have much the same effect and the result may be that your drug won't be as effective as it could be. Doctor-prescribed diarrhea medications may increase drug absorption by slowing down gastric motility, but over-the-counter preparations that contain **Kaolin/pectin** combinations may prevent the drug from doing its job.

If a person who is consuming Kaolin/Pectin combos:

(Kaopectate, Kalpec, Kay-Pec, KBP, Kaoparic, Kapectin, Keotin, Pargel, Pecto-Kalin, Pectokay, etc.)

ALSO TAKES:	THIS COULD RESULT:

DIGITALIS HEART MEDICINE
Digitoxin
    Crystodigin
    Digitaline
    Purodigin
Digoxin
    Lanoxin
    Masoxin
	Anti-diarrhea drugs that contain **kaolin** and **pectin** may reduce **Digoxin** absorption. This in turn could lead to reduced effectiveness. For someone who must be controlled carefully the loss of activity on the part of their **Digitalis** heart medication could have dangerous consequences. If you have to use a drug like **KAOPECTATE** take it at least six hours after your **Digitalis.**

LINCOMYCIN Lincocin	Here is a sad paradox. **LINCOCIN** is an antibiotic that can cause severe diarrhea. But if you use anti-diarrhea medicine like **KAOPECTATE** the drug won't be absorbed and won't be as effective. If diarrhea or stomach cramps occur, check with your doctor. It could be an omen of more serious side effects to come including life-threatening colitis.

DIARRHEA MEDICATION (continued)

If a person who is consuming Kaolin/Pectin combos:

ALSO TAKES:	THIS COULD RESULT:

PSEUDOEPHEDRINE/EPHEDRINE
  Actifed
  Asthmaspan
  CoTylenol
  Dimacol
  Emprazil-C
  Fedrazil
  Novahistine Sinus tabs
  Novafed
  Phenergan-D
  Sudafed
  Tussend
	There is some evidence that **Kaolin** may prevent proper absorption of the decongestant **Pseudoephedrine**. This is no big deal—it just means your stuffy nose may not open up. If, however, the asthma medicine **Ephedrine** is blocked, it will be less effective in preventing an asthmatic attack. If you have to use this kind of diarrhea medicine space it out at least two hours before the **Ephedrine** or four hours after.

DIGITALIS HEART MEDICINE

Digitalis is a magnificent drug. It is one of the oldest of therapeutic agents, having been used by the ancient Egyptians and the healers of Rome as a diuretic and heart tonic. Today it is still the mainstay in the treatment of congestive heart failure and is one of the most commonly prescribed drugs on your doctor's prescription pad. But despite its benefits, **Digitalis** can be quite dangerous. The dose at which the drug is effective is very close to the dose where it can be toxic. More than most medications, **Digitalis** requires continued vigilance, especially when it comes to interactions with other drugs. While some products can reduce its effectiveness, others may make it more dangerous. Unless you take some extra precautions you may find yourself in serious trouble.

If a person who is prescribed Digitalis:

(Acylanid, Cedilanid, Crystodigin, Digitaline, DIGITOXIN, DIGOXIN, Gitaligin, Gitalin, Lanoxin, Nativelle, Purodigin, SK-Digoxin)

ALSO USES:	THIS COULD RESULT:

ANTACIDS
  Aluminum Hydroxide
  Magnesium Hydroxide
  Magnesium Trisilicate
	Digitalis will be less effective in combination with these antacids. For full information turn to **Antacid** heading in non-prescription drug interactions.

ANTIFUNGAL ANTIBIOTIC
Amphotericin B
  Fungizone
  Mysteclin-F
	This powerful antifungal agent can produce serious potassium loss from the body. This in turn may cause dangerous **Digitalis** toxicity. Frequent blood checks are a must.

BARBITURATES
  Butabarbital
  Butalbital
  Butisol
  Mebaral
  Nembutal
  Pentobarbital
  Phenobarbital
  Secobarbital
	The **Digitalis** drug to worry about here is **Digitoxin.** Barbiturates increase its metabolism and may lead to a diminished effect. Be alert for the need to alter the dose with a doctor's supervision.

DIGITALIS HEART MEDICINE (continued)
If a person who is prescribed Digitalis:

ALSO USES:	THIS COULD RESULT:
COLD REMEDIES, DECONGESTANTS, ASTHMA DRUGS, DIET AIDS *Adrenaline* *Amphetamine* *Ephedrine* *Isoproterenol* Etc.	Very sticky! These over-the-counter drugs may sensitize the heart to beat irregularly—about the last thing someone with heart failure needs. For more information on this interaction turn to the **Cold Remedy** heading under non-prescription drug interactions.
DIARRHEA MEDICINE Kaolin/Pectin	Possibly reduced effectiveness. Turn to the **Diarrhea Medicine** heading under non-prescription drug interactions.
DIURETICS (POTASSIUM WASTING) Edecrin Hygroton Lasix Zaroxolyn *Thiazides* Aldoril Anhydron Diuril Enduron Esidrix Hydrochlorothiazide HydroDIURIL Etc.	This is a biggie, so hold on tight! It is very common for people who are taking **Digitalis** drugs to receive a diuretic as well, especially **LASIX**. The hidden danger is that these water pills almost inevitably deplete the body of potassium and that in turn makes **Digitalis** very dangerous. (If you eat licorice you are in even bigger trouble for the same reason). No matter what, have frequent blood tests to monitor potassium levels. Eat foods high in this mineral (see chart on page 105). and if your doctor insists you swallow those foul tasting potassium supplements you better follow her advice.
LAXATIVES/CATHARTICS You name them . . . thousands . . .	Very messy . . . Depending upon the type of laxative or cathartic, you could experience either an increased effect or a decreased effect from your **Digitalis** drug. Check with your doctor before you start playing around with your digestive tract.

DIGITALIS HEART MEDICINE (continued)

If a person who is prescribed Digitalis:

ALSO USES:	THIS COULD RESULT:
PROPRANOLOL Inderal	**Digitalis** drugs and **INDERAL** can be combined under careful supervision. Heart rate can slow to dangerously low levels. Your doctor really has to know what he is doing to pull this one off.

QUINIDINE
  Cardioquin
  Quinaglute
  Quinidex
  Quinora
  Etc.
	Quinidine is often used to treat irregular heartbeats and so it is not uncommon for a digitalized patient to receive this medication. The danger is that it can increase the **Digitalis** effect and produce toxic reactions such as nausea and vomiting. Periodic blood checks would be an excellent idea.

SPIRONOLACTONE
  Aldactazide
  Aldactone
	A recent investigation has demonstrated that **Spironolactone** can significantly slow the elimination of **Digoxin.** If the doctor doesn't make a dosage adjustment, a toxic **Digitalis** response could occur.

ULCER MEDICINE
  Propantheline
  Pro-Banthine
  Robantheline
  Ropanth
  Spastil
	These ulcer drugs slow down the stomach and in so doing may increase the absorption of **Digitalis**. This in turn leads to increased effectiveness and may cause unexpected toxicity. Keep on the lookout for halos around lights, loss of appetite, and nausea—early symptoms of a **Digitalis** overdose.

HIGH BLOOD PRESSURE MEDICINE
If a person who is prescribed:

Aldomet or Aldoril (Methyldopa)

ALSO USES:	THIS COULD RESULT:

ANTIDEPRESSANTS
Amitriptyline
  Amitril
  Elavil
  Endep
  Etrafon
  Limbitrol
  SK-Amitriptyline
  Triavil
	Amitriptyline antidepressants may reverse the blood-pressure-lowering effect of **ALDOMET**. In fact pressure may actually rise. The combination of these two drugs may also produce some very unpleasant side effects including an increased heart rate and the shakes. This package could put a strain on your head as well as your heart.

MAO Inhibitors
  Marplan
  Nardil
  Parnate
	MAO Inhibitor antidepressants also may increase blood pressure. Even worse, they may bring on severe headaches and in some cases hallucinations. This is an interaction that should be avoided.

LEVODOPA
  Bendopa
  Dopar
  Larodopa
  Parda
  Sinemet
	The anti-Parkinson drug **Levodopa** may be rendered much less effective if you are also on **ALDOMET** or **ALDORIL** for high blood pressure. If this combination is necessary it will require careful supervision from a physician.

NERVOUS SYSTEM DEPRESSANTS *Anesthetics* (General) *Alcohol* *Barbiturates*	With this combination blood pressure could fall too far, especially during surgery. If you have to go in for an operation, make sure the doctors know you have been on **Methyldopa**.
METHOTRIMEPRAZINE Levoprome	This is an unlikely interaction, but if it does occur watch out for a drop in blood pressure. If you stand up too quickly you may land flat on your face.
ASTHMA DRUGS	Watch out! If you have asthma, **INDERAL** is extremely dangerous. It should be taken, if at all, only with careful supervision. **INDERAL** can cause severe breathing difficulties.

HIGH BLOOD PRESSURE MEDICINE (continued)

If a person who is prescribed:

INDERAL (Propranolol)

ALSO USES:	THIS COULD RESULT:
Aminophylline	Messy—the two drugs work at cross purposes and are basically incompatible.
Epinephrine Adrenalin Asthma Nefrin Vaponefrin	This interaction could be bad! Blood pressure can go up and heart rate can go down. Damn serious!
Isoproterenol Isuprel Medihaler-Iso Norisodrine	**INDERAL** may counteract the effect of these aerosols. If you need this kind of asthma medicine you probably should not be using **INDERAL** at the same time.
ANTACIDS Aluminum Hydroxide Amphojel Gaviscon Gelusil Maalox Mylanta Etc.	Aluminum-containing antacids taken at the same time as **INDERAL** may seriously interfere with proper absorption of the heart drug. The drugs should be taken at different times or an adjustment in dose might be necessary.
DIGITALIS HEART MEDICINE Digitoxin Digoxin Lanoxin	Heart rate could slow to dangerously low levels. This interaction is a little bit like tiptoeing through the tulips. With caution you can make it but the doctor really has to know his or her stuff.
DIABETES DRUGS Diabinese Dymelor Insulin Orinase	1 + 1 may well = 3 on this one. The combination of **INDERAL** and diabetes drugs could reduce sugar levels much too low. These drugs should generally not be taken together.

HIGH BLOOD PRESSURE MEDICINE/DIURETIC

If a person who is prescribed:

LASIX (Furosemide)

ALSO USES:	THIS COULD RESULT:

ANTIBIOTIC
Cephaloridine
  Loridine
  Cephalomycine
  Ceporin
  Keflodin
  Kefloridin
	This strong antibiotic is known for its ability to do damage to the kidney. This potential is greatly increased if you take **LASIX** simultaneously. Only under extreme situations should these two drugs be combined and then with utmost caution.

ASPIRIN/SALICYLATES
  Alka-Seltzer
  Anacin
  Ascriptin
  Bufferin
  Cope
  Coricidin
  Darvon Compound
  Dristan
  Excedrin
  Vanquish
  Etc.
	For your average headache victim, there will probably be no problem if you mix and match your **LASIX** and your **aspirin**. For arthritis sufferers it's a different story. **LASIX** may increase the likelihood of **aspirin** toxicity when the drug is taken in the larger quantities necessary to achieve inflammatory relief. Be on the alert for ringing in the ears as an early warning sign of danger.

CHLORAL HYDRATE
  Aquachloral
  Noctec
  SK-Chloral Hydrate
	This can be a nasty interaction. If you combine this sedative/sleeping pill with your potent diuretic you may experience hot flushes, high blood pressure, rapid pulse, and severe sweating.

CORTISONE STEROIDS
  Aristocort
  Cortef
  Decadron
  Kenacort
  Prednisone
  Prednisolone
	Both **Cortisone** and **Lasix** drive potassium from your body. When these two drugs are combined it is only natural that this unfortunate side effect would be magnified. Frequent blood tests should be called for if it is necessary to maintain this combination, especially if you also must take a digitalis heart medicine.

GOUT MEDICINE *Allopurinol* Zyloprim	One of the unfortunate side effects of **Lasix** is its habit of raising uric-acid levels in the body. This is bad

HIGH BLOOD PRESSURE MEDICINE/DIURETIC
(continued)

If a person who is prescribed:

LASIX (Furosemide)

ALSO USES:	THIS COULD RESULT:
Bloxanth Foligan Zyloric *Probenecid* Benemid ColBENEMID Urocosid *Sulfinpyrazone* Anturane Anturidin Enturen	news for people with gout because that is what generally causes them their misery in the first place. Given in combination with these gout medications, **Lasix** may reduce their effectiveness.
LITHIUM CARBONATE Eskalith Lithane Lithonate Lithotabs	**Lasix** may seriously increase the toxicity of **lithium**. The diuretic can increase the levels of the drug used for manic/depression and the result could be dangerous. Symptoms of **lithium** toxicity include weakness, diarrhea, vomiting, drowsiness, and incoordination. If they occur, get to a doctor fast!

PAIN RELIEVERS

If a person who is prescribed Propoxyphene:

(Darvon, Darvon Compound, Darvocet, Dolene, Pro-Pox 65, Progesic, Ropoxy, Scrip Dyne, SK-65, Stogesic, Wygesic, Etc.)

ALSO USES:	THIS COULD RESULT:
ALCOHOL Beer Wine Liquor	Oof. This is a potential killer, especially if you get in your car and try to drive. The interaction of alcohol and **DARVON** could lead to Zombieville.
EPILEPSY MEDICATION Tegretol	**DARVON** may increase the likelihood of side effects from **TEGRETOL**. Watch out for fatigue, nausea, headache, and dizziness.
OPHENADRINE Disipal Norflex Norgesic	These antiparkinson and anti-spasmodic drugs can get you into trouble in conjunction with **DARVON**. Reports of anxiety, confusion, and tremors have been noted, so play it safe.
SEDATIVES, TRANQUILIZERS, SLEEPING PILLS Barbiturates Dalmane Doriden Equanil Librax Librium Miltown Nembutal Phenobarbital Quaalude Seconal Tranxene Valium Etc.	The FDA and Eli Lilly, the drug company that makes **DARVON**, have recently issued strong warnings about mixing these nervous system depressants and the pain relievers. Driving ability may be impaired and too many pills may lead to an unwanted suicide. There is growing concern by many health professionals that **DARVON** has a significant risk in combination with drugs like **VALIUM**, **LIBRIUM**, and **NEMBUTAL**. Given the fact that there is little if any evidence that **DARVON** is any better than aspirin it seems hardly worth taking the risk.

ARTHRITIS MEDICATIONS

If a person who is prescribed:

Motrin (Ibuprofen)

ALSO USES:	THIS COULD RESULT:

ASPIRIN
  Alka-Seltzer
  Anacin
  Ascriptin
  Bufferin
  Cope
  Darvon Compound
  Empirin Compound
  Excedrin
  Vanquish
  Etc.
	As with many potent arthritis medications, the effectiveness of **MOTRIN** may be slightly compromised by **aspirin**. We know that sounds ridiculous since both drugs are supposed to relieve inflammation, but that is one of those strange paradoxes. This is not terribly serious, but if you want the most for your money (and **MOTRIN** is expensive) you better make up your mind what it will be—one drug or the other.

ANTICOAGULANTS
  Coumadin
  Dicumarol
  Panwarfin
  Sintrom
	For a change, we have some good news. While many other arthritis medications really interfere with blood thinners, preliminary data seem to indicate that **MOTRIN** has a minimal effect. Nevertheless, caution is the better part of valor. We recommend that you have a blood test periodically.

If a person who is prescribed:

Indocin (Indomethacin)

ALSO USES:	THIS COULD RESULT:
ANTACIDS Pick your brand among the 8,000.	There goes the anti-inflammatory effect. Antacids may significantly interfere with the benefits of **Indocin**. What a shame, too; the arthritis drug can be very irritating to the stomach. Always take **Indocin** with food.

ARTHRITIS MEDICATIONS (continued)

If a person who is prescribed:

Indocin (Indomethacin)

ALSO USES:	THIS COULD RESULT:

☠ ANTICOAGULANTS
  Coumadin
  Dicumarol
  Panwarfin
  Sintrom
	Here is an arthritis drug that does interact with anticoagulants in a most dangerous manner. Be extraordinarily careful if you end up on this combination. You could hemorrhage if the dose of blood thinner rises too high. Frequent blood tests are a must. Better yet, avoid the interaction.

THYROID HORMONE

If a person who is prescribed:

(Cytomel, Euthroid, Letter, Proloid, Synthroid, Thyrolar, etc.)

ALSO USES:	THIS COULD RESULT:
ANTICOAGULANTS Coumadin Dicumarol Panwarfin Sintrom	Watch out for hemorrhage. **Thyroid hormones** can increase the "effectiveness" of anticoagulants. Your doctor may have to make a dosage adjustment.
ANTIDEPRESSANTS Aventyl Elavil Norpramin Pertofrane Presamine Sinequan Tofranil Triavil Vivactil	**Thyroid** may enhance the ability of these drugs to relieve psychological depression. It may also increase the possibility of toxicity. If you notice a rapid pulse, nervousness, or any heartbeat irregularities, check with your doctor.
DIABETES MEDICINE (ORAL) Diabinese Dymelor Orinase Tolinase	No sweat. **Thyroid** therapy may elevate blood sugar levels in a diabetic. It may be necessary to increase the dose of your medication. Better yet, check with your doctor and see if a dietary program may not do the trick.
QUESTRAN	This cholesterol-lowering drug can really foul up your thyroid therapy. The interaction will reduce the absorption of **thyroid** and you may start to notice some of those old symptoms recurring. If it is necessary to use **QUESTRAN**, make sure you take your **thyroid hormone** at least an hour before or five hours after the cholesterol medication.

4

Graedon's Grab Bag of Wonderfully Wacky Weirdness and Helpful Home Remedies

Taking care of your heart: don't let joggers intimidate you; poor Mr. Cholesterol; the dangers of ATROMID-S • The benefits of Booze, Onions, and Garlic: bad breath can be beautiful! • Aspirin: when less is more • The earlobe is connected to the heart • Surviving the Common Cold: Three cheers for chicken soup! • The Fight for the Fart! • Searching for an authentic aphrodisiac • Sexual downers: The sins of **Saltpeter** • Soap: Claims for gentleness are mostly banana oil • Help for Hangovers • The fruit salad cure for skin • Airplane Ears • Home remedies from readers • Helping the medicine go down • A handy Table of the Sexual Side Effects of Drugs.

This chapter is dedicated to the principle that watching out for your health doesn't always have to be unpleasant or boring. We will destroy some myths and offer some surprising suggestions. We have scoured the medical literature for tantalizing tidbits, sexy trade secrets, and unusual occurrences. And thousands of readers of *The People's Pharmacy* have sent in some pretty interesting (and often bizarre) home remedies that we now have an opportunity to share with everyone. So here is a chance to relax, put your feet up and Enjoy! We can't vouch for the effectiveness of some of this craziness but we sure hope you'll find it fascinating.

TAKING CARE OF YOUR HEART

Americans put up with an awful lot in the name of preventing heart attacks and clogged arteries. Doctors exhort us to stop eating all those delicious desserts. Mr. Cholesterol is a bad guy even though he tastes yummy. We're supposed to cut back on the ice cream, the scrumptious souffles, and those succulent steaks. They tell us to use less butter and less salt and get more exercise. And we take them seriously. We've given up using real cream in our coffee. We eat only a few eggs each week and we do our best to avoid the cakes and pastries. And of course we jog. A nation of runners is out there pounding the pavement and galloping on grass and gritting their teeth through the early-morning smog.

Are all these heroic efforts worth it? Certainly exercise is good for you. It gets the juices flowing, reduces excess flab, assists in lowering blood pressure, promotes sleep, helps relieve constipation, improves outlook, and just generally makes you feel better. But lack of exercise does very little to increase your risk of heart disease. Whoops!—that sounds like heresy. With tens of millions jogging and thousands competing in marathon races the runner is king and he is a powerful evangelist. One of his strongest selling points has been the claim that long-distance runners never develop coronary-artery disease and don't drop dead from heart attacks. But in 1979 investigators reported eighteen people who died of heart attacks during or shortly after jogging. And these weren't weekend warriors either. "They were seasoned, veteran runners who had no previous heart trouble."[1] Research has also proved that "coronary-artery disease does develop in at least some marathon runners."[2] Does this mean you should give up exercise? Of course not, but the good news is that if you absolutely hate to jog, you can use the findings of these studies so that runners won't intimidate you or make you feel guilty. Rest your weary feet and relax.

All right, one myth shot down. Are you ready for another? Cholesterol has received a lot of bad press over the last twenty years. It's supposed to plug your pipes and bring on an early demise. One television commercial starred an ugly, fat little "Mr. Cholesterol" gremlin who had a nasty habit of popping up out of nowhere to ruin people's dinners. Lots of folks took him seriously and cut out milk, eggs, butter, shrimp, and liver, because these foods have high levels of the evil stuff. One of our faithful readers wrote in to ask the following questions:

**I'm healthy, 45 years old and happily married.
I'd be even happier if only my wife would stop**

trying to reform my diet "because she loves me." Her latest kick is eggs—I love them and used to eat one or two for breakfast every day. Now she's cut me back to two a week. My cholesterol levels have always checked out normal. Is there any good reason for me to give up my eggs?

B.D., Detroit, Mich.

The answer is No. B.D. doesn't have to give up his eggs. Dietary cholesterol doesn't deserve its bad reputation. The evidence is mounting that the cholesterol you eat is not the major factor that determines the cholesterol levels in blood or whether your arteries will clog with fatty build-up. Now don't misunderstand us, diet is crucial. The prudent person would do well to reduce *total* fat in the diet, especially saturated fats found in beef, pork, lamb, cream, and coconut oil (often found in non-dairy creamers), which in themselves can raise blood cholesterol levels. However, researchers at the University of Missouri recently found that serum cholesterol and triglyceride levels in 116 healthy men were no different after three months of one or two eggs every day from what they were after three months of no eggs at all.[3]

There goes myth number two. But lowering blood cholesterol levels is still a good idea, isn't it? Well, the answer isn't in on that one either. The respected journal *Medical Letter* summarized current thinking on this subject: "Lowering of markedly elevated blood cholesterol by diet is generally considered desirable even though it remains to be proven that such a reduction decreases the risk of coronary heart disease."[4] Apparently there just isn't any positive proof that lowering blood cholesterol through diet (or drugs) reduces the risk of heart attacks or prolongs life. In fact, one large study undertaken by the World Health Organization uncovered some amazing information. A cholesterol-lowering drug called ATROMID-S (clofibrate) may actually increase the risk of death from causes other than heart attacks (gallbladder, liver, and digestive tract diseases).[5] In a surprisingly candid editorial that appeared in the British journal *Lancet,* a doctor summarized the research results with ATROMID-S this way: "the treatment was successful but unfortunately the patient died."[6]

HOORAY FOR BOOZE

Bah humbug! Here we promised good news and all we've given you is grief. Don't give up and don't get disheartened. There really is reason to rejoice. You know how you've often heard that life's little pleasures are bad—salt is a killer, saccharin can cause cancer, and tobacco is just plain suicide. Unfortunately, all of that is probably true. But at long last we can report that something pleasurable may actually be good for you for a change. Alcohol in moderation seems to reduce the risk of coronary artery disease and heart attacks. So Grandma, in her infinite wisdom, was right all along when she said a shot of whiskey or a little sherry after dinner was good for the heart. As usual, it took the medical profession many years and a lot of money before they could accept her advice. The most recent research comes from investigators at Harvard Medical School. They found that:

> **The lowered risk of coronary death among light to moderate drinkers [2 oz or less of alcohol daily], which we reported previously, is remarkably similar for beer, wine, and liquor after adjusting for the different alcohol content of each of these types of beverage. [2 ozs of alcohol is comparable to 40 ozs of beer, 12 ozs of wine or 4 ozs of liquor.] Thus, it seems probable that a protective effect in coronary disease is actually due to alcohol itself rather than to other substances found in each type of drink.**[7]

This is only the latest confirmation in a long list of impressive research from around the world.[8-16] Doctors from the Honolulu Heart Study project found that Japanese men living in Hawaii who consumed moderate quantities of beer had less coronary heart disease and fewer heart attacks than non-drinkers.[17] Epidemiologists from Cardiff, Wales, reviewed data from eighteen different countries and concluded that there "is a strong and specific negative association between ischemic heart-disease deaths [heart attacks] and alcohol consumption. This is shown to be wholly attributable to wine consumption."[18] (Translated from medicalese, that means wine drinkers had fewer heart attacks.) These wonderful Welshmen concluded their research report with some wise advice for their colleagues:

> **If wine is ever found to contain a constituent protective against I. H. D. [ischemic heart disease] then we consider it almost a sacrilege that this constituent should be isolated. The medicine is already in a highly palatable form (as every connoisseur will confirm). We can only regret that we are as yet unable to give**

information to our friends about the relative
advantages of red, white or rose wine. [19]

Needless to say, this sort of good news makes many doctors very
nervous. At a recent meeting of the American Heart Association
physicians and researchers debated the significance and impact of the
alcohol data. One of the leading experts, Dr. William Castelli,
Director of the Framingham Heart Study remarked: "Can you tell
people to take two drinks a day and stop? I can't see telling someone
to start. That person could be prone to alcoholism, and you could end
up destroying his family." [20]

Of course heavy drinking is harmful! No one is suggesting that the
new scientific information be used as an excuse to start hitting the
bottle or to induce someone who dislikes alcohol to take it up. With
seventeen million alcoholics in this country the last thing we intend
is to encourage them to continue drinking or to add to their numbers.
But it is refreshing to know that if you like a glass or two of wine with
dinner, a few beers, or an occasional cocktail, you may be doing your
heart some good. One participant at the American Heart Association
Meetings offered what we think is a reasonable perspective on the
whole issue:

Dr. Arthur Klatsky (Chief, Division of Cardiology, Kaiser-
Permanente Medical Center, Oakland, California.)

> *"I think the evidence is strong that nondrinkers are at
> greater risk of coronary heart disease. I don't think
> it's the function of the medical profession to tell
> everyone what to do; patients should just be told the
> facts . . . [I] occasionally see patients in their 40s who
> have 'gone clean,' becoming teetotalers not because
> of a drinking problem but because of the fear that
> moderate social drinking is bad for their hearts.
> When such a patient asks what he can do to reduce
> his risk of a heart attack, [I] tell him to stop smoking,
> to exercise, to watch his diet, and to resume having
> one or two drinks a day."* [21]

How is alcohol exerting its beneficial effect on your heart and
arteries? That is a zillion-dollar question. There are many theories,
but the prevailing opinion has it that alcohol rearranges the
cholesterol levels in your blood. Your body manufactures something
called High Density Lipoprotein (HDL) which acts a little like a
scavenger. It runs around the bloodstream removing nasty cholesterol
build-up from arteries. Then it carries the gunky stuff to the liver

an answer. The latest research is exciting indeed because it suggests that one-half tablet (160 mg) daily is all that's necessary to obtain a beneficial anti-clotting action. Dr. Hershel Harter and his colleagues at the Washington University School of Medicine concluded that "low dose aspirin is effective, is of theoretically greater benefit than higher doses and will almost certainly be associated with less toxicity."[40] In fact, these same researchers think that even 80 mg (one-quarter tablet) might do the job. When asked if he took his own research to heart, Dr. Harter confessed that he is now taking half an aspirin tablet daily:

> **There's fairly clear evidence that at my age—38—I've got coronary vessel disease. We don't have any direct evidence, but my assumption is that if I can prevent platelet aggregation by taking half an aspirin, maybe I won't have a heart attack. We feel it's like going to church: we don't know whether it'll help, but it sure won't hurt.**[41]

As tempting as all this may seem, it would be foolish for anyone to start taking aspirin prophylactically for the rest of his or her life without checking first with a doctor. Even simple aspirin can have side effects, such as irritating the stomach lining, and it can interact in a dangerous way with many prescription medications. But if the investigators continue to report favorable results perhaps at last we can label good old aspirin a "wonder" drug and maybe it will receive the respect it deserves!

THE ENIGMATIC EARLOBE CREASE

Who should consider heart insurance? If the plumbing is in great shape and you're fit and frisky as a flea it would be foolish to reach for the garlic, onion, alcohol, or aspirin. But if you have some reason to be nervous—close members of your family who have died from heart attacks or strokes, or if the bod is in bad shape—you might want to have a heart-to-heart talk with a cardiologist. You might also want to look in the mirror and check out your earlobes. Say What? That's right, take a look at your earlobes. Some years back some doctors from the division of Cardiology at the Mount Sinai School of Medicine in New York discovered that patients with coronary artery disease frequently showed up with a "diagonal earlobe crease."[42]

In *The People's Pharmacy* we mentioned that "For reasons that are not entirely clear (genetic? physiological?), people with clogged arteries seem to have a greater chance of having a diagonal fold,

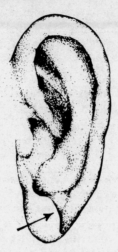

crease, or wrinkle in one or both of their earlobes. This is not to say that everyone with a crease is a candidate for a coronary, just that it could serve as an early warning sign of coronary artery disease and might merit further study." In response to that little paragraph we received an extraordinary letter from one reader who recounted his own personal experience:

> I bought "The People's Pharmacy" on the recommendation of a friend. I thought, what the heck, I've paid my money, I may as well read it. I couldn't put that book down. I was just about ready to go to sleep, maybe 2 in the morning, and I came to the heart attack part about ear lobe creases, wrinkles, and so on. I damn near fell out of bed laughing. I'd read almost all the way through and then I discover this guy Graedon has been blowin' smoke all along. Doctors from Mt. Sinai Hospital, indeed. I rolled over and went to sleep.
>
> The next morning, late (it was a Saturday) I looked into the shaving mirror and there was an old diagonal crease across my left ear lobe. Aw, . . . bull shit, I thought to myself. Sure I had experienced some chest pains off and on and I got winded easily but no big deal.
>
> But a strange magnetic force propelled me to the Nashville VA Hospital. Well, they put me on a treadmill, noting that I was 45 pounds

overweight. (I never did smoke, but I do like my beer, and I don't exert myself unduly) ... I crapped out in less than two minutes. They ran those colored dye tests on me and discovered that I had two heart arteries completely blocked and two more about 80 percent clogged. Man I was *ready!* They hospitalized me immediately.

To make a long story short, I'm home recuperating from open heart surgery. They tore hell out of my legs to get new tubes to stick up around my heart. Man, it was misery. But I reckon it beats being dead. Next week I'll be back on my sitting-on-my-ass job. I've also dropped 50 pounds and I've been walking about two miles every day.

Thanks to you and that wild-assed theory my beautiful wife and my six-year-old son, both of whom I am absolutely nutty about, will have to put up with me for a good many more years! I say "wild-assed" because a close friend of mine, after my experience, saw that he had those slanting creases on *both* ears. He went on the treadmill and the dye test and got a clean bill of health!

E.M., Nashville, Tenn.

Gadzooks! Now if that isn't an amazing story we don't what is. Do not, we repeat, DO NOT freak out just because you might have a little wrinkle in your earlobe. You read what the man said, his friend had slanting creases on both ears and "got a clean bill of health." So clearly this is not a sure thing and no one needs to rush off to the emergency room of their local hospital for a stress test, an electrocardiogram, or an angiogram (a dye test). And you certainly don't need to plan on open-heart surgery just because you have a little fold in your earlobe. But, there may be something to this weird earlobe thing after all, and it might merit a talk with a cardiologist.

Since the earliest reports quite a few articles and letters have appeared in the medical journals.[43-48] It would be only fair to state that there is no unanimity on the significance of this phenomenon. One group of researchers believes that a diagonal earlobe crease is merely associated with getting older and has nothing at all to do with heart disease.[49] However a recent review of the medical literature seems to confirm "the appearance of these creases significantly more often in CHD (coronary heart disease) patients than in age-matched controls.[50, 51] And in one study it was reported that "121 of 133 patients (90%) with a diagonal earlobe crease had angiographic evidence of CHD, while 10 of 11 (91%) of those without a diagonal crease had a normal coronary angiogram."[52]

The point of all this earlobe discussion is not to scare you out of your wits, but merely to encourage you to start taking care of your body. Prevention is the key. Our recommendations for good health: (1) Lose that tummy roll, (2) exercise—it will get your juices flowing, (3) keep the blood pressure under control, (4) relax—avoid stress whenever possible, (5) pass up the salt shaker—sodium sucks, (6) skip those saturated fats (steaks, coconut oil, bacon, etc.), (7) take tea and see—keep coffee drinking down, (8) keep up with Vitamin C—it's a friend, (9) try those onions and garlic—if you have understanding friends, (10) enjoy a drink or two with meals, and (11) last, but not least, check with your doctor about half an aspirin a day to keep the heart attack away.

SURVIVING THE COMMON COLD

Sniffle, sneeze, cough. At the first sign of a cold the collected wisdom has it that you're supposed to take two aspirins, drink plenty of fluids, and rest in bed. Baloney! Flaking out is fine, but not everyone belongs in bed with a cold. In our hustle-bustle world lots of folks just can't afford to sandbag for two or three days with a snuffly nose and a scratchy throat. And even if you do decide to treat yourself to some time off there is no evidence the cold will disappear any faster whether you climb under the covers or just keep on truckin'. All right, suppose you do skip the "rest in bed" part of the traditional advice—surely taking aspirin for a cold is a sound suggestion? Not so fast, sweetheart. Aspirin is okay if you intend to quarantine yourself, but definitely poor form if you intend to interact with your family, friends, or business associates.

Popular wisdom to the contrary, aspirin is not all that great for relieving cold symptoms. Some researchers at the University of Illinois College of Medicine undertook a truly scientific study of aspirin for the treatment of colds and found that while some people experienced a little benefit the overall effect was "disappointing."[53] Even worse than that was the totally unexpected discovery that aspirin might actually make matters worse by turning you into a walking virus-shedding "factory" that would be more likely to spread those nasty viruses around to the folks in your vicinity, sort of like a "Typhoid Mary." The doctors found that aspirin increased "virus shedding" in nasal secretions by as much as 38 percent:

> The increase in virus shedding must be considered an adverse event . . . It is probable that its occurrence in association with some relief of symptoms makes the person a better candidate to increase the spread of virus to contacts . . . Aspirin treatment, which permits the person to stay on the job with more infectious secretions, should make him a greater epidemiologic hazard. Whether the enhanced rhinovirus [cold virus] replication has any adverse effects on the individual host is not known, but it is possible . . . If so, it could influence the course of the disease, perhaps enhance the spread of virus within the host as well as to contacts, and prolong or perpetuate the infectious process.[54]

No one knows why aspirin causes this increased "virus shedding" but some investigators have hypothesized that it may reduce the natural inflammatory reaction and prevent white blood cells (your body's defenders) from mobilizing their attack against the invaders. If the ability to fight the infection is diminished this may account for the increased multiplication of the cold viruses.

Well, good golly, Miss Molly, if bed rest and aspirin aren't particularly beneficial for a cold surely plenty of fluids are a good idea? Yes and no. It sort of depends a little on what you go with. Cool liquids may actually be counterproductive.

THREE CHEERS FOR CHICKEN SOUP

It took medical science only a few hundred years to catch up with what any good grandmother knew all along—chicken soup is where it's at for colds. Three doctors from the division of Pulmonary Disease at the Mount Sinai Medical Center in Miami Beach, Florida, finally proved that hot chicken soup is tops:

> We decided to assess whether chicken soup might have a therapeutic rationale other than its good taste. We measured nasal mucus velocity, since transport of nasal secretions serves as a first line of host defense in removal of pathogens [nasties like viruses]. It was not possible to design a double blind study because the placebo could be distinguished by taste from chicken soup, but we did randomize the various treatments.

Drinking hot chicken soup either by sipping or by straw increased nasal mucus velocity compared to the sham procedure... An increase of nasal mucus velocity should be beneficial in acute rhinitis [stuffy nose] since the contact time of a pathogen on the nasal mucosa would be shortened, thereby minimizing its penetration and multiplication... Finally, the delayed suppression of nasal mucus velocity 30 minutes after drinking cold water suggests that hot rather than cold liquids might be preferable in the recommendations for fluid intake in patients with upper respiratory tract infections [colds].[55]

What these doctors are trying to say is that if you have a cold, hot chicken soup is much better for your nose than cold water. As we've said, any grandmother could have told them that. We hope they won't try to figure out what the "aromatic compound" is that produces this therapeutic effect. Like our wonderful Welshmen said when they concluded their report on the value of wine in helping to prevent coronary heart disease, "we consider it almost a sacrilege that this constituent should be isolated. The medicine is already in a highly palatable form." Any connoisseur of chicken soup would heartily agree.

THE FIGHT FOR THE FART

Flatulence is not something polite people are supposed to talk about. Although intestinal gas is a normal part of living, about the best we can do is try to pretend it doesn't exist or make jokes that are, as the neighbor's son would say, gross. But gas is gas and gross though it may be, it is hard to ignore. Flatus can be *uncomfortable,* especially when restrained, *embarrassing* when you are at a party, and ultimately *smelly.* Given all those unpleasantries, plus a cultural taboo against talking about the subject, it's no wonder that a lot of people suffer in smelly silence. Well it's time we opened the window, pulled back the blind, and fought the fight for the fart.

Now some folks might be offended by the use of this Anglo-Saxonism. But really now, is the more acceptable "breaking wind" or "flatus" any better than this simple, more common word? A recent letter to the editor of the prestigious *New England Journal of Medicine* suggests that the word fart is a perfectly appropriate term and not offensive when used clinically:

Speaking The Unspeakable

This letter is to make it official. The word fart was used factually, without embarrassment at 1310 hours (1:10 PM) on Wednesday, May 17, in Lecture Room B, University Hospital, during a lecture to the second-year medical class on "Gaseousness." I was encouraged to use the term by the recent correspondence on the matter in the *Journal.* I am essentially a God-fearing man, an avoider of obscenities, and a lover of the English language. On due reflection I was persuaded of the intrinsic value of this word and of its non-offensiveness. The students have been encouraged to use it freely where clinically appropriate. Not unnaturally, there were a few titters; indeed it would be true to say there were even a few guffaws at first. But once the word had been used a few times, it came to sound natural and as unremarkable as any other suitable clinical term.

I hope that all other clinicians, men of honor and upright standing, will follow this lead. A spark has been struck, a torch has been lit. Let it shine forth and illumine the dark recesses of what has hitherto been that unspeakable thing.

I am acknowledging the encouragement of the *Journal,* with fart healt thanks.[56]

W. C. Watson, M.D.
Victoria Hospital
London, Ontario, Canada

Dr. Watson has opened the door to liberation. Perhaps if we follow his lead and destroy some of the myths and blow away some of the hot air surrounding this topic we would all be a little less nervous or offended. Everyone makes gas—it's a normal part of the digestive process. The average amount varies from about a little less than a pint to almost two quarts per day, and some poor souls can produce significantly more than that, especially after pigging out on certain notorious foods.

Despite all the "How do You Spell Relief" ads, there is little evidence that antacid ingredients like sodium carbonate (ROLAIDS), sodium bicarbonate (ALKA-SELTZER, BISODOL, ENO, SODA MINT, etc.) or simethicone (DI GEL, FLACID, GELUSIL, MYLANTA, RIOPAN, SILAIN-GEL, etc.) will relieve intestinal gas problems. While they may have some effect on stomach bubbles, that hardly seems helpful since flatus is formed mainly in the large intestine, at the end of the track, so to speak. Bacteria in the large intestine continue to break down whatever food or residue is left after the small intestine gets done doing its digestive thing. Depending upon your particular constitution and the type of food you eat, a fermentation process begins that leads to the production of gas. In a marvelous article titled "Passing Gas," Drs. Eugene Silverman and Eric Rabkin describe the process this way: "In champagne, fermentation produces bubbles; in the large intestine—flatus."[57] When the pressure mounts, out it comes, sometimes with impressive force.

There are basically five different kinds of gas that contribute to flatulence. Oxygen and nitrogen are swallowed in the process of eating, chewing, and drinking but are relatively less important than carbon dioxide, hydrogen, and methane, which are by-products of bacterial fermentation in the large intestine. By the way, not everyone makes methane (otherwise known as swamp gas). For reasons that are totally obscure, only about one-third of the population are methane producers. The quickest way to tell whether you belong in that category is to check on whether you make floaters or sinkers. A stool that floats is often caused by methane gas.

Once upon a time doctors told people that if farting was a problem it must be because they were swallowing too much air when they ate. Better research by experts in this field (flatologists) now seems to indicate that while a few folks do gulp excessive amounts of air while eating, the gas they pass is generally unrelated to the air they swallow and probably results more from their own fermentation factory than anything else.[58] One quick way to determine the origins of the problem is the sniff test. Swallowed air does not produce an unpleasant odor.

If you do suffer from smelly flatulence, dietary discretion might help. A large-scale study undertaken by Dr. Walter Alvarez in 1942 revealed that onions give most people trouble. (Good for the heart, but they'll make you fart.) He also found that after onions, "the foods most commonly blamed were cooked cabbage, raw apples, radishes, dried beans, cucumbers, milk, fatty or rich foods, melons, cauliflower, chocolate, coffee, lettuce, peanuts, eggs, oranges, tomatoes and strawberries."[59] In a more recent and more quantitative test, scientists at the University of California, Berkeley, actually analyzed the gas that was passed after some extremely cooperative human guinea pigs consumed selected fruits and juices. They discovered that apple juice and raisins significantly increased output while orange juice and apricot nectar had no effect at all.[60]

How can a flatulator get relief? Unfortunately, the medical profession has a pretty poor track record when it comes to treatment. One of the readers of *The People's Pharmacy* offered a real tale of woe:

> **I happen to be inflicted with the irritating and embarrassing problem of excessive gas. I have had everything from VALIUM to psychiatric help, but nothing has helped. I have had different diets that excluded gas-producing foods (like beans, peas, cabbage, pizza, carbonated beverages, etc.), but included foods rich in bulk, bran and roughage. I took LIBRIUM, VALIUM, DI-GEL, MAALOX, MYLANTA, GELUSIL, SERUTAN, PHAZYME, ACTIVATED CHARCOAL TABLETS, etc., etc., etc. I have seen countless medical doctors, internists, gastroenterologists, x-ray technicians, laboratory personnel, etc. I was even given advice on table etiquette; that is, eating my meals slowly with moderate morsels, so as not to swallow too much air into my stomach. Along the way I also went to a "reputable" hypnotist. To sum it all up: Nothing worked!**
>
> **W. N., Elmhurst, N.Y.**

Our friend from Elmhurst certainly has been through the wringer. Even though he has not had any success with diet we would recommend that he keep a food diary and try to correlate any improvement or worsening in his condition with particular foods, especially milk. A surprisingly similar case history was reported by Dr. Michael Levitt, a sensitive and knowledgeable flatologist from the University of Minnesota Department of Medicine:

> **The physician seldom deals rationally with a patient complaining of excessive flatus.... Evaluation usually consists of X-ray and endoscopic studies, when, in truth, there is no known cause of excessive flatus that such procedures might identify. As a result, psychologic or medical therapy (or both) is administered without knowledge of the cause of the problem. We studied an unusual patient who**

documented his flatulence by means of a meticulous recording of the time of each passage of gas.

A 28-year-old man had a five-year history of passing excessive flatus for which he had consulted seven different physicians. Repetitive X-ray and endoscopic studies of the gastrointestinal tract gave normal results. His problem was attributed to air swallowing, and he was counseled to eat slowly with his mouth closed and to reduce the pace of his life. This advice and a variety of medications were of no benefit.

In 1974 he began to keep "flatographic" recordings of the time of each passage of flatus ... Over a one-year period he passed flatus an average of 34 times a day ... His food recordings suggested that the high gas excretion might be related to milk ingestion. When he ingested nothing but milk (2 liters per day for two days) his daily flatus frequency rose to 141, including 70 passages in one four-hour period ... Daily flatus frequency on a lactose-free diet has averaged 25, which is significantly less than that on his previous milk-containing diet ... [61]

It is hoped neither you nor any of your friends suffer like Dr. Levitt's patient. But if flatulence is a problem we recommend that you keep a "flatographic" record and try to match food intake with gas outflow. You may find to your surprise that certain unsuspected foods will be particularly gassy. If you are one of the millions of people who are unable to digest lactose, the major sugar in milk, that could explain problems of bloating, cramping, flatulence, or diarrhea after consuming milk or milk-containing foods. If it does turn out that "lactose intolerance" is causing you grief that doesn't necessarily mean you have to give up milk. There is a product available called LACT-AID (available from the Sugarlo Company, P.O. Box 1017, Atlantic City, New Jersey 08404) that contains an enzyme which predigests a large proportion of the milk sugar when it is added to milk. For most people who use this powdered enzyme symptoms caused by undigested lactose all but disappear.

There is also good news on the bean front. If you are like many other people beans can really do you in. A recent update in our favorite magazine (*Mother Jones*) offers the following optimistic report:

> **Now that you've presumably adjusted to the concepts of the square tomato and the burpless cuke, get ready for the gasless bean. Dr. Bent Skura, a food scientist at the University of British Columbia, reports that he's been signing up student volunteers at $25 a day to test for potentially non-gas-producing beans. Skura claims that a nutritious bean that would not cause its eaters "subsequent embarrassment" would be "a significant dietary breakthrough."[62]**

We wish Dr. Skura lots of luck in this crucial research. But if he is unsuccessful or if dietary discretion is a bore, if activated charcoal doesn't bring relief and if bran is a bust, then all we can say is **DON'T FIGHT THE FART**. Some experts blame diverticular disease on our passion for polite restraint.[63] If you suffer the consequences of overindulgence, an understanding spouse should appreciate the need for relief, though we agree, a certain distance would be welcomed.

SUCCULENT SEX:
SEARCHING FOR AN AUTHENTIC APHRODISIAC

Ever since humans discovered what a good thing sex was it seems they've been trying to improve on it. The endless search for aphrodisiacs and sex enhancers dates back to ancient times. Artichokes, asparagus, truffles, oysters, ginseng, garlic, ground-up rhinoceros tusk, and crocodile kidneys are just a few of the agents that have been used to perk desire or improve performance. There is little evidence that any of these "delicacies" did anything more than stimulate the imagination. Supporters, however, are enthusiastic. Take ginseng, for example. Folklore surrounding this root stretches back at least two thousand years. Current claims for its ability to promote sexual potency are puny at best and only semi-substantiated in animal research. Some studies report that ginseng facilitates mating behavior in rats, increases gonadal weight, accelerates ovulation in frogs, and stimulates egg-laying in hens. But whether enhanced egg-laying or faster frog ovulation has any relevance for human sexuality is yet to be established.

The one drug with the hottest but least deserved reputation is still SPANISH FLY. Tales of phenomenal sexual exploits with this alleged aphrodisiac have circulated in men's locker rooms and at fraternity parties for years. Although there are minor variations, the recycled stories imply that if a woman is slipped some SPANISH FLY she will become wild with desire. Not only will she be unable to resist any man's advances, she will go to great lengths to satisfy her need for gratification. As usual, the stories are pure poppycock. Even the name is a misnomer.

SPANISH FLY or cantharides doesn't come from a fly at all but rather from a beetle and Spain is not its primary territory. The bug ranges from southern Europe to western Siberia and into parts of Africa.[64] In the eighteenth and nineteenth centuries the beetle extract was prized for its medicinal properties. It is a counterirritant and in fact is still occasionally employed today as the ointment cantharidin when it is applied to blister warts in order to make them disappear. The drug got its undeserved reputation as an aphrodisiac because when the liquid is swallowed it irritates the digestive and urinary tract, dilates genital blood vessels, and causes a painfully persistent penile erection that is unrelated to sexual pleasure or arousal. Nevertheless, the myth persists and there are still occasional "cases of self-poisoning by men or poisoning of women by men in anticipation of producing sexual arousal."[65] Side effects include vomiting, diarrhea, severe stomach pain, and shock. Too large a dose can even be fatal.

POPPERS

The latest candidate in the continuing quest for an aphrodisiac is an unlikely heart drug called AMYL NITRITE. This prescription medication is a close cousin of nitroglycerin and is used to relieve the acute pain of angina. Instead of taking the medicine orally or dissolving a tablet under the tongue, patients squeeze open a capsule between their fingers and inhale the vapors. Amyl Nitrite is a fast-acting drug that goes to work in about thirty seconds to diminish chest pain. The effect lasts about three to five minutes.

How can a medication that was designed for older people with clogged coronary arteries improve sexual pleasure? Although no one seems to know exactly how the rumors got started, the current craze apparently originated about a decade ago within the gay community in California. AMYL NITRITE or "POPPERS" (named because of the popping sound heard when the capsule was broken) were reported to bring on "increased awareness and intensified orgasm or a sense of prolonged orgasm and increased sense of excitement or involvement."[66] Although AMYL NITRITE could hardly be categorized a drug of abuse and banned, drug companies did make it more difficult for people to get it without a prescription. To fill the void another chemical was created called ISOBUTYL NITRITE and sold at discos and head shops under such unlikely names as LOCKER ROOM, CRYPT, and BULLET. Pretty soon the movement spread to the heterosexual community but there is some doubt POPPERS can live up to expectations. A letter we received from one reader points up some of the problems that you can run into with this so-called aphrodisiac:

> Last week my husband came home with a surprise he said would really add zest to our sex life. Someone at work gave him something called POPPERS. I thought the whole idea was pretty dumb but my husband was all excited and so I figured what the heck. Well, all I have to say is that the big event turned into a big disaster. First, taking time out in the middle of love making to sniff some horrible smelling drug was a little like having a coffee break in the middle of a roller coaster ride. Second, I found the experience far from pleasant or exciting. I got a terrible, pulsating headache almost immediately. My heart started beating very fast, I felt nauseous and I almost fainted. Fortunately, these unpleasant side effects didn't last too long but they had just the opposite effect my husband was anticipating. All that got stimulated was my urge to sock him. Our big love making episode ended up in an argument.
>
> **T.L., Buffalo, N.Y.**

What a bummer! POPPERS may still be big in the gay community but the side effects (headaches, racing heartbeat, nausea, and dizziness) and the interruption in the middle of lovemaking seem about as conducive to sex as forty lashes with a wet noodle. If it's your thing, great, but don't push it onto anyone else. Although serious adverse reactions have been rare there are reports that some sensitive persons can experience a drop in blood pressure that might precipitate circulatory collapse. In our opinion a good dose of TLC (Tender Loving Care) would be a whole lot more effective in adding zest to your sex life.

PLACEBO POWER

And the beat goes on. Today's list of alleged aphrodisiacs includes VITAMIN E, QUAALUDE, (methaqualone), MARIJUANA, L-DOPA, and an experimental drug called PCPA (p-chlorophenylalanine). At the risk of being called party poopers all we can say is that there is little evidence that any of these agents will truly restore lost libido or enhance lovemaking. Mental attitude is much more important than anything else and if expectations are high it is entirely possible that performance will follow even if the substance provides no actual physical benefit. Remember that simple foods like asparagus, artichokes, and sweet potatoes, which we now take for granted, were once thought to be powerful aphrodisiacs. The lowly prune was considered so sexually stimulating by Shakespeare's contemporaries that "owners of brothels distributed them free to clients so that the customers' performance would match their passion."[67]

GET WHAT EVERY MAN NEEDS
WITH FANTASTIC PLACEBO SEX AIDS

**For A Better Erection That Will Astound
You and delight Your Partner
ERECTION PILLS**

**Do You Measure UP? You Can.
IMITATION SPANISH FLY & GINSENG**
Unbelievable In Their Effect

Not Getting It Up Lately?
STA-POWER PILLS
For A Terrific Rise

Do You Need Help?
INSTANT ERECTION CREAM
Create a New Dimension of Sexual Delight[68]

Today, the advertisements in men's magazines tell the story best. Obviously, these manufacturers are counting on the fact that their readers aren't familiar with the scientific term for the inactive sugar pill (placebo) when they promote their "PLACEBO SEX AIDS." If a person believed that one of these drugs really worked it is conceivable he would experience some benefit, but it's sad to see people with problems that might be truly helped with adequate counseling left to drift with an expensive placebo preparation. And some erection creams could cause problems. These products which are designed to delay ejaculation almost inevitably contain local anesthetics that can cause allergic reactions and skin irritation both for the man and the woman. Take a hard look at any erection preparations before you waste good money. Impotence can be caused by many things, including a number of prescription medications, and the root cause should be treated rather than the symptom.

NEARING THE GOLDEN FLEECE

We promised good news in this chapter and so far our search for the elusive aphrodisiac has been a bust. Before we give up the quest entirely there is some hope for the future. It has been known since 1973 that a natural hormone called LRH (luteinizing releasing hormone) has a stimulating effect on sexual behavior. Respectable researchers at the Salk Institute "custom-designed" a similar chemical that apparently "turns on the sex drive."[69] The drug is currently being studied by Dr. Robert Moss at the Southwesten Medical School and preliminary testing on animals is tantalizing.[70,71] However, a lot more work has to be done before this experimental drug makes it out of the preliminary stage and is judged safe for humans. In the meantime we recommend big doses of TLC.

SEXUAL DOWNERS

The classic complaint of soldiers, prisoners, boarding-school students, and university undergraduates alike has been, "They're putting SALTPETER in the food." The collective paranoia assumed that the "authorities" were trying to turn everyone off. Well, you can relax. We've got some good news. There is no evidence that anyone ever put potassium nitrate (SALTPETER) in anything and even if they did it is unlikely to have had any effect. Dr. Thomas Benedek, a professor of medicine at the University of Pittsburgh, researched the matter and came up with some comforting information:

> **Saltpeter has no effect on sexual function. The origin of this myth is obscure ... The most generally accepted nontoxic medicinal effect of saltpeter in the 18th and 19th centuries was that it "cools," even though no temperature lowering effect was demonstrated objectively. For instance, according to the** *American Dispensatory* **(1806): "... It diminishes the heat of the body, and the frequency of the pulse ..."**
>
> **The most plausible conclusion that may be drawn from the small amount of information available is that since sexual excitement is equated with "heat," the lore about the anaphrodisiac [anti-sexual] effect of saltpeter has resulted from the belief in its refrigerant action.**[72]

The male population should probably give a collective sigh of relief after discovering that SALTPETER is harmless. Actually, harmless is not quite the right word. SALTPETER is pretty hot stuff seeing as how it's the primary ingredient in gunpowder and fireworks. While it won't make your sex life blast off it shouldn't make it fizzle either.

Folklore aside, however, there are many drugs that *can* affect in a negative way not only sexual desire but also performance. Although doctors are reluctant to discuss the sexual side effects of the drugs they prescribe, reduced libido, impotence, inhibition of ejaculation in men, and failure to achieve orgasm in women are some of the sexual dysfunctions associated with many of the medications in the physicians' arsenal. But before we tackle the heavy stuff, here's a gentle word of caution for the candy connoisseurs. Bizarre as it may seem, the licorice lover who overindulges (gorges might be a more appropriate term) may suffer various side effects including libido loss and impotence.[73] If that sounds too incredible for words here is a recent case report from the Department of Endocrinology of the famed Karolinska Hospital in Stockholm, Sweden (published in *Lancet*, 1979):

> A 22-year-old gymnastics teacher without any previous serious illness or medications was investigated in 1973 because of secondary amenorrhea [loss of periods] and impaired libido . . .
>
> In 1977, she attended [the] hospital because of attacks of severe headache for 1½ years. During attacks, which occurred about once a month, the pain began in the forehead and then spread, ending in vomiting and photophobia [sensitivity to light]. Blood pressure during attacks and during observation period on the ward was 240-210/130-100 . . . with a pulse rate of 44-60/min.
>
> On careful questioning the patient said that she had for several years been eating excessive amounts of liquorice. When the liquorice was withdrawn, the blood-pressure returned to normal within 2 weeks . . . After 6 months, when the hormone levels had gradually returned to normal, menstruation returned. She has had no headache attacks . . . The symptoms of this patient—headache, vomiting, and photophobia—indicate liquorice toxicity . . . [74]

Presumably, the elimination of licorice restored her libido and ended an intriguing medical mystery. Would that all cases of impaired sexuality could be cured so easily. A surprisingly large number of prescription drugs can muck up a person's love life. Drugs used to treat high blood pressure are the worst offenders when it comes to interfering with sex, but they are by no means the only ones. Medications used to treat psychological depression and anxiety may also adversely effect sexuality. Anti-psychotic medications, especially the major tranquilizers, can produce a range of unpleasant reactions. For example, MELLARIL (thioridazine) can make achieving and maintaining an erection very difficult and it may totally interfere with ejaculation. In addition, the drug may cause breast engorgement and milk secretion. Even some medicine used to relieve ulcers can lead to impotence or infertility.

It is time for the silence surrounding sexual side effects to stop. Doctors are reluctant to warn or ask their patients about these drug-induced disabilities because they are afraid that the mere mention that a medicine could produce libido loss or cause impotence might produce a psychosomatic response. While it's true that suggestion by itself can sometimes cause a side effect we can think of nothing more devastating than the feelings of self-doubt and marital discord that could be created if a patient developed impotence or had difficulty achieving orgasm and did not know the reason. A reader of our newspaper column, *"The People's Pharmacy,"* anonymously sent the following letter which points up the kinds of problems that may occur:

> **Three years ago my doctor discovered I had moderately high blood pressure. He put me on a drug called ALDOMET (methyldopa) that he said would control it and would have few side effects. I haven't noticed any bad reactions, but over the last couple of years I have occasionally experienced some difficulty in having sexual relations with my wife. This was making me more and more depressed so when I told my doctor I was feeling pretty low, he prescribed TOFRANIL (imipramine), an anti-depressant medication. I started taking the new drug six weeks ago and now I can't make love at all. I even have had trouble urinating. My doctor never mentioned sexual problems when he gave me my prescriptions, but I am starting to wonder whether my troubles in bed are all in my head or might be caused by my medicine.**
>
> **Anonymous**

If doctors were only more upfront about side effects this sort of situation would never have occurred. ALDOMET can indeed interfere with sexuality, and to compound the problem, the drug that was prescribed to deal with this poor fellow's depression (TOFRANIL) has also occasionally been associated with impotence. No wonder his troubles got worse! People have a right to know about all adverse reactions, including sexual ones. And men are not the only victims. Although there has been much less effort devoted to discovering how women react, there is evidence that some prescription medications can limit their libido and cause a failure to achieve orgasm.

Fortunately, people need not suffer in silence because they're too embarrassed to mention their problem. Doctors have a number of alternative medications that can achieve the same therapeutic benefit but may not have these unpleasant consequences. Usually the symptoms disappear when the drug is stopped. Perhaps switching from one medication to another may well eliminate the difficulty. By no means, however, should anyone cease taking a medicine without a doctor's supervision. At the end of this chapter you will find a brief chart that will help you find out which commonly prescribed medications have the potential to cause sexual side effects. If you have been using one of these drugs without experiencing any problems, don't start looking for any now, just count your blessings. It is hoped this guide will serve as a general reference that will encourage doctors and patients to start communicating about a sensitive but crucial subject.

Since we promised strangeness, here is one final bizarre word of caution about sexual side effects from drugs. If you are allergic to penicillin it may not be enough to avoid taking the drug yourself. Dr. Larry Millikan, a professor of dermatology at the University of Missouri, was reported as cautioning that "A woman who is allergic to penicillin may •acquire urticaria [itchy hives] after having intercourse with a man who is taking the drug. This phenomenon occurs because penicillin levels in seminal fluid can be as high as those in the blood, causing the hypersensitivity reaction."[75]

SOFT AS A BABY'S ARSE

Wouldn't it be lovely if we could all keep our baby skin forever? Soft, smooth, and beautiful. No such luck, but the kind of soap you use may make a difference. Most of the soap- makers' ads are nothing but a lot of froth. According to our favorite dermatologist, Dr. Albert M. Kligman, Professor of Dermatology at the University of Pennsylvania, advertisements that claim a particular soap is mild, soothing, softening, or gentle "are baloney, totally without substantiation."[76] Writing in the *Journal of the American Academy of Dermatology,* Dr. Kligman recently stated, "The average American is having a love affair with cleansing agents, consuming over 28 pounds of soaps and detergents yearly. Little is known about the safety of soaps ... The naked truth is that physicians, dermatologists included, have no more knowledge than their spouses or patients concerning which soaps to recommend for 'sensitive' skins." [77]

Dr. Kligman set out to remedy that situation by scientifically studying eighteen popular brands. He discovered that many of the expensive, highly respected soaps we thought were gentle were no better than cheaper bar soaps. Here are some of his conclusions: "ZEST, CAMAY and LAVA were the most irritating," and most likely to induce redness, scaling, chapping and cracking in sensitive individuals. Faring better but still tough on tender skin were IRISH SPRING, BASIS and CUTICURA. IVORY was not the super-mild soap we expected, but rather, according to Kligman, ranks "somewhere in the middle" of the pack. "NEUTROGENA, a supposedly neutral soap, was no different than IVORY."[78]

Where's the good news? One soap stands proud. Much to our amazement, DOVE was the big winner. It received Kligman's golden-ring award for mildness. It wasn't just good, it was in a league all its own, and of the eighteen soaps he tested DOVE was the only brand that consistently satisfied the dermatologists' standards for gentleness. Personally, we find the smell of DOVE a little overwhelming but we discovered a trick to overcome that drawback, at least to a degree. Take the bar out of its box a few weeks before you expect to use it and stash it away in a corner someplace. When you get around to washing with it the smell won't be so noticeable. One other problem—DOVE seems to melt away very quickly, but that may be the price you pay for a mild soap. Although nothing else approached DOVE for gentleness, AVEENOBAR, PURPOSE, and DIAL (in that order) came the closest of the remaining seventeen brands.

Naturally, the major soap manufacturers got all in a lather over Dr. Kligman's results. A representative of Procter and Gamble claimed that his study "involved an exaggerated and unrealistic laboratory test ... We do not believe that this research is at all representative of the way consumers use bar soap."[79] We'll put our chips on Kligman any day. When buying soap it's easy to be seduced by claims of germ-killing potency on one hand or mildness on the other. But you don't have to use an antibacterial soap to smell clean and you can't rely on the manufacturers' ads for proof as to which soap is gentle. Of course if your skin is not sensitive you can probably use just about any brand you want and never suffer the consequences.

ODDS AND ENDS

As we said at the beginning of the chapter we have received lots of fascinating home remedies from readers all across the country. Although we can't guarantee the effectiveness of any of these sometimes bizarre suggestions we did find some of them either so entertaining or potentially helpful that we felt like sharing. A pharmacy student sent in the following suggestions:

> **I would like to pass along to you a few "cures" which I know of. The first one has worked for me many times and also for the people I recommend it to. It is simply to put LISTERINE on mosquito bites to relieve itching. If this doesn't work, at least you will have a mosquito bite that doesn't have bad breath.**
>
> **The second "cure" is to take moderate to large doses of vitamin B complex before you consume large amounts of alcohol. This remedy is to avoid a hangover the following day.**
>
> **M.K., East Brunswick, N.J.**

To be perfectly honest, we didn't find LISTERINE all that great, but you may want to give it a shot. However, as we said in *The People's Pharmacy* we have had good luck with hot water for itchy bug bites. The trick is to use water that is slightly painful but not so hot that it burns. Application for a few seconds can provide relief for hours.

EYE OF NEWT AND HAIR OF DOG

Hangover remedies are a whole other kettle of fish. Ever since humans discovered the process of fermentation they have been searching for a quick solution to the aftereffects of intoxication. The humorist H. Allen Smith offered a rather drastic antidote: "The only known cure for a hangover is to lie face down in a snow drift." If that sounds too extreme you could always go with one of the totally untested hair-of-the-dog folk remedies that get passed around on New Year's day. Our Mexican friends swear by tripe soup first thing in the morning. If you ever tasted tripe you'd swear too. Texans tend toward the dramatic. One self-proclaimed authority from Dallas assured us that spicy hot chili smothered with chopped onions and topped off with tequila will make you forget your headache instantly. It will probably make you forget everything else as well. The late

Toots Shor, a renowned restauranteur in New York City, offered his debauched clients a "bull shot"—beef bouillon, two teaspoons Worcestershire, two teaspoons ketchup, a dash of pepper, two dashes of vinegar, and the yolk of a raw egg. The glop is then swallowed in one gulp, taking extra care not to let the egg break on the way down. Anything that tastes that terrible almost has to be good for you.

As for the vitamin-B hangover remedy that our friendly pharmacist from East Brunswick, New Jersey, recommended earlier, we admit that we've heard about such a "cure" from other sources. It certainly seems healthier than some of the folk tales we just mentioned but we're reluctant to (1) endorse the consumption of "large amounts of alcohol" or (2) promote something that hasn't been proved. However, if you are wont to overindulge from time to time, you may wish to give this home remedy a try. Please do let us know if it works.

We can eliminate one other home remedy for hangovers. A reader from Phoenix, Arizona, suggested large quantities of apple juice or other high-level fructose beverages to relieve inebriation. But an article in the *Annals of Internal Medicine* shot that one down pretty fast. The researchers discovered that "Not only was fructose found ineffective in treating acute alcohol intoxication, but there were also indications it could be potentially harmful: it increased serum levels of uric acid and lactate in all patients."[80, 81]

If what you need is a sober-up pill, there's hope on the horizon. And we don't mean coffee. Popular wisdom to the contrary, caffeine is totally ineffective in clearing up the cobwebs. At best it can make you only an awake drunk, even more dangerous behind the wheel because you might think you could really drive. Okay, enough suspense. The good news we're referring to comes from the University of California at Irvine where medical researchers have successfully tested three common drugs that will rapidly reverse some of the effects of alcohol on the brain. Dr. Ernst Noble, a neurobiologist and psychiatrist, and his colleague, Dr. Ronald Alkana, experimented with two drugs used to treat asthma—ephedrine (50 mg) and aminophylline (200 mg). They found that both medications could improve motor coordination and balance by almost 50 percent within 30 minutes."[82, 83] They also obtained good results with the drug L-Dopa which is used to treat Parkinson's disease, but it had the drawback of causing nausea in some of the test subjects. Although there is no clear explanation of how ephedrine or aminophylline reverse the effects of alcohol, Dr. Noble offers the following hypothesis:

> They work in the same way adrenaline does
> when a motorist with a few drinks under his
> belt sees flashing red police lights approaching.
> They stimulate chemicals in the brain that
> reverse the effects of alcohol and help sober you
> up.[84]

Ephedrine is available in the over-the-counter asthma remedy BRONKAID tablets, or generically as straight ephedrine. We are, of course, not actually recommending the use of such a drug to sober up. For one thing it could have negative effects on people with high blood pressure or diabetes. And for another, moderation is the best policy. A wise woman once said that dilution is the solution to pollution. What she meant is that if you keep your drinks low in alcohol content and high in mixer you won't get polluted. That way there won't be any intoxication and better yet, no hangover.

PAPAYA—GOOD FOR THE TUMMY
AND GREAT FOR THE SKIN

A reader in Durham, North Carolina, sent us an intriguing clipping that told of a "fruit salad" cure for resistant skin infections. A British surgical team discovered that they could cure post-operative infections by "laying strips of raw papaya or paw paw fruit on the wound in a technique borrowed from African folk medicine ... We have treated at least 10 patients with infected wounds of various sorts, and it works. We do not know why, but there appears to be something in the fruit that stimulates the wound to heal."[85] Papaya contains an enzyme called papain which is the primary ingredient in meat tenderizer. In the past we have recommended this remedy for the treatment of bee stings (add a few drops of water to a teaspoon of the powder, make a paste, and spread it over the sting). You can buy a commercial product (with a prescription from your doctor) called PANAFIL OINTMENT that contains the pure papain enzyme. It is unlikely that your pharmacist will ever have heard of PANAFIL but she can order it from the Rystan Company (470 Mamaroneck Ave., White Plains, New York 10605). Interestingly, it is specifically intended for "promotion of normal healing of surface lesions, particularly where healing is retarded by local infection."[86] The "fruit salad" cure is not as strange as it sounds. Here is one home remedy that may really work.

ALOE VERA FOR BURNS

Another possibility comes from a woman in Texas who says:

I've been using the juice of a cut aloe vera plant to treat common household burns. I notice immediate relief from the pain and I swear that the burn goes away much faster. I have passed this home remedy around to friends, neighbors and relatives and everyone agrees that it is much better than anything you can buy in a drugstore.

When I told my doctor about aloe vera the other day he just laughed. He said that it had been tested and proved ineffective. Adding insult to injury he told me that if I believed in it hard enough it probably would work, but that it wasn't any better than a cream or an ointment. I don't care what he says. My experience tells me that aloe vera does work!

D. G., El Paso, Tex.

This wasn't the first letter we received telling us about the successful use of aloe vera to treat burns. It has been a popular home remedy for this and other skin problems for many years. In fact, there is even some evidence that aloe vera was used as long ago as the sixteenth century for treating burns and wounds. The doubting doctor was probably referring to an article he saw in the *Journal of the American Medical Association (JAMA)*. A few years ago Dr. Martin C. Koenig from Gila Bend, Arizona, wrote a letter to the "Question and Answer" section of *JAMA* requesting information from the journal's expert on such matters:

Q Many desert-area residents of Arizona use the mucus of a freshly cut leaf of the aloe vera plant as a home remedy for first- and second-degree burns. They claim that its application to the burn provides immediate pain relief and speeds the healing process, with no infection or systemic symptoms resulting. What are the ingredients of this plant that cause users to claim immediate pain relief, a result not achieved by medications such as Mafenide cream?

The answer to Dr. Koenig's question came from Dr. Arthur George Ship of the Albert Einstein College of Medicine in New York. Here is an excerpt from his reply:

A ...Aloe Vera appears to be a widespread home remedy used in the Southwest. A number of people cultivate this plant in their yards to use the juices for scrapes, minor cuts, nicks, bites, abrasions, and burns. Lay users are convinced of the plant's definite beneficial properties as a home remedy for relieving pain . . .

In the late 1950s Dr. Truman Blocker was given a contract by the U.S. Army Medical Research and Development Command to do an extensive study on aloe vera. This was the result of what Col. Harold Hamit described as "like the legendary Phoenix in crab grass; aloe vera comes back to haunt us again." Dr. Blocker showed that without a doubt aloe was of no meaningful value in the treatment of burns.[87]

Although Dr. Blocker's research may have shown that the aloe plant was ineffective, common sense and practical experience do have a place in this dispute. Even though we prefer to stick with scientific proof and avoid testimonial reports, there is some justification for trying aloe vera. The juice from the aloe vera plant will keep air away from the wound and that will reduce the pain. Whether there is some special property about the plant that speeds recovery has yet to be proven "scientifically," but if it works for you, great! Some doctors even use aloe vera to treat poison ivy and we have used aloe vera for burns and think it works, too. At the very least, this home remedy is safer than most of the sprays, lotions, and creams you can buy in a drugstore for minor burns and scratches. Most of these products contain local anesthetics and antihistamines which can cause an allergic skin condition in sensitive persons.

For mild household accidents it is always a good idea to get the burn under cold water as fast as possible. If you act quickly enough not only will the pain disappear but the seriousness of the burn can be dramatically reduced. Keep the burned skin under water until the pain is gone. Then give the aloe vera a try. In our book, experience is as good a teacher as anything else.

AIRPLANE EARS

Several months ago a friend of ours, who has to fly around the country a lot on business, asked us if there wasn't something he could do about "airplane ears." During the hay-fever season he was in agony during every descent. And even after landing he claimed the dizziness and disoriented feeling could last up to an hour. Our friend suffered from what the doctors call "barotitis." When the plane descends from a high altitude a partial vacuum develops within the ear and the resulting pain can be unbearable, especially if your eustachian tubes or sinuses are blocked because of a cold or hay fever.

Experienced travelers often chew gum, swallow frequently, or pinch their nostrils and blow air out of the nose while keeping their mouth shut. These maneuvers tend to equalize pressure and reduce the pain of the vacuum. A reader from Florida sent in a "stewardess" remedy that may prove to be the best one of all. We don't guarantee this one but our friend said it worked like a charm:

> **As an airplane traveler I used to suffer with an excruciating ear problem on every descent. Many years ago an airline stewardess gave me the following remedy that really works. It is a simple device that consists of a wooden bead with a balloon covering one of the holes. The bead should be a size that cannot be drawn or inserted into the nostril. And it is helpful to blow up the balloon a couple of times before it is placed on the bead.**
>
> **Place the bead to one nostril and while holding the other nostril closed, attempt to blow up the balloon by blowing through the open nostril. The relief is fantastic and immediate.**
>
> **F.M.C., Fort Lauderdale, Fla.**

A more traditional "medical" approach might be to use an oral decongestant before taking off. In addition, some doctors recommend using a small amount of nasal spray before the pilot starts his descent. In theory this is supposed to keep the tubes open and allow the pressure to equalize. We rather like the bead-and-balloon idea since if you overdo with the nasal spray it could, paradoxically, cause drug-induced congestion and stuffiness and just add to the problem. But if you can't find a bead and a balloon, nasal decongestants used cautiously can make flying the unfriendly skies bearable.

Here is an odd assortment of home remedies that we do not endorse but leave up to your good judgment to review. Pick and choose and have fun.

From *H.G. in Winthrop, Massachusetts*: "For cold sores apply an ice cube to the lip as soon as the tingling warning symptom occurs. Patience is the key to success. You have to keep the ice on the lip for at least an hour (1½ hours is best). That may seem like a drag but if you do it while watching television the time passes easily. By the next morning the blisters should be gone."

From *Mrs. D.M.C. in Bishop, California*: "For hemorrhoids make daily applications of ice and after each bowel movement wipe gently with witch hazel. The ice reduces the swelling and the witch hazel eliminates the itching. True, it is a little uncomfortable but much less so than having surgery."

From *R.E.S. in Minneapolis, Minnesota*: a cure for hiccups: "If a teaspoon of sugar doesn't do the trick, try peanut butter—never fails. If that doesn't work place hand over nose and mouth and do not breathe for a few minutes." (That sounds more than a mite drastic to us—it would probably cure the hiccups and just about everything else—permanently!) We still stand by the sugar cure: a teaspoon of dry granulated sugar will stimulate the phrenic nerve when it is swallowed dry and cut off those hiccups pronto. *A.L. in Huntington Park, California,* testifies to the power of sugar: "My store manager today came up with a really bad case of hiccups. After listening to it for a couple of hours I went to a market close by where I bought a one pound box of sugar. As I walked back in the door I called out, 'Hey, catch,' and tossed the box to the poor sufferer. He hiccuped just at that moment, missed catching the box, which hit him in the head. INSTANT CURE! A Miracle! He didn't even have to open the sugar, so strong a cure it is. This is honest truth, I swear it." We believe.

From *T.D. in Temples, Florida*: "Use vanilla extract over a sore tooth. A temporary relief from pain that lasts fifteen minutes to several hours."

G.B. in Rahway, New Jersey, offers the following: "I've had a foot odor problem for years. My whole family used to complain whenever I took my shoes off. A friend suggested baking soda. Plain old, everyday household baking soda. It's the greatest thing since pantyhose! Just apply it liberally to socks and shoes and sprinkle between toes. For double protection add a little ZEASORB POWDER It will keep those tootsies cool, calm and dry. A combination of baking soda and corn starch are also a great underarm deodorant. Best of all it's cheaper than anything you can buy in a drug store."

OH, THOSE PILL-TAKING BLUES

Not too long ago we received an anguished cry for help from a woman in St. Louis, Missouri. She wrote: "I have always found it hard to swallow pills. Most of my life I've just avoided tablets and capsules by asking the doctor to prescribe a liquid instead. Just recently, though, I've been put on a blood pressure medicine and the daily struggle to get these horse pills down is turning my life to agony. They stick in my throat and the roof of my mouth. I have to take these things the rest of my life, but I can't go on like this. What can I do?"

We searched high and low for an answer and discovered that millions of people go through the same misery every time they try to gulp down a pill. Even if they're successful at swallowing the darn thing, they may be left with the nasty feeling that the capsule got stuck halfway down. And they may often be right. Two doctors from Cardiff, Wales, undertook a fascinating investigation to determine how long it takes for pills to make it down through the esophagus and into the stomach. They discovered that more than 50 percent of the people who took the aspirin-sized test tablets retained the pills in their esophagus from five minutes to an hour and a half (especially if they were lying down).[88] This is more than just uncomfortable; many drugs can be dangerous if they don't reach the stomach quickly. Arthritis medication, potassium supplements, and even some antibiotics can irritate the esophagus or cause ulceration if their passage is delayed. This danger is especially important when taking expandable laxatives like dry psyllium seed preparations.

What's the answer to this problem? It's not often that we can recommend a simple solution for such a distressing plea for help. However, we recently came across a special drinking glass that takes the trauma out of swallowing pills. Called Pill Taker or Drink-A-Pill this nifty plastic cup has a slotted shelf built into the side on which the tablet is placed. The person then drinks the water and the medicine is washed down with hardly any notice. The pharmacist should be able to order this special kind of cup either from Robbins Associates in Burnsville, Minnesota, or Apex Medical Supply in Minneapolis. It may also be possible to order directly from "Family Medical Aids," Box 2974, Philadelphia, Pennsylvania 19126.

There is another possibility as well. We have received many letters from people who offered commonsense suggestions on how to make swallowing pills easier. *R.K. from North Freedom, Wisconsin,* wrote to say, "I was one of the millions unable to swallow drugs. The answer is take your medicine with food. Chew the food well, and just before you are ready to swallow it press the pill into the food on your tongue, swallow and you will never know you are taking medicine."

A great grandfather, *W.L.B. from Dunedin, Florida,* had this to say: "My mother taught me to take a spoonful of jelly, jam or preserves—insert the pill—swallow with one gulp and follow with water. For a variation try applesauce." Another contributor swears that milk is the answer. She **says** that even large pills will "slide down easily, especially if you tilt your head back and swallow." A mother, *Mrs. E.M.A., from Covington, Virginia,* says that drinking the liquid through a straw is the solution. "I put my pills in the front of my mouth and take a big drink through a straw and you will never know when they go down the hatch." And *J.M. from Beaumont, Texas,* reports that you can make the medicine go down a whole lot easier if you cut a slit in a piece of canned peach or pear and insert the pill in the fruit. Then swallow the whole thing quickly. She says that a piece of banana will also do the job.

Many of these helpful hints make good sense to us, and if you ever have occasion to give a tablet to a youngster one of them might come in handy. Some medicine should be taken on an empty stomach, however, and in this case the inexpensive pill-taking cup might be just the answer. It would also be an excellent idea to check our drug-and-food-interaction chart before taking any medicine. But we hope you and your family will stay nice and healthy and never need to take any pills and that these home remedies will be unnecessary.

TAKING IT ON HOME

Well, that is the end of our "Grab Bag of Wonderfully Wacky Weirdness and Helpful Home Remedies." We hope it was a refreshing change from all the problems and unpleasant news that we have presented in other places in this book. The moral of this chapter is that "Taking care of your health can be fun and creative!" ENJOY!

The following table summarizes many of the reported problems associated with specific drugs. Some effects are rare and others are hard to document. It is practically impossible to find reliable information on the actual incidence of adverse sexual reactions for most medications because of the traditional secrecy surrounding this topic. Many disorders can themselves cause impotence and loss of libido.

SEXUAL SIDE EFFECTS OF DRUGS

HIGH BLOOD PRESSURE MEDICATIONS

GUANETHIDINE (Esimil, Ismelin)	This is a heavy-duty anti-hypertensive that can throw a monkey wrench into your sexual machinery: impaired ejaculation and loss of sexual potency are possible.
METHYLDOPA (Aldomet, Aldoclor, Aldoril)	Less trouble than with guanethidine but it can decrease libido and make it hard to maintain an erection.

SEXUAL SIDE EFFECTS OF DRUGS (continued)

HIGH BLOOD PRESSURE MEDICATIONS (continued)

	Although rare, something called "gynecomastia" may occur where a man's breasts may become developed and even secrete milk.
RESERPINE (Serpasil, Diupres, Exna-R, Rau-Sed, Regroton, Sandril, Salutensin, Ser-Ap-Es)	While most commonly associated with psychological depression this drug can also cause sexual side effects: reduced desire, decreased potency, and delayed ejaculation. Breast enlargement has occasionally been reported in both men and women.
CLONIDINE (Catapres)	The most common side effects are drowsiness and dryness of the mouth, but it can also produce sexual disability: impotence and impaired ejaculation in men; failure to achieve orgasm in women. Less common than with other high-blood-pressure medications.
PARGYLINE (Eutonyl, Eutron)	It can cause impotence, difficulty in urinating, delayed ejaculation in men, and delayed orgasm in women. People taking this drug *must* avoid many foods such as aged cheese (cheddar, camembert), pickled herring, ripe bananas, chicken livers, avocados, beer and wine.
PROPRANOLOL (Inderal, Inderide)	Sexual side effects are really quite rare and this may be an ideal alternative to some of the other drugs. Some susceptible persons may have trouble with their erections. Loss of hair may occur but it is a reversible side effect. Never discontinue taking this medicine abruptly.

ANTI-PSYCHOTIC DRUGS

THIORIDAZINE (Mellaril)	Employed for a wide range of mental disturbances including schizophrenia, depression accompa-

SEXUAL SIDE EFFECTS OF DRUGS (continued)

ANTI-PSYCHOTIC DRUGS (continued)

	nied by anxiety, and severe agitation. It may make achieving and maintaining an erection most difficult and can delay or totally interfere with ejaculation. Less common reactions may include breast engorgement, absence of menstruation, and secretion of milk.
MESORIDAZINE (Serentil)	This anti-psychotic medication is primarily used for treating schizophrenia. The manufacturer suggests that it's useful for dealing with problems of alcoholism and anxiety. It's similar to **MELLARIL** in its ability to interfere with sexuality. May impair ejaculation and cause impotence. May also cause incontinence and bed wetting.
HALOPERIDOL (Haldol)	Although primarily used for schizophrenia, **HALDOL** can reverse the strange and little-understood Gilles de la Tourette's syndrome where a person manifests a tic and involuntarily emits some rather startling swear words, often at embarrassing moments. The drug can produce lactation, breast engorgement, menstrual irregularities, impotence, and increased libido.

OTHER ANTI-PSYCHOTICS

CHLORPROMAZINE (Thorazine) FLUPHENAZINE (Prolixin) PERPHENAZINE (Trilafon) PROCHLORPERAZINE (Compazine) TRIFLUOPERAZINE (Stelazine)	Adverse sexual or hormonal side effects have been associated with many drugs used to treat mental illness. It is very difficult to estimate which medicines produce which reactions. Symptoms that may occur include impotence, inhibition of ejaculation, abnormal lactation, irregular menstruation, increased and decreased libido, and false positive pregnancy tests.

SEXUAL SIDE EFFECTS OF DRUGS (continued)

TRICYCLIC ANTI-DEPRESSANTS

AMITRIPTYLINE
(Elavil, Endep, Etrafon, Triavil)
DESIPRAMINE
(Norpramin, Presamine)
DOXEPIN
(Adapin, Sinequan)
IMIPRAMINE
(Imavate, Janimine, Presamine, Tofranil)
NORTRIPTYLINE
(Aventyl, Pamelor)
PROTRIPTYLINE
(Vivactil)

These drugs save lives by preventing people from jumping off bridges and out windows and performing other nasty acts to do away with themselves. They have revolutionized the treatment of chronic depression. Although depression can itself cause a reduction in sexual activity, these medications may also produce sexual side effects. There may be significant differences from one drug to another among these but such variations have not been well studied. As a result, we are listing all potential problems even though they may not have been reported with a specific drug. Both increased and decreased libido have been detected. Difficulty with urination is not uncommon. Men may experience testicular swelling, impotence, and breast development. Women may note breast enlargement and milk secretion. If sexual disabilities occur with any of these medications the patient should get in touch with the doctor and definitely NOT stop taking the drug. Remember, psychological depression itself can mess up a person's sex life.

MAO-INHIBITOR ANTIDEPRESSANTS

ISOCARBOXAZID (Marplan)
PHENELZINE (Nardil)
TRANYLCYPROMINE (Parnate)

These antidepressants are used relatively infrequently because of their side effects and because they are incompatible with many other medications and certain foods (see Drug Interaction table). Sexual dysfunctions associated with MAO-inhibitor antidepressants include impotence, problems with urination, impaired ejaculation in men, and delayed orgasm in women. People taking these drugs must avoid foods such as aged cheese (cheddar, camembert), pickled herring, ripe bananas, chicken livers, avocados, beer and wine.

SEXUAL SIDE EFFECTS OF DRUGS (continued)

ANTI-ANXIETY AGENTS

CHLORDIAZEPOXIDE (Librium) DIAZEPAM (Valium)	These drugs are the most popular medications in the world today. They are prescribed almost like candy. It is unclear how often sexual side effects occur but the manufacturer claims both drugs may increase as well as decrease libido. Any "improvement" in sexuality is probably due to a reduction of inhibitions through a tranquilizing-type of action.

ANTISPASMODICS AND DRUGS FOR DIGESTIVE-TRACT DISORDERS

ATROPINE (Antispasmodic Elixir) BELLADONNA (Donnagel, Donnatal) DICYCLOMINE (Bentyl) METHSCOPOLAMINE (Pamine) TRIDIHEXETHYL (Pathibamate) METHANTHELINE (Banthine) PROPANTHELINE (Pro Banthine)	These medications are promoted for the treatment of assorted stomach trouble including irritable bowel, irritable colon, and ulcer. They tend to reduce secretions (dry mouth, etc.) and decrease movement within the digestive tract. They may also cause problems with urination, impotence, and suppress lactation.

BIRTH-CONTROL PILLS

ASSORTED BRANDS	No one has a good understanding of this. Some researchers report that the Pill increases libido by separating sexual activity from fear of pregnancy. Others suggest that libido is reduced by interfering with ovulation and suppressing a woman's hormonally increased sexual desires. You "pay your money and take your chances."

REFERENCES

1. AMA News Release. "Health and Medical Events in 1979—A Review by the American Medical Association." Dec. 3, 1979, p. 2.

2. Editorial. "Cardiomythology and Maratons." *N. Engl. J. Med.* 301:103–104, 1979.

3. Flynn, M. A.; Nolph, G. B.; and Flynn, T. C. "Effect of Dietary Egg on Human Serum Cholesterol and Triglycerides." *Am. J. Clin. Nutr.* 32:1051–1057, 1979.

4. "Margarines and Other Dietary Fats." *Med. Letter* 18(20):81–83, 1976.

5. Editorial. "Cholesterol, Coronaries, Clofibrate and Death." *N. Engl. J. Med.* 299:1360–1362, 1978.

6. Editorial. "Clofibrate: A Final Verdict?" *Lancet* 2:1131–1132, 1978.

7. Hennekens, Charles H., et al. "Effects of Beer, Wine, and Liquor in Coronary Deaths." *JAMA* 242:1973–1974, 1979.

8. Shurtleff, D. "Some Characteristics Related to the Incidence of Cardiovascular Disease and Death: Framingham Study, 16-year follow-up, in Kannel, W. B., and Gordon, T. (eds): *The Framingham Study,* section 26. Government Printing Office, 1970.

9. Klatsky, A. L.; Friedman, G. D.; and Sigelaub, A. B. "Alcohol Consumption Before Myocardial Infarction." *Ann. Intern. Med.* 81:294–301, 1974.

10. Stason, W. B., et al. "Alcohol Consumption and Nonfatal Myocardial Infarction." *Am. J. Epidemiol.* 104: 603–608, 1976.

11. Hennekens, C. H.; Rosner, B.; and Cole, D. S. "Daily Alcohol Consumption and Fatal Coronary Heart Disease." *Am. J. Epidemiol.* 107:196–200, 1978.

12. Castelli, W. P., et al. "Alcohol and Blood Lipids." *Lancet* 2:153–155, 1977.

13. Berecochea, J. E. Report of "Health Consequences of Drinking Practices: Kind of Beverage and Subsequent Mortality," prepared for the Wine Institute, California. Berkeley, 1978.

14. Myrhed, M.; Berglund L.; and Bottiger, L. E. *Acta Med. Scand.* 202:11, 1977.

15. Paul, O.; Lepper, M. H.; Phelan, W. H.; Dupertius, G. W.; MacMillkan, A.; McKean, H.; and Park, H. *Circulation* 28:20, 1963.

16. Wilhelmsen, L.; Wedel, H.; and Tibblin, G. *Circulation* 43:950, 1973.

17. Yano, K.; Rhoads, G. G.; and Kagan, A. "Coffee, Alcohol and Risk of Coronary Heart Disease Among Japanese Men Living in Hawaii." *N. Engl. J. Med.* 297:405–409, 1977.

18. St. Leger, A. S.; Cochrane, A. L.; and Moore, F. "Factors Associated with Cardiac Mortality in Developed Countries With Particular Reference to the consumption of Wine." *Lancet* 1:1017–1020, 1979.

19. Ibid.

20. Medical News. "Unresolved Issue: Do Drinkers Have Less Coronary Heart Disease?" *JAMA* 242:2745–2746, 1979.

21. Ibid.

22. Goldbourt, Uri, and Medale, Jack H. "High Density Lipoprotein Cholesterol and Incidence of Coronary Heart Disease—The Israeli Ischemic Heart Disease Study." *Am. J. Epidemiol.* 109:296–308, 1979.

23. Castelli, W. P. (editorial) "How Many Drinks a Day?" *JAMA* 242:2000, 1979.

24. Barboriak, J. J., et al. "Alcohol and Coronary Arteries." *Alcoholism* 3:29–32, 1979.

25. Jain, R. C. "Onion and Garlic in Experimental Cholesterol Induced Atherosclerosis." *Indian J. Med. Res.* 74:1509–1515, 1976.

26. Jain, R. C., and Konar, D. B. "Onion and Garlic in Experimental Atherosclerosis in Rabbits. II. Effect on Serum Proteins and Developments of Atherosclerosis." *Artery* 2(6):531–539, 1976.

27. Jain, R. E., and Konar, D. B. "Effect of Garlic Oil in Experimental Cholesterol Atherosclerosis." *Atherosclerosis* 29:125–129, 1978.

28. Sharma, et al. *Indian J. Nutr. Diet.* 12:288, 1975.

29. Quantum Sufficit. *Am. Fam. Physician 10:22, December, 1977.*

30. "Heavy Garlic Intake Lowers Serum Lipids." *Med. Tribune* 19(39):2, 1978.

31. Ibid.

32. Jain, R. C. "Effect of Garlic on Serum Lipids, Coagulability and Fibrinolytic Activity of Blood." *Am. J. Clin. Nutr.* 30(9):1380–1381, 1977.

33. Outlook. "Antistroke Recipe: Onions and Garlic?" *Med. World News,* Sept. 3, 1979, p. 33.

34. Cobb, Sidney, et al. "Length of Life and Cause of Death in Rheumatoid Arthritis." *N. Engl. J. Med.* 249:533–536, 1953.

35. Elwood, P. C. "A Randomized Controlled Trial of Acetylsalicylic Acid in the Secondary Prevention of Mortality from Myocardial Infarction." *Br. Med. J.* 1:436–440, 1974.

36. Boston Collaborative Drug Surveillance Group. "Regular Aspirin Intake and Acute Myocardial Infarction." *Br. Med. J.* 1:440–443, 1974.

37. The Canadian Cooperative Study Group. *N. Engl. J. Med.* 299:53–59, 1978.

38. Pick, R.; Chediak, J.; and Glick, G. "Asiprin Inhibits Development of Coronary Atherosclerosis in Cynomolguys Monkeys (*Macaca fascicularis*) . . . Fed an Atherogenic Diet." *J. Clin. Invest.* 63:158–162, 1979.

39. News. "Aspirin May Prevent Heart Attacks, Strokes." *Am. Fam. Physician* June, 1979, p. 183.

40. Harter, Herschel, R., et al. "Prevention of Thrombosis in Patients on Hemodialysis by Low-Dose Aspirin." *N. Engl. J. Med.* 301:577–579, 1979.

41. "To Prevent Clots, Less Aspirin is Better than More." *Med. World News* October 15, 1979, pp. 27–28.

42. Lichstein, Edgar, et al. "Diagonal Ear-Lobe Crease: Prevalence and Implications as a Coronary Risk Factor." *N. Engl. J. Med.* 290:615–616, 1974.

43. Ben Halim, M. M. M. D. thesis, Bristol University, 1976.

44. Christiansen, J. S.; Mathiesen, B.; Andersen, A. R.; and Calberg, H. *N. Engl. J. Med.* 293:308, 1975.

45. Andresen, A. R.; Christiansen, J. S.; and Jensen, J. K. "Diagonal Ear-Lobe Crease and Diabetic Retinal Angiopathy. *N. Engl. J. Med.* 294:1183, 1976.

46. Moncada, B.; Ruiz, J. M.; Rodriguez, E.; and Leiva, J. L. "Ear-Lobe Crease." *Lancet* 1:220–221, 1979.

47. Wiedemann, H. R. "Ear-Lobe Creases, Congenital and Acquired." *N. Engl. J. Med.* 301:111, 1979.

48. Burton, J. L. "Ear-Lobe Crease." *Lancet* 1:328, 1979.

49. Mehta, J., and Hamby, R. I. *N. Engl. J. Med.* 291:260, 1974.

50. Wyre, L. H. Jr. "A Cutaneous Manifestation of Coronary Artery Disease." *Cutis* 23:328–331, 1979.

51. Abstracts. "Does a Diagonal Earlobe Crease Really Predict CHD." *Mod. Med.* 47(14):85, 1979.

52. Ibid.

53. Stanley, Edith, D., et al. "Increased Virus Shedding with Aspirin Treatment of Rhinovirus Infection." *JAMA* 231:1248–1251, 1975.

54. Ibid.

55. Sakethhoo, K.; Januskiewicz, A.; and Sackner, M. A. "Effects of Drinking Hot Water, Cold Water, and Chicken Soup on Nasal Mucus Velocity and Nasal Airflow Resistance." *Chest* 74:408–410, 1978.

56. Watson, W. C. "Speaking the Unspeakable." *N. Engl. J. Med.* 299:494, 1978.

57. Rabkin, Eric S.; and Silverman, Eugene M. "Passing Gas." *Human Nature* 2(1):50–55, 1979.

58. Levitt, M. D. "Comment." *Am. J. Dig. Dis.* 17(5):388–389, 1972.

59. Alvarez, Walter, C. "What Causes Flatulence?" *JAMA* 120(1):21–24, 1942.

60. Hickey, C. A.; Calloway, D. H.; and Murphy, E. L. "Intestinal Gas Production Following Ingestion of Fruits and Fruit Juices." *Am. J. Dig. Dis.* 17(5):383–388, 1972.

61. Levitt, M. D.; Lasser, R. B.; Schwartz, M. A.; and Bond, J. H. "Studies of a Flatulent Patient." *N. Engl. J. Med.* 295:260–262, 1976.

62. Frontlines. "Next, The Atonal Fruit." *Mother Jones* 5(1):12, 1980.

63. Wynne-Jones, Geoffrey. "Flatus Retention is the Major Factor in Diverticular Disease." *Lancet* 2:211–212, 1975.

64. Benedek, Thomas, G. "Aphrodisiacs: Fact and Fable." *Medical Aspects of Human Sexuality.* December, 1971, pp. 42–63.

65. Ibid.

66. Everett, Guy M. "Effects of Amyl Nitrite ('Poppers') on Sexual Experience." *Medical Aspects of Human Sexuality* 6(12):146–151, 1972.

67. Donegan, Frank. "Lovable Feasts." *Viva* February, 1978, p. 70.

68. Advertisement for "Potent Pharmaceutical Products, Inc." *Penthouse* 11(3):224, 1979.

69. "...And One Might Prove the Ideal Aphrodisiac." *Med. World News,* September 17, 1979, p. 4.

70. Ibid.

71. News Front. "Brain Hormone Increases Sexual Behavior." *Mod. Med.* 46(16):21, 1978.

72. Benedek, Thomas G. "Saltpeter as Anaphrodisiac." *Medical Aspects of Human Sexuality* March, 1974, pp. 131–132.

73. Langeman, M. J. S. "Liquorice Derivatives," in *Meyler's Side Effects of Drugs,* vol. 8, ed. M. N. G. Dukes, New York: American Elsevier, 1975, pp. 792–793.

74. Werner, Sigbritt; Brismar, Kerstin; and Olsson, Sigvard. "Hyperprolactinemia and Liquorice." *Lancet* 1:319, 1979.

75. Meeting Highlights. "Two Unusual Causes of Urticaria." *Modern Medicine* 46(20):33, 1978.

76. Silberner, Joanne. "Expensive, 'Gentle' Soaps no More Mild." *Med. Tribune* September 27, 1979, p. 6.

77. Frosch, Peter J., and Kligman, Albert M. "The Soap Chamber Test." *J. Am. Acad. Dermatol.* 1:35–41, 1979.

78. Ibid.

79. Silberner, op. cit.

80. General Medicine. "Fructose Treatment for Alcoholism Not Effective." *Mod. Med.* March 15, 1978, p. 85.

81. Levy, Richard; Elo, Tom; and Irwin, B. Hannenson. "Intravenous Fructose Treatment of Acute Alcohol Intoxication: Effects On Alcohol Metabolism." *Arch. Intern. Med.* 137:1175−1177, 1977.

82. Alkana, R. L.; Parker, E. S.; Cohen, H. B.; and Noble, E. P. "Reversal of Ethanol Intoxication in Humans: An Assessment of the Efficacy of L-Dopa, Aminophylline, and Ephedrine." *Psychopharmacology* 55:203−212, 1977.

83. Alkana, Ronald L., and Noble, Ernst P. "Amethystic Agents Reversal of Acute Ethanol Intoxication in Humans," in *Biochemistry and Pharmacology of Ethanol*, vol. 2, eds. Majchrowicz, Edward, and Noble, Ernest, P. New York: Plenum, 1979, pp. 349−374.

84. Medicine. "A Sober-Up Pill?" *Newsweek* November 1, 1976, p. 63.

85. London (AP). "Fruit Salad Cure Revealed by Doctor." *Durham Morning Herald* April 14, 1977.

86. Huff, Barbara B., ed. *Physicians Desk Reference* 33rd ed., Oradell, N. J.: Medical Economics, Inc., 1979, p. 1500.

87. *Questions and Answers* "Is Topical Aloe Vera Plant Mucus Helpful in Burn Treatment?" *JAMA* 238:1770, 1977.

88. Evans, K. T., and Roberts, G. M. "Where do All the Tablets Go?" *Lancet* 2:1237−1238, 1976.

vita . . . Vita . . . VITAMINS

The Great Vitamin War rages on: Vitamin enthusiasts versus the nutrition establishment ● **RDA: R**ecommended **D**ietary **A**llowances or **R**idiculous **D**ogmatic **A**ssertions? ● Let's hear it for nutritional individuality! ● The myth of the "balanced diet" ● Nutrition Insurance: is it a good buy? ● Vitamins as drugs: **Vitamin A**—retinoids to the rescue. The complicated **B-Complex** plus a unique table of foods. **Vitamin C**—Cholesterol, Cancer and Common Colds. Dazzling **D**—Calcium and strong bones. The Mystery of **Vitamin E**. Coagulating with **Vitamin K** ● Vitamin and Drug Interaction Tables.

There is a war going on—a messy, grubby, ugly war with lots of injuries on both sides. Fortunately, the injured all survive because there hasn't been any blood shed. But the psychic wounds are real and the level of hostility keeps increasing. What we're talking about of course is the Great Vitamin War. It's been fought by the doctors, biochemists, and physiologists of the nutrition "establishment" on one side and the health food "freaks" and the vitamin scientists of the nutrition "counter-establishment" on the other. Reason and logic have gone by the board. The cheap shots, petty bickering, and low blows delivered by both camps have been extraordinary.

Why in the world should so much emotional energy be expended on what should be one of your basically boring subjects? Come on now, admit it, high school health class was downright dreadful. If your school was at all like ours you were force fed a lot of dull information about green leafy vegetables, brown rice, beriberi, and rickets. If you had a hard time keeping your eyes open through these classes you were not alone. So why should such a ho-hum topic lead to major controversy? What is it about this stuff that turns friends into raging lunatics when they start arguing about the virtues of vitamin E or C at a cocktail party? Well, it is a long and complicated story and we certainly don't claim to have all the answers, but we're going to give it our best shot.

Have you ever asked yourself what a vitamin is? If you're like most folks you probably take vitamins on faith, but what are they and what do they do? Bear with us for a moment while we draw a crude analogy and compare your beautiful body to an automobile. Any fool knows that a car needs gas to run, and it's pretty obvious that your body needs food to serve as its fuel. Protein, fats, and carbohydrates provide energy that make your personal engine run. But vitamins are a lot more subtle. They don't supply calories, but they do keep the body functioning normally. If you think of vitamins as the oil and grease and even the spark plugs that assist in moving the car you won't be too far off the mark. Your car can go pretty far with inadequate lubrication. It may squeak a little and it will definitely wear out faster, but even with poor maintenance it will get you around town, after a fashion. Even if your spark plugs aren't firing perfectly, the car will run. You may not even realize that good old Betsy's engine is not running efficiently without some sophisticated tests at the garage.

Vitamins act much the same way. You can abuse your body with inadequate nutrition, but it'll still get you around, after a fashion. Without some sophisticated tests, you might not even realize that you're not firing on all cylinders. Like your car, your body may deteriorate pretty far before these deficits become blatantly obvious. In summary, vitamins themselves provide no "fuel" or energy, but act as catalysts to keep all those biochemical reactions running smoothly.

The initial discovery of vitamins around the turn of the century was met with considerable enthusiasm. The whole idea that there were life-giving natural substances in food captured the public imagination. People were ready to believe all sorts of things about them. They became, in a sense, a substitute for the old-timey "tonics" which were supposed to cure all ills and promote general vim and vigor. Oh sure, there were a few diehards who got annoyed when the vitamin researchers pulled the rug out from under their pet theories of certain diseases. Let's face it, when you've got your scientific reputation built upon a certain hypothesis you don't like to have some upstart prove you're all wet. And that is exactly what the vitamin investigators did. For example, one doctor claimed that pellagra was caused by a contagious infection. His proof of infection was based on the clear "fact" that when poor black people were herded together in a mental institution they all developed the three D's—Dermatitis, Diarrhea, and Dementia—we now know that these are classic symptoms of niacin (vitamin B3) deficiency, and it was the inmates' shared diet, and not a communicable germ, which caused the disease. Although there was some resentment and resistance it was hard to refute the obvious improvement dietary supplementation made and ultimately solid data won out over opinion and guesswork.

By the late 1940s, however, excitement began to wane. Although it was clear that vitamins are essential in facilitating many of the body's crucial reactions, they had not turned into the miracle cure for every ill that everyone had been hoping for. There were still some enthusiasts and some hard-core researchers fascinated by these compounds but the introduction of antibiotics grabbed the limelight and became the new magic bullets that would rid mankind of all disease. There were some skirmishes between the "hard" researchers and the "enthusiasts" but the level of their hostility was kept under control and mostly they kept to their own turf. But in the sixties an undeclared war started heating up.

Part of the battle was caused by backlash. A lot of folks were turned off, bummed out and generally disgusted by all the plastic garbage that fronted for food. Emulsifiers, stabilizers, flavor enhancers, texturizers, colorizers, preservatives, and artificial everything took over the food industry. In order to sell, the products had to be sexed up and the processors and the preparers managed to create a chemical feast that could have choked an elephant. The golden archers multiplied and their chemically tipped arrows jammed the taste buds of gillions of gullible young people. A generation of junk food junkies became hooked on burgers, fries, and shakes.

But a few responded to the chemical onslaught by going "natural." Soon "health food" blossomed and along with it came the Vitamin Revolution. As folks started rejecting artificial flavors and colors they started embracing the religion of the Organic and with it high-potency "megavitamins." The counter-establishment began to flourish. "Nutrition centers" began competing with McDonald's and started cropping up in practically every mall in the country. Mail-order vitamin hucksters replaced the traveling medicine showmen of a bygone era. With the right combination of supplements you were guaranteed the regrowth of hair, a bigger bust, and a more satisfying sex life. The nutrition network needed a guru and Adelle Davis fit the bill. Her message was that vitamins and other nutritional supplements could cure a multitude of ills. If you wanted to be really, really, really, **REALLY** healthy you needed to gorp down huge quantities of this or that super-potency combination.

The establishment got nervous. Nutrition "experts" in academic centers often served as advisors to the gigantic food industry. They had a vested interest in preservatives, food coloring, and a host of other "Generally Recognized As Safe" (GRAS) ingredients. Their pride was at stake along with their professional reputation. The upstarts were treading on sacred territory and making a good profit at someone's expense. The know-nothings were dictating dogma on what was rightfully the turf of "professionals." The battle lines were drawn. The nutrition establishment had a lot of power and profit that it was unwilling to share. For one thing it helped shape the opinions of the health care establishment—doctors, nurses, pharmacists. But even more important, the experts influenced policy makers. They whispered sweet nothings in the ear of the bureaucrats and these people in turn issued the "sacred stone tablets"—RDAs, otherwise known as Recommended Daily Allowances. The Word was given to the masses. If you want to be healthy you shall consume x amount of vitamins and minerals each day—no less, no more. Most important of all, these power brokers determined who got research money. The ability to influence funding profoundly affects the knowledge that is harvested. Never let anyone tell you that basic research isn't a political battle. Them's that got, gets, and them's that don't got, well, tough luck, Charlie. Unfortunately, this same rule applies to cancer research.

Well, what's the fight all about anyway? To boil it down to the bare·bones, the battle is all about how much of what is appropriate. The establishment is hooked on the RDA philosophy. Their emphasis is deficiency disease. Their needle is stuck in a groove which says "All you need is enough vitamin C to prevent scurvy or enough thiamine (vitamin B_1) to avoid beriberi. A well-balanced diet (whatever that may be) will do the trick nicely." They are so worried about your pocketbook that they warn you not to throw away good money on a vitamin supplement and by all means steer clear of high-potency preparations.

The vitamin enthusiasts, on the other hand, claim that you need more than just the RDA to maintain good health. For one thing, they· have serious reservations about the average diet, and for another, they suggest that occasional large doses of some vitamins can actually provide health benefits by preventing disease or speeding recovery if you do become sick. Since the medical establishment has traditionally tended to concentrate more on illness than on wellness and since it is easier to detect deficiency diseases than to measure optimal health you can see that the battle lines are clearly drawn.

Nowhere was the war waged more vigorously (and ruthlessly) than on the battleground of the common cold and vitamin C. Dr. Linus

Pauling, winner of two Nobel prizes, one for chemistry and one for peace, was the principal scientific advocate for large doses of ascorbic acid. The Food and Nutrition Board of the National Research Council recommended in 1974 that the proper amount of vitamin C should be 35 mg per day for infants, 40 mg for children, and 45 mg for adults. Actually, the establishment was being "generous." They concluded that 10 mg was all that was really needed to prevent scurvy and so just to be on the safe side they added a little extra. Dr. Pauling, on the other hand, believes that "the optimum daily intake is somewhere between 250 mg and 10 g (10,000 mg)."[1] Although we will discuss in much more detail the role of this vitamin later in the chapter, suffice it to say that Linus Pauling stirred up a hornets' nest when he recommended megadoses of ascorbic acid for the common cold. You would have thought that he was storming the battlements. The medical establishment, the nutrition experts, and the policy makers were outraged. Letters to the editors of medical journals were filled with emotional and often vitriolic attacks upon Dr. Pauling's credibility. Physicians who had never once raised their voices to criticize drug companies that manufactured expensive over-the-counter cold remedies that not only offered questionable benefits but significant risks for millions and millions of Americans devoted undue energy to criticizing vitamin C, which even in large doses appears to be relatively non-toxic.

When Dr. Pauling suggested that instead of inoculating people with a swine-flu vaccine during the winter of 1976—1977 they should be encouraged to take vitamin C, the establishment was incensed. Medical authorities and the policy makers had placed all their eggs in the vaccine basket. The result was a fiasco. The predicted swine-flu epidemic never occurred, but many people suffered a rare and potentially deadly paralytic disease called Guillan-Barre syndrome from the vaccine. Millions of dollars in lawsuits were filed against the drug companies and the federal government.

It is not our intention to joust in the lists of the Great Vitamin War. We cite the Pauling example in order to provide some insight on the areas of conflict and the intensity of the hostility. In the following pages we will attempt to objectively provide some solid nuts-and-bolts type of information and some gee-whiz material that you probably have never heard before. We have reviewed the scientific literature and will try to separate the fact from the fiction as much as possible.

Unfortunately, the state of the cold (and occasionally not so cold) war between the enthusiasts and the establishment types makes it difficult for the "non-aligned" person to get good information on the clinical usefulness of vitamins, particularly with respect to promoting optimal health. The standard establishment line labels the counter-establishment claims "quackery" or "hogwash"[2] and views the individuals concerned as faddists or worse.

For their part, the counter-establishment vitamin enthusiasts tend to rely heavily on testimonials which have no scientific validity, and at times even stretch credulity. Adelle Davis used this technique frequently in her books. In one typical case, she described in great detail a young man who had been severely burned, and claimed, "Without vitamin E his back would have been a mass of scars, yet it healed rapidly and not a trace of a scar formed."[3] The clear implication is that smearing vitamin E on the skin will prevent the formation of scar tissue. There is no reliable scientific evidence supporting this claim, and "would have beens" are almost impossible to prove in such individual cases. (On the contrary, there is substantial evidence demonstrating that topical application of vitamin E can cause a nasty skin irritation in sensitive individuals.) Animal research can also be misleading. Just because some researchers back in the 1940s discovered that rats made deficient in vitamin E could not function sexually does **NOT** mean that whopping doses of vitamin E will improve human libido or cure impotence. In this chapter, we're going to look beyond the testimonials ("I would have been dead six months ago if I weren't taking vitamins X, Y, and Z") so we can evaluate the research on the use of vitamins and minerals as drugs and examine some of the interactions they may have with each other and with other drugs.

One reason many people "self-dose" with vitamins and minerals is their skepticisms of their doctor's nutritional expertise. In some cases, perhaps too many, this lack of confidence is justified. Although some physicians have taken enough interest in the subject to become well-versed, by and large medical education in nutrition is "wholly inadequate," according to Keith B. Taylor, M.D., Barnett Professor of Medicine and Co-Chairman of the Stanford University Committee on Human Nutrition.[4] Other people are not reassured by the usual admonition to "eat a balanced diet," because they are not sure they know what a "balanced diet" is. Robert Rodale, writing in *Prevention*, a "counter-establishment" publication, presents their point of view:

> **If you know which foods are good and which aren't, and have the will-power and the means to eat more of the good ones and fewer of the bad, you can stay thin and be healthy eating a diet**

> that the chairman of the nutrition department
> at Harvard wouldn't think is too strange. But
> most people can't do that ... So they grow fat
> and die young while eating foods that their
> families, friends, neighbors and even their
> dietitians think is O.K.—even all-American.[5]

Well, just what *is* a balanced diet? Won't we be all right if we follow the home economists' advice to select some foods from each of the "basic four" food groups* every day? As it turns out, no one answer holds for everybody. For most people, a diet selected from the "basic four" does provide most nutrients at levels high enough to prevent deficiencies. And a diet which emphasizes just one food, say grapefruit; or one type of nutrient, say protein; or excludes some type of food, such as bread and grain products, is far less likely to supply needed vitamins and minerals, without making a valiant effort to make up for what is lacking. But there are about forty known nutrients with different roles in the body's chemistry, far too many even for a biochemist to keep close tabs on all at once. Many of them have complex interactions with each other and with other body constituents. Take iron, for example. If you eat your egg-salad sandwich with a glass of iced tea none of the egg's iron will be absorbed into the bloodstream, whereas if you ate it all by itself a small fraction of the iron would be absorbed. However, if you drank a glass of orange juice with the egg the percentage of iron that would be absorbed is increased dramatically.[6] The reason is that vitamin C improves iron absorption while the tannin in tea prevents iron absorption. Tea can also interfere with the utilization of thiamine. The requirements for vitamin D and calcium are linked to each other as well and interact with hormones and other minerals and vitamins. If all this sounds somewhat complicated, it is, but we assure you it's fascinating and understandable.

The whole situation is muddied further by the fact that each of us is a unique individual. A truism, you say? Yes, but the usual medical attitude is that every person is believed "normal," that is to say, average, until proven otherwise. It stands to reason, however, that since every protein, enzyme, or hormone is determined by a

---

* For anyone who has forgotten that horrible high school health lesson, the "basic four" includes: (1) milk and milk products; (2) meat, poultry, fish, and legumes; (3) vegetables and fruits; and (4) bread, cereals, and other grain products (excluding *distilled* grain products, which supply calories but no other nutrients).

particular genetic blueprint, our inner workings should all be as unique as our faces or our fingerprints. Dr. Roger J. Williams, the biochemist who has written about this concept of nutritional individuality for the past twenty-five years, cites a study which determined the calcium requirement in nineteen healthy men. One man required only 220 mg per day, while another needed 1,018 mg daily.[7] A "balanced" diet providing 800 mg of calcium daily would have been inappropriate for these men on the extremes; the second would have been in a state of "calcium deficiency." Williams goes on to describe twenty-one healthy young men who were chosen for study because their diets seemed adequate and they were knowledgeable about nutrition. An enzyme test for vitamin B_6 revealed, however, that they all had some degree of vitamin B_6 deficiency.[8]

RDA

Recommended Dietary Allowances

or

Ridiculous Dogmatic Assertions

The National Research Council, a branch of the National Academy of Sciences, appoints the fifteen members of the Food and Nutrition Board. If all that sounds bureaucratic and respectably "establishment" to you, you hit the bull's eye. These eminent research-oriented scientists meet every five years to review their Recommended Dietary Allowances. Since 1941, when the first RDAs were issued, these documents have been used for planning and evaluating the diet of the American population. They carry a lot of weight. The Food and Drug Administration uses the RDA information to establish nutrient labeling for packaged foods. Vitamin companies use this information when formulating new products. And "experts" use this data as ammunition in their fight against the counter-establishment folks. What few people realize is that the sacred stone tablets are far from the final word. To some extent, as our understanding evolves, the RDAs also change. For example, the Recommended Dietary Allowances for the United States included only ten nutrients in 1964; by 1974 the thrice-revised recommendation published values for eighteen nutrients and mentioned twelve more.[9] The 1980 revision includes values for all thirty nutrients listed.

The Food and Nutrition board is made up of reasonable people. The 1974 report has been characterized as a "moderate document that reflects a current consensus . . . among a group of rational scientific thinkers. They profess no ultimate dietary wisdom, admit their uncertainties about many questions, and confess that establishing nutritional recommendations is not unlike working a jigsaw puzzle with many of the pieces missing."[10]

Unfortunately, policy makers and health professionals seem unaware of the Board's continuing evolution and reservations and certainly fall down in their responsibility to inform the consumer of them. And, while averages may hold nicely for large populations, they fall apart very quickly for real people. We have already seen that there can be a considerable degree of variation in nutritional requirements between individuals. The Recommended Dietary Allowances will not tell you if your diet is "just right" for you. And they were never meant to. If you smoke or use birth control pills or suffer heavy-duty stress your needs will differ dramatically from those of a laid-back surfer. Despite these considerations, the Food and Drug Administration maintains a dogmatic and uncompromising attachment to their U.S. Recommended Daily Allowances. Don't forget, these are the people who are responsible for approving the artificial flavors and colors and all the preservatives (like nitrite in hot dogs) that the health food folks have railed against. One way to get back at the revolutionaries is to control their "supply lines" by regulating permissible levels, establishing "appropriate allowances," and dictating labeling requirements. Our point is that RDAs were not designed to determine whether *your* diet is right for you. They may have some use as a flexible guideline but only you can attempt the task of approximating what your body's needs really are.

THAT WELL-BALANCED DIET?

According to *Consumer Reports,* Americans are eating almost half their meals outside the home. Fast-food chains alone rake in over $10 billion each year from Americans on the run.[11] We are a society that is moving so fast we can't find time to relax and enjoy our food. In the morning it's a cup of coffee and a Danish. Lunch may be a Big Mac or one of the Colonel's plucked chickens. Supper may be a TV dinner or a hot dog at the ball park. The experts for Consumer's Union discovered some fascinating facts about Americans' favorite foods.

> **The six nutrients most commonly in short supply in fast-food meals are: biotin, folacin, pantothenic acid, total vitamin A, iron and copper. These nutrients, which perform a variety of functions in growth and life-support,**

are derived from many food sources, some of
which would usually be part of almost any
standard diet that includes a variety of foods. If
you eat at a fast-food chain regularly, it would be
wise to make sure that your other meals include
such nutritious foods as beans, dark green leafy
vegetables, yellow vegetables, and a variety of
fresh fruits.[12]

A lot of people may be skating closer to a deficiency state than the
nutrition establishment is willing to admit. They make the assumption that most people are eating well most of the time and
automatically assume a "balanced" diet. How many times have you
heard the recommendation to eat "dark green leafy vegetables?"
This is an often-repeated litany in health classes, popular articles,
and as you just read, even the experts for *Consumer Reports* toss out
the phrase without even thinking. But have you ever stopped to ask
yourself what green leafy vegetables are in the first place? Oh, sure,
we can hear you saying, no big deal, you eat lots of salads, right.
Wrong, wrong, wrong! Lettuce is not a green leafy vegetable, at least
not according to the experts. It has little in the way of nutrients or
food value to speak of. When the big boys refer to dark green leafy
vegetables they are talking about collard *greens,* beet *greens,* mustard
greens, turnip *greens,* kale, Swiss chard and last, but not least, spinach.
And the reason these *greens* are good is because they are high in
vitamins A and C as well as in folic acid and iron.

Now we ask you, when was the last time you sat down to a real
meal of greens? If you are white, middle class, and live anywhere
other than the South our bet is that it's been a good long while. Oh,
you may eat some spinach now and again and if you have a garden
you may even get some kale and swiss chard in the summer, but the
average family has a hard time finding real greens and even if they did
locate some good old collards, chances are they'd have a devil of a
time acquiring a taste for them. So that mythical "balanced" diet may
be even more elusive than everyone imagines.

Although it's usually assumed that Americans don't suffer frank
nutritional deficiency diseases, that's not necessarily so. We found a
surprising concession in a traditional medical reference book
(*Current Medical Diagnosis and Treatment*):

Scurvy is usually due to inadequate intake of
vitamic C, but may occur with increased
metabolic needs. The disease is seen *frequently*
in formula-fed infants, elderly bachelors and

**widowers, and food faddists. Vitamin C concen-
tration in tissues has been reported to be
decreased in healthy women taking oral contraceptives.**[13] **[italics ours]**

Signs of scurvy include swollen or bleeding gums, easy bruising, pinpoint red spots under the surface of the skin, and weakness. Other symptoms caused by a lack of vitamin C are dry itchy skin, loss of hair, dryness of the mouth and eyes and loosening of teeth or fillings. In some people this deficiency may be associated with regular aspirin use since as little as two tablets a day can keep vitamin C from getting into cells.

Older people on fixed incomes have a hard enough time making ends meet without balancing their nutrient requirements. Add to that the fact that they are often taking many different prescription drugs which can profoundly interfere with nutrient levels and the conditions are ripe for real deficiency diseases. Even the teenager who could care less about diet (except to keep a sexy bod) could end up a borderline case of vitamin deficiency.

NUTRITIONAL INSURANCE

Okay, enough beating around the bush. Who needs what and how much do they need? Well, that is an impossible question to answer. If you live in the country, grow your own vegetables, have a fruit orchard, and eat a varied diet the chances are excellent that you don't need any "nutritional insurance" in order to prevent a deficiency disease. (Let's put aside the whole issue of pharmacological effects from vitamins, such as the use of vitamin C for the treatment of colds, till later). If, on the other hand, you are a fast-food fanatic and would rather pop a pill to insure adequate nutrition than change your frenzied life style, then maybe you had better invest in a little insurance. While we can't recommend this approach to a decent diet, we can give you some advice on selecting a supplement. You will probably need a pencil and paper to find the product you want at a price that's right. There are well over two hundred vitamin/mineral preparations on your pharmacy shelves and the formulas vary considerably. You will want to check different brands to see whether they contain the kinds of vitamins and minerals you want in the dose you'd like to take; you'll also have to dust off your long division or carry a pocket calculator to figure out which of the multitudinous brands costs less on a daily basis.

We offer two recommended formulas for you to choose from. Both are, we think, moderate and sensible. Both are designed for general adult use rather than for specific populations with special needs; but one is derived from a slightly more conservative source, while the other one is somewhat "counter-establishment" in flavor. The first was published in *Nutrition & the M.D.,* a monthly newsletter for physicians and nutritionists. For patients who "want a vitamin-and-mineral supplement as 'insurance' against poor eating habits," the author recommends a preparation which provides all of the vitamins and some essential minerals in amounts ranging from a third or a half of the RDA up to the entire RDA, but not much beyond.[14] He suggests that you buy the cheapest brand that meets the formulation, and offers the hint that the deterioration of these preparations is quite slow, so a bargain on a bottle that has passed its expiration date is a good deal. His recommended formulation:[15]

Vitamin A:	5,000 IU
Vitamin D:	400 IU
Vitamin E:	15 IU
Vitamin C:	45 mg
Thiamin:	1.5 mg
Riboflavin:	1.8 mg
Niacin:	20.0 mg
Pyridoxine:	2.0 mg
Folacin:	0.4 mg
Vitamin B$_{12}$:	3.0 mcg
Calcium:	200 mg
Iron:	10 mg
Magnesium:	100 mg
Zinc:	10 mg
and possibly	
Potassium:	100 mg
Copper:	1 mg
Manganese:	1 mg
Pantothenate:	5 mg

We recommend that you take this list to shop for the best product at the best price. We haven't found any supplements that fit the recommendations exactly, but the following formulations come close: CHOCKS, DAYALETS, FEMIRON WITH VITAMINS, FLINTSTONES, MULTIVITAMIN SUPPLEMENT WITH IRON (FISON), ONE-A-DAY, ONE-A-DAY PLUS MINERALS, PALADAC, STUART FORMULA, VIGRAN, VI-SYNERAL, ONE-CAPS, VITAGETT, VITAMIN-MINERAL CAPSULES (NORTH AMERICAN), VITERRA, and ZYMACEP CAPSULES. Most of these supplements are made by the big drug companies, and may be more expensive than products with limited distribution. Very few of these contain the recommended minerals, and almost none supply the "optional" ingredients at the recommended levels.

Because many minerals are needed in fairly large quantities, it would be impractical to include the entire recommended intake in a pill: the thing would be so large it would choke a giraffe. So both this formulation and the following should be taken as they were intended, "nutritional insurance" to make sure that an ordinary or lackluster diet will be adequate, and not as a license to commit dietary iniquities of gross proportions. Dr. Roger J. Williams, a respectable biochemist who does not always share the establishment view, recommends a formulation of twenty-nine nutrients, pointing out that no one vitamin or mineral works in isolation, but that they all work together, "like cogs in a metabolic assembly line."[16] His suggested supplement would include the following vitamins: [17]

Vitamin A:	7500 IU	
Vitamin C:	250 mg	(ascorbic acid)
Vitamin D:	400 IU	
Vitamin E:	40 IU	
Vitamin K:	2 mg	
Vitamin B$_1$:	2 mg	(thiamin)
Vitamin B$_2$:	2 mg	(riboflavin)
Vitamin B$_6$:	3 mg	(pyridoxine)
Vitamin B$_{12}$:	9 mcg	(cobalamine)
Niacinamide:	20 mg	
Pantothenic Acid:	15 mg	
Biotin:	0.3 mg	
Folic Acid:	0.4 mg	
Choline:	250 mg	
Inositol:	250 mg	
P-Aminobenzoic Acid:	30 mg	
Rutin:	200 mg	

Dr. Williams' recommendations for minerals include:

Calcium:	250 mg
Phosphate:	750 mg
Magnesium:	200 mg
Iron:	15 mg
Zinc:	15 mg

Copper:	**2 mg**
Iodine:	**0.15 mg**
Manganese:	**5 mg**
Molybdenum:	**0.1 mg**
Chromium:	**1.0 mg**
Selenium:	**0.02 mg**
Cobalt:	**0.1 mg**

Few commercial preparations of vitamin/mineral supplements closely resemble Williams' formulation. Bronson Pharmaceuticals, 4526 Rinetti Lane, La Canada, California 91011, puts out a Vitamin and Mineral Formula based on Williams' recommendations. Other more widely available supplements only approximate more or less roughly his recommended levels of vitamins. These include ENGRAN-HP, GERILETS, MYADEC TABLETS AND CAPSULES and NATALINS. FEMINAID, FEMININS, and STUART PRENATAL straddle the fence between our two suggested formulations. If you decide that you like the formula—and the price!—of a supplement marketed for pregnant women, don't worry: you don't have to be pregnant to take them. But do shop carefully for the formula you choose. Many "high-potency" supplements carry an outrageous price tag, even when they don't include all the nutrients you want. Comparison shopping is the name of the tune.

Okay, there you have it—two different kinds of insurance policies. Keep in mind that the FDA generally opposes vitamin supplementation on the grounds that such protection is unnecessary and serves only to make the manufacturers richer and the consumer poorer, without improving health. We laud the feds their public-minded spirit, but their compulsion to spread the "word" rings a little flat. Manufacturers of many over-the-counter remedies—from sleeping pills to acne remedies—have been getting richer and making the consumer poorer with a lot less scientific support than the vitamin enthusiasts can muster. Apparently FDA's evangelism is not completely objective. And while many studies have established a strong association between nitrite preservatives, nitrosamines, and cancer the FDA prefers to ignore this danger while scaring people about "harmful" or "unnecessary" vitamin intake. And we didn't intend to get lured into this fight! We definitely do not want to imply that everyone needs a "potent" vitamin supplement. But if you are worried that your diet may not be all it could be, we have provided some basic guidelines that should make shopping easier. And look for the best bargain you can find. No sense paying through the nose for some big drug company's snazzy advertising campaign (where they show a frazzled consumer burning the candle at both ends), when an unadvertised brand may provide essentially the same nutritional value.

VITAMINS AS DRUGS

Up to now, we have stuck to fairly straightforward questions about vitamins to insure adequate nutrition. But the bloodiest battles of the Great Vitamin War have been fought over the use of vitamins to prevent or cure diseases—and we're not talking about scurvy or pellagra, which have the nutrition establishment's Seal of Approval as preventable by vitamins. On the issue of megavitamins, emotions run so high that neither side can hear what the other is saying: they're both screaming too loud. Unfortunately, all the din leaves room for plenty of charlatans and hucksters to prey on the public in this no-man's-land.

A wonderful example of this sort of pitch caught our eye just recently. A large ad in one of the supermarket tabloids announced in headlines, "**Doctor discovers method of regaining lost hair.**" The advertisement goes on to tout the miracle of Biotin. Here is a small sampling of the fantastic hype:

> **Scientists nation-wide are raving about a special treatment of Biotin, the H vitamin, and absolutely fantastic test results that have been attained by a city doctor using Biotin as the reactivating agent in the revival of dormant hair roots!**
>
> **Now, you can do it for yourself right at home for hundreds of dollars less. With the same results.**
>
> **If your hair is only "sleeping," biotin solution will wake it up, and you'll be on your way to the most fabulous head of hair you can possibly have!**
>
> **Are you finding hairs on your pillow? On your suitcoat? Are too many hairs coming out in the wash? You had better get biotin solution to work on the problem right away!**
>
> **In the intensive research done with biotin, in addition to proving biotin able to catalyze hair growth in dormant scalps, biotin brought**

excessive hair loss under control in 9 out of 10 cases!

You can get biotin solution to use and apply by yourself. You don't need any special training. You don't need any special, expensive equipment . . .

Rush _____ jar(s) of biotin solution at $14.95 each plus $1.00 shipping.

If that ad weren't for real we would give it the prize for best parody of the year. If "scientists nation-wide are raving about a special treatment of Biotin, the H vitamin," they sure haven't been mentioning it in any of the major scientific journals.

In case you're wondering, biotin is actually a little-known vitamin. Although it was discovered in the 1920s it never made the big time quite the way thiamine and riboflavin did and it never got its own number such as B_1 or B_6. Perhaps because there is no sexy deficiency disease associated with a lack of biotin the average person never paid much attention to it. It really is hard as the devil to develop a deficiency. It is possible, but you would have to work at it in a most unpleasant way. Turns out uncooked egg white globs on to biotin and prevents its absorption so you would have to put away a pile of raw eggs before problems would be detectable. Now it is conceivable that if you ate, oh, about sixty raw eggs or kept up a regular regimen of six a day for eighteen months you could develop a pretty blatant biotin deficiency characterized by skin rash, loss of appetite (you'd lose your appetite too after that many Humpty Dumpties) and loss of hair.[18] And biotin supplements *would* miraculously bring back your lovely locks. And, of course, if your hair loss had a different origin, biotin would do nothing for it. There is scant evidence that this wonder vitamin as advertised will "wake up 'sleeping' hair."

Inflated claims and out and out quackery aren't the only reasons the feds are freaked. There are many vitamin promoters who virtually guarantee that if vitamins are taken in large enough doses and in appropriate combinations they can restore health even if one has cancer or heart disease. The FDA is justifiably worried that people with serious illnesses will attempt to "cure" their conditions with vitamin self-medication, thus allowing the underlying disease to progress further and reducing their chances of eventual recovery when they finally do seek medical care. The regulators caution that these high-potency special preparations should only be used to treat specific, medically diagnosed deficiencies, and then only under a physician's recommendation.[19]

The battle cry of the rebels is that this illness-oriented doctor-centered approach is what has been wrong with the health care system all along and that many physicians are less likely to be knowledgeable about nutrition than educated laymen who have gone to the trouble of becoming informed. Now that sounds like a pretty presumptuous assertion. But just hear what Dr. Jean Mayer, one of the world's most renowned nutritionists and President of Tufts University has to say:

> **Our studies at Harvard suggest that the average physician knows a little more about nutrition than the average secretary — unless the secretary has a weight problem. Then she probably knows more than the physician.**

Megavitamin doses won't cure everything that ails you and in some instances they could cause harm. But at the same time, there is some very valid scientific research done by eminently respectable investigators that establishes therapeutic or potentially useful application of some vitamins in large doses for some special problems. Sometimes the research is just tantalizing, in other cases it's downright exciting. In the next section we are going to bring you up to date on the most recent advances in the use of vitamins for specific health problems.

VITAMIN A:

RETINOIDS TO THE RESCUE

Do you ever remember hearing that eating carrots would help you see in the dark? Although such popular wisdom is often of dubious veracity, this particular gem is actually a very simplified summary of the discovery for which George Wald was awarded the Nobel Prize. What Wald found out was that vitamin A is part of the chemical (rhodopsin) in the retina of the eye which is essential for black-and-white vision when there's not enough light to see colors.

This effect is tremendously important, but vitamin A, which actually is a name that stands for a family of chemicals called for obvious reasons Retinoids, has a couple of other functions in the body which are just as crucial. Vitamin A is needed to promote the proper structure and function of cell membranes; it controls the orderly development and differentiation of skin cells, even those called "epithelium" which are found inside the mouth, the lungs, and several other internal organs. Lately we are learning that it plays a significant role in the immune system as well.

But so what? Who really cares about all that stuff besides a handful of biochemists and physiologists? YOU should! New research on vitamin A is exciting and dramatic and may affect your life. Some of it concerns the treatment of several unpleasant and tenacious skin diseases, of which psoriasis is the most common and best known. But even more thrilling is research on the role of synthetic retinoids in "chemoprevention"[20] of certain cancers! "Synthetic" is a key word here as you will soon discover.

Vitamin A first stirred up excitement in the medical community in 1923 when scientists discovered it could prevent a dreadful eye disease called xerophthalmia which once blinded millions of children. Since then the fortification of milk with this vitamin has made xerophthalmia an unknown disease nearly everywhere in Europe and North America. (Unfortunately, children in developing countries where nutrition is inadequate aren't quite so lucky.)

Twenty or thirty years ago, some clinicians who were aware that vitamin A was necessary for healthy skin tried to use it to treat disorders such as acne and psoriasis. Their experiments never really got off the ground because of an insurmountable obstacle: to get a therapeutic benefit from natural vitamin A compounds the dose had to be so great that undesirable toxic effects quickly set in. This problem arose because vitamin A is stored in the liver, so doses above the daily requirement soon accumulate. This can lead to liver damage similar to cirrhosis.[21] Other unpleasant symptoms of vitamin A overdose include dry, cracked skin; poor appetite and weight loss; brittle fingernails and hair loss; abnormal bone metabolism and joint pain; anemia, fatigue, and lethargy; restlessness, insomnia, and severe throbbing headaches.[22, 23] Now that ain't just whistling Dixie! Who said vitamins are innocuous? Babies and children are less capable of metabolizing large doses of the vitamin than are adults, so they are more susceptible to undesirable effects, with fever and increased pressure inside the skull also showing up occasionally in young children.[24] Although inadequate levels of vitamin A in a mother's diet can lead to birth defects, overdose has been reported to cause malformations in lab animals.[25]

The nasty syndrome that we have been describing is called "hypervitaminosis A." It has occurred whenever natural retinoid compounds have been used therapeutically for anything other than preventing or correcting a vitamin A deficiency. It is almost impossible to get too much of the vitamin from food, although starving Arctic explorers who ate polar-bear livers soon learned more than they ever wanted to know about hypervitaminosis A. Taking as little as 40,000 IU every day over a period of months has resulted in toxic reactions in adults. For this reason, and because each of us has such individually determined nutritional needs, the findings of a group of dentists are encouraging though they cannot be recommended as a general guideline for vitamin A intake. The dentists found that the "healthiest" individuals in their study sample—those with the fewest symptoms of poor health—had an average vitamin A intake of nearly 33,000 IU.[26] This is probably dangerously near the toxic level for some people, but it does suggest that daily intakes *somewhat* in excess of the Recommended Dietary Allowances of 4,000 IU for women and 5,000 IU for men may be beneficial.

To flip the coin for a moment, nutritionists were surprised to discover that *marginal* vitamin A deficiency is far from rare:

> **The ten-state nutrition survey of 1972 detected low plasma vitamin A levels in a surveyed population . . . [including] 10% of white children, 20% of black children, and almost 40% of all Mexican American children between the ages of 2-5 years.**
>
> **Furthermore, autopsy specimens of human livers showed widespread occurrence of dangerously low liver reserves . . . in 12-35% of the various age and geographic groups examined, regardless of social or income levels.[27]**

What Dr. George Wolf of the Massachusetts Institute of Technology means by those statistics is that up to one out of every three Americans may be deficient in vitamin A, even without the flamboyant signs of vitamin A deficiency so often seen in underdeveloped countries. It could mean that *you* have almost one chance in three of a marginal vitamin A deficiency. Now, obviously, it does you no good to wait for an autopsy analysis to find out if you are in that minority; and a liver biopsy, which could reveal it while you are still alive, is both expensive and very traumatic. Definitely not worth the trouble. But if the following vitamin A super-all-stars don't rank high on your list of favorite foods, you could be in trouble. If you are one of those obsessive types this list should help you to get compulsive and calculate your weekly vitamin A intake and compare it to your recommended allowance.

Beef liver (2 ounces supply 30,280 IU)*

Dandelion greens (1 cup supplies the equivalent of 21,060 IU)

Pumpkin (1 cup has 14,590 IU)

Spinach (1 cup of cooked spinach: 14,580 IU)

Sweet potato (1 boiled sweet potato has 11,610 IU)

Collards (1 cup of cooked greens: 10,260 IU)

Dried hot peppers (1 tablespoon has 9,750 IU)

Winter squash (1 cup has 8,610 IU)

Kale (1 cup of cooked kale: 8,140 IU)

Mustard greens (1 cup of cooked greens has 8,120 IU)

Beet greens (1 cup, cooked, gives 7,400 IU)

Cantaloupe (1/2 melon provides 6,500 IU)

Carrot (1 medium-sized carrot has 5,500 IU)

Bok choy (1 cup of cooked greens has 5,270 IU)

Broccoli (1 cup of cooked broccoli: 4,500 IU)

Papaya (1 cup of sliced fresh fruit contains 3,190 IU)

Chicken pot pie (1 pie: 3,020 IU)

Plums (1 cup of canned plums has 2,970 IU)

Apricots (3 fresh apricots give you 2,890 IU)

Watermelon (1 medium-sized wedge has 2,510 IU)

Beef and vegetable stew (1 cup homemade stew, USDA's recipe: 2,310 IU)

Lettuce (1 head of Boston lettuce gives you 2,130 IU)

Endive (2 ounces of this curly stuff has 1,870 IU)

Swordfish (3 ounces broiled with butter or margarine: 1,750 IU)

Cherries (1 cup: 1,660 IU)

Tomato (1 medium tomato: 1,640 IU)

Peach (1 yellow peach has 1,320 IU)

Green peas (1 cup cooked peas contains 860 IU)

Summer squash (1 cup, cooked: 820 IU)

Oysters (1 cup—about 15 medium oysters: 740 IU)

Corn (1 cup of canned yellow corn will give you 690 IU)

---

*IU means International Units

Eggs (1 boiled egg has 590 IU, all in the yolk)
Butter or margarine (1 tablespoon has 470 IU)
Whole milk (1 cup has 350 IU; skim has vitamin
    A value only if the label says it has been
    fortified.)

If your usual diet doesn't include some of these foods on a regular basis, you might want to consider changing your eating habits or taking out a little "nutrition insurance."

By now you are probably pretty confused about vitamin A, and we don't blame you one bit. When we described a few pages back all the terrible things that could happen if you overdo this vitamin you probably thought you'd be better off staying "light" rather than risk the consequences of going "heavy." Unless your fridge is stocked with polar-bear liver you don't need to worry about getting too much vitamin A from food. But swallowing an abundance of those little golden footballs that you buy in your local health food store could get you into a heap of trouble.

But there's great news! The chemists have been working busily on creating synthetic equivalents of vitamin A. These "artificial" retinoids are not nearly as toxic as the "natural" vitamin A chemicals and don't do such a heavy number on the liver. They are being used experimentally with some success on a variety of skin diseases which have not responded to previously available treatments. If you think "ichthyosis" sounds icky, you're right; it's the name for a group of diseases which make the skin look like fish scales. Some of the new synthetic retinoids have shown a lot of promise in treating these diseases as well as some other serious skin conditions called Lichen planus.[29-33] The chemical used most often in these clinical trials is called Ro 10-9359, so you can see how far removed it is from plain old vitamin A (retinol). We want to emphasize that the great advantage of the synthetic compounds is their ability to produce therapeutic benefits without causing the terrible toxicity that is associated with natural retinoids.

The treatment is not completely free of undesirable side effects. Many people using the drugs find that it makes the mouth, lips, and tongue feel dry, and they get cracks at the corners of the mouth. Some have scaling and thinning of the skin on the palms of the hands and the soles of the feet and a few find that their hair falls out. Fortunately, all these problems fade when they stop taking the drug.

Now if you have psoriasis, we don't suggest that you rush to your doctor and demand Ro 10-9359. For one thing, it is an experimental drug, and the physicians using it at this point are still testing it. If you lived near a big medical center and your doctor referred you to someone who was using the drug on his patients, you would have to agree to be a guinea pig before you could receive it. For another thing, even the synthetic retinoids don't work on all cases of severe psoriasis. Most of the clinical trials so far have found good responses in 50—60 percent of the psoriasis patients, at most.[34–37] Unfortunately, the beneficial effects often don't last much more than a few months after stopping the drug: evidently the retinoids can "shape up your skin" only in fairly high concentrations. And that is why it would be foolishness itself to try to self-treat psoriasis or any other serious skin condition with high doses of natural vitamin A. Anyone who did would find him or herself in the hospital with some very nasty problems long before there was any noticeable improvement in the skin disease.

As exciting as these breakthroughs sound, they are not the only area where the retinoids are making a big splash. Some cancer researchers are convinced that retinoids can provide "chemoprevention" from some forms of cancer. A five-year Norwegian study of a large group of middle-aged men found that many more smokers than non-smokers developed lung cancer; but vitamin A intakes of these men were known. **Three times** as many heavy smokers with low levels of vitamin A in their diets developed cancer, as compared with the heavy smokers with normal vitamin-A intakes.[38]

Although other studies of vitamin-A intake and cancer patients have been less conclusive,[39, 40] laboratory animals deficient in vitamin-A compound are most susceptible to induced cancer.[41] Dr. Michael G. Sporn, Chief of the Lung Cancer Branch, National Cancer Institute, concludes from these data:

> **that no human population at risk for development of cancer should be allowed to remain in a vitamin A-deficient state. Considering the relatively trivial cost of supplementation of the diet with a minimal daily requirement of retinyl acetate or retinyl palmitate, this is certainly a goal which should be met for the entire population.**[42]

When Dr. Sporn says "at risk" what does he mean? Normally, this would refer to people who have been exposed to some carcinogen (asbestos, cigarettes, etc.) or who, perhaps because of heredity, run a greater-than-usual chance of developing cancer. In mice, rats, and hamsters scientists create a "population at risk" by taking animals genetically susceptible to a certain type of cancer, then exposing them to a chemical, virus, or tumor cell known to "kick the cancer off." What they have found, in so many studies it would be impossible to mention them all, is that chemicals in the vitamin-A family will help prevent[43-50] or slow the growth of the tumors that were induced.[51-59]

So how are the retinoids doing their "chemoprevention" thing? Scientists believe that there are two functions of the vitamin that are involved in this cancer prophylaxis. First, as we said in plain English on page 193, they play a critical role "in controlling the normal differentiation of many epithelial tissues."[60, 61] Secondly, retinoids appear to stimulate the immune system, especially in combination with other immune "energizers."[62-66] At this point, there is ample evidence that synthetic retinoid compounds can help prevent a wide variety of cancers from growing in epithelial types of tissues, and these include the most important types of cancer in the United States: lung, colon-rectum, breast, pancreas, prostate, stomach, liver (bile duct), and bladder.[67] (The uterine cervix is also made up of epithelial tissue.)

We can now be certain, as Dr. Sporn pointed out at an important meeting of biologists in 1976 that:

> We are not dealing with a nutritional fad, but rather with a serious attempt to modify either: 1) the initiation phase, or 2) the progression phase (otherwise known as the latent period or the period of preneoplasia) of the development of cancer, by means of pharmacological agents that are synthetic chemical derivatives of a naturally occurring vitamin.[68]

Some good results have already been obtained in human beings when synthetic retinoids were employed to prevent "precancerous lesions" from developing into tumors.[69] A study that was heralded in the *Journal of the American Medical Association* tested the ability of retinoids to prevent recurrence of bladder cancer in people who have small superficial tumors removed.[70] This large investigation and others to follow may lend some support to Dr. Sporn's opinion that:

> Chemoprevention of epithelial cancer by synthetic retinoids eventually may provide a practical approach to the cancer problem in man.[71]

If an ounce of prevention is worth a pound of cure, this should prove welcome news indeed. But, and this is a very large BUT, the value of retinoids will most probably be in prevention, not treatment. There are no strong indications that vitamin A compounds (natural or synthetic) will be of any use in curing established cancers.[72]

So, dear reader, are you completely befuddled? Is this too complicated for words? Well, we grant you, there is more than a little contradiction in what you have just read. Let's summarize. Too little vitamin A can cause problems including an increased susceptibility to cancer. Too much vitamin A can cause problems including a whole range of serious side effects from dry, cracked skin to cirrhosis and headaches. Careful nutrition planning can provide an adequate level of vitamin A, but as many as one out of every three Americans may be deficient in the crucial vitamin. "Nutrition insurance" may be appropriate for people with inadequate diets, but if overdone, could put you in the hospital with a dangerous case of hypervitaminosis A. Exciting new research with synthetic retinoids may serve as powerful tools in the treatment of severe skin disorders such as psoriasis, acne, Lichen planus, and "fish-scale" disease when other, more traditional therapies have proved unsuccessful. Cancer researchers are really turned on by the synthetics, too. Used prophylactically by high-risk patients these retinoids may be able either to prevent the occurrence of some very common cancers or prevent a recurrence once the tumors are treated successfully.

So, vitamin A and its kissing cousins, the synthetic retinoids, are pretty hot stuff. Establishment types who say that you don't have to worry about sufficient vitamin A levels clearly haven't done their homework. Their eminently respectable medical colleagues (especially Dr. Michael Sporn) think differently. And vitamin enthusiasts who tell you to gobble down huge quantities of natural vitamin A could put you in the hospital with a toxic reaction. If you chart a middle course, eat well (don't forget to keep an eye on the food chart on page 195) and rely on your own common sense, the chances are pretty good you won't go wrong.

THE COMPLICATED B-COMPLEX

When Casimir Funk first discovered "vitamin B" in his lab in Poland, he thought he had hold of a pretty neat substance. It later turned out, however, that Funk's "water-soluble B" extract was not one compound, but many—just how many is still being debated. At first the extracts were given numbers by their proud discoverers in the order that they were announced to the world. This led to an incredible mishmash of tricky terminology, where we have vitamins B_1, B_2, and B_3, which are more commonly known by their chemical names: thiamine, riboflavin, and niacin. Vitamins B_4 and B_5 were discredited and have been dropped from the list, leaving only B_6 and B_{12} to be generally referred to by number. There are many other members of the B-complex, including folic acid and pantothenic acid which long ago earned the Nutrition Establishment's seal of approval as true vitamins; our hairy pal, biotin, which gained that status more recently; and a number of other substances still being contested as essential vitamins.

You would think, after nearly seventy years that we would have a pretty good handle on the B-complex, but the fact is that although members of the B-complex are used in practically every cell in the body, we still don't know the exact metabolic functions of many of these vitamins. There is even some dispute as to whether or not some of these compounds are truly necessary for bodily function.

The various members of the B-complex are not variants of the same chemical (as in the case of vitamin A and retinoids). Rather, they are all different chemicals, many with their own families of chemical variations, which tend to appear together in foods and work together in the body. They are necessary factors in many of the complex chemical reactions that are the molecular basis of activities we take for granted: breathing, eating, using energy, just plain living. Fortunately, the B vitamins are widely distributed in foods, so that a "normal, well-balanced" diet (at least according to the nutritionists) will keep most of us free of deficiency disease. Here is a useful table that will enable you to tell at a glance which foods are richest in the B-complex vitamins. The list is ranked in order of total B-vitamin value.

FOODS RICH IN VITAMIN B

	FOOD	B_1 (mg)	B_2 (mg)	B_3 (mg)	B_6 (mcg)	Folic Acid (mcg)	B_{12} (mcg)
1.	Liver (2 oz)	.15	2.37	9.4	479	168	45.6
2.	Peanuts (1 cup)	.46	.19	24.7	576	82	0
3.	Chicken (3 oz)	.05	.16	7.4	581	2.5	.4
4.	Split peas (1 cup, cooked)	.37	.22	2.2	325	127.5	0
5.	Avocado (1)	.33	.61	4.9	420	30	0
6.	Collards (1 cup)	.27	.37	2.4	370	194	0
7.	Brewer's yeast (1 tb)	1.25	.34	3.0	200	162	0

FOODS RICH IN VITAMIN B (continued)

FOOD	B_1 (mg)	B_2 (mg)	B_3 (mg)	B_6 (mcg)	Folic Acid (mcg)	B_{12} (mcg)
8. Cooked prunes (1 cup)	.08	.18	1.7	648	13.5	0
9. Pork (lean) (2.4 oz)	.73	.21	4.4	306	1.4	.5
10. Beef (lean) (2.5 oz)	.04	.16	3.3	313	7.9	1.3
11. Sweet potatoes (1 cup, canned)	.10	.10	1.4	475	26	0
12. Mushrooms (1 cup, canned)	.04	.60	4.8	146	9.8	0
13. Broccoli (1 cup)	.14	.31	1.2	264	84	0
14. Spinach (1 cup)	.13	.25	1.0	234	135	0
15. Cowpeas (1 cup, cooked fresh)	.49	.18	2.3	152	66	0
16. Green peas (1 cup, cooked)	.44	.17	3.7	80	40	0
17. Bran flakes (1 cup)	.14	.06	2.2	134	—	0
18. Potatoes (1 medium, boiled)	.13	.05	2.0	237	9.5	0
19. Cauliflower (1 cup)	.11	.10	0.7	228	25	0
20. Turnip greens (1 cup)	.15	.33	0.7	145	61	0
21. Yogurt (1 cup) (skim)	.14	.06	2.2	134	—	0
22. Milk (1 cup) (whole)	.07	.41	0.2	98	2.4	1.0

Even with a normal diet that supplies adequate B-complex vitamins, certain drugs can interfere with your body's use of these agents and get you into trouble. This is especially true when the requirements for these vitamins are increased, such as during the so-called stress situations of an accident or injury, diarrhea or digestive-tract illness (that prevents proper absorption of food), major surgery, or periods of rapid growth.[73] Drugs that are prescribed for tuberculosis, such as isoniazid (INH, NICONYL, NYDRAZID, etc.) or arthritis, such as CUPRIMINE (penicillamine) work against vitamin B_6.[74] Oral contraceptives increase a woman's requirement for both B_6 and folic acid.[74] Folic acid is depleted by epilepsy medication such as DILANTIN (phenytoin), but watch out, there's a "catch 22" here — taking large amounts of folic acid to correct the deficiency may induce seizures. A commonly prescribed drug for high blood pressure called hydralazine (APRESAZIDE, APRESOLINE, DRALSERP, DRALZINE, SER-AP-ES, SERPASIL-APRESOLINE, UNIPRES, etc.) can interfere with B-complex vitamins. So can booze—so watch out, all you after-five drinkers—you may be burning out your brains and your B's.

Even as innocent a substance as plain tea can have an adverse effect: the tannic acid in tea has anti-thiamine activity which could lead to thiamine deficiency in people whose dietary intake is marginal.[75] Picture Aunt Martha who at age eighty-three favors tea and toast, or maybe Cousin Brucie who is about twenty pounds overweight. He is constantly dieting by cutting back on bread and cereals (which provide at least one-third of the thiamine in most diets). At the same time he drowns himself in iced tea to quiet his inner urges. Both Brucie and Aunt Martha could be in trouble because the tea is zapping what little thiamine they take in.

NIACIN: NICOTINIC ACID, NIACINAMIDE, B3

While we have a good idea how much thiamine you need to keep you from getting beriberi, and how much niacin will keep you from coming down with pellagra, there has been, as usual, very little research devoted to determining the optimal intake of the B vitamins. One exception, done in the Department of Oral Medicine at the University of Alabama and published in the *International Journal of Vitamin and Nutrition Research,* utilized a survey of 1,053 dentists and their wives. Although not very sophisticated, the study demonstrated that those with high dietary intake of niacin had significantly fewer symptoms or medical complaints.[76] The average daily niacin intake in these "super-healthy" people was over 80 mg, considerably above the recommended dietary allowances for grown men and women suggested by the National Research Council (which range from 16–20 mg daily for men and from 12–16 mg for women).

Niacin (also called nicotinic acid) is not toxic in doses that are significantly higher than the RDAs. However, if you consume more than 1,000 mg over a period of time you could damage your liver, aggravate an existing stomach condition (ulcer or gastritis), upset sugar metabolism, and if you are susceptible, you could trigger asthma attacks.[77, 78] Niacinamide, another chemical form of vitamin B3, is as effective as niacin, or nicotinic acid, in producing two drug-type effects of nicotinic acid in high doses: dilating blood vessels (giving a sensation of tingling and flushing) and lowering serum cholesterol.[79] Although nicotinic acid reduces blood cholesterol, it doesn't appear to substantially reduce the chance of death from a heart attack.[79]

One of the most intriguing things about niacin is that it has been used in the treatment of schizophrenia. Remember pellagra, the disease which results from severe niacin deficiency? We already talked about the three D's (Diarrhea, Dermatitis, and Dementia). Well, it's not surprising that somebody decided to try high doses of niacin in other cases of mental illness. Some doctors in Canada used big doses of nicotinic acid on schizophrenics in 1952,[80] and controversy about its effectiveness has been raging ever since. Its proponents claim that nicotinic acid has been proven successful in clinical use and some "double-blind" studies[80] where psychological bias is eliminated from the experiment. This was accomplished by keeping both the investigators and the subjects in the dark as to who received a sugar pill placebo and who received the active vitamin until after the study was completed. We respect these researchers but, quite honestly, we have to admit that theirs is a minority opinion and the more widely acceptable view is that "most controlled studies do not show significantly different results [of megadoses of niacin for schizophrenia] when compared with placebo."[81]

Although niacin may not be a magical cure for schizophrenia, it is clear that B-complex vitamins in general are essential for the health and proper functioning of the nervous system. Two British investigators, who found that 30 percent of the geriatric hospital patients they studied were deficient in thiamine, discovered that low thiamine levels were associated with confusion in these older people.[82] Severe thiamine deficiency can lead to an evil-sounding disease called the "Wernicke-Korsakoff syndrome." In the later stages, the resulting psychosis is irreversible, and many of the affected individuals (burned-out alcoholics mostly) end up in mental hospitals for the rest of their lives. Folic acid, too, has been implicated in mental disturbances. A study at the Medical University of South Carolina found that psychiatric patients are more likely to have low serum folate levels than are normal people, even though the diet of both groups was essentially similar.[83] There are some other hints that B vitamins are important for the nervous system. Remember that folic acid can counteract anticonvulsant medications and vitamin B_6 (pyridoxine) can reduce the effectiveness of levodopa (BENDOPA, DOPAR, LARODOPA, PARDA, RIO-DOPA) a drug for Parkinson's disease.

There is, however, no evidence whatsoever that taking ultra-high doses of the B-complex vitamins will keep all your mental cylinders clicking and ward off senility or even stupidity. In fact, high doses of folic acid are usually considered dangerous—because, although folic acid and vitamin B_{12} (cobalamin) work together to prevent anemia, folic acid alone can mask important symptoms of vitamin B_{12} insufficiency, without stopping the associated nerve degeneration. As a result, the deficiency may not be discovered until it is too late to help the patient much. Some conditions do demand more folic acid than usual: periods of rapid growth such as infancy and pregnancy; infections; conditions of chronic blood loss or increased metabolic rate; and rheumatoid arthritis.[84] People with one of these conditions, and of course boozers, should probably be taking a vitamin supplement which includes folic acid.

PRECOCIOUS PYRIDOXINE (VITAMIN B_6)

Pyridoxine has had researchers hopping recently just to keep up with the wild claims that are being made for it. An international flurry of letters in the prestigious *New England Journal of Medicine* discussed at some length the merits and demerits of using vitamin B_6 to suppress lactation in mothers who do not wish to breast-feed their babies—the principal demerit being that it apparently is ineffective for that purpose.[85] While the recommended dietary allowance for vitamin B_6 is slightly greater for pregnant and lactating women, these higher amounts can usually be provided through diet (including meats, cereals, lentils, nuts, bananas, avocados, and potatoes).[86]

Okay, that's not very exciting. But wait, here comes the "good" stuff. Two obstetricians intrigued the American Fertility Society with their report that "12 of 14 women with premenstrual-tension syndrome who had been infertile for 18 months to seven years were finally able to conceive during a course of high-dose vitamin B_6 therapy."[87] The women took 100 to 800 mg of B_6 daily until they conceived—a dose of some 50 to 400 times greater than the recommended dietary allowance. While the doctors have some speculations about why this treatment may have been effective on these women with premenstrual-tension syndrome, they really don't know what's going on here. And, of course, a dozen women are just too few to be able to tell if the results were more than some kind of fluke. But if it's hot, other doctors may be interested enough to pick up on the research, and we should know within a few years whether B_6 can be used effectively for cases of infertility.

Here is another biggie for pyridoxine. Researchers at the University of Wisconsin—Madison are suggesting that B_6 may be useful in treating cancer.[88] In a study of 121 patients with bladder cancer it was found that the vitamin B_6 therapy was as effective as the usual chemotherapy treatment. A different study in the same medical center discovered that women with advanced stages of breast cancer have depleted levels of B6 in their bodies, even though their diets are normal and contain adequate amounts of the vitamin. Dr. David Rose, the endocrinologist in charge of the study, believes that "large doses of vitamin B6 may not prevent the onset of breast cancer but, as with bladder cancer, the vitamin might be beneficial to those women who already have the disease."[88] Further studies to test this theory are currently underway. It is tantalizing because any effective and non-toxic addition to the anti-cancer armory will be welcome indeed. Unfortunately, it will take a few years before we will know whether this approach has promise.

Ready for another hot potato? A couple of doctors at the Massachusetts Institute of Technology are tackling heart disease, and B6 is the defense they propose. Drs. Stephen Raymond and Edward Gruberg hypothesize that the true culprit in arteriosclerosis (hardening of the arteries) is a product resulting from protein metabolism, an amino acid called homocysteine. And they claim that a daily intake of 10 to 25 mg of vitamin B6 (about 5 to 10 times the amount recommended by the feds) will help the body clear extra homocysteine out of the bloodstream, and help keep your arteries flexible and clear, if not young and beautiful.[89] They have a reasonably well-developed theory, and some other medical honchos agree that it has merit. What's more, Dr. Gruberg says that Dr. Gyorgy, the original discoverer of the vitamin, has recently concluded that everyone should be getting close to 25 mg daily, rather than the 2 mg recommended by the National Academy of Sciences—National Research Council.[90] If you want to hedge your bets against heart attack, you might want to try a B6 supplement of 10 to 25 mg every day; but don't *count* on it to work. Clinical studies to test the theory have not yet been conducted.

VITAMIN B12

Vitamin B12 is different. Unlike other B complex vitamins it is derived uniquely from microorganisms, and therefore is found concentrated only in animal products such as organ meats, shellfish such as clams and oysters which filter those B12 beasties out of seawater, eggs, muscle meats, and good old smelly fermenting cheeses like Camembert or Limburger.[91] B12 is also unique in that, although it is water-soluble like the other B-complex vitamins, it is stored in the body (in liver and muscle) for quite extended periods of time. In fact, it may be years after starting on a vitamin-B12 deficient diet before the absence becomes severe enough to interfere with health. (Remember that it only takes a couple of weeks for other B vitamins to be depleted.) But once there is a deficiency, watch out; you can get into big trouble. Complications include pernicious anemia and progressive nerve degeneration—both highly unpleasant if not fatal. Because it *is* stored in the body, the amount needed every day is very, very small, and even vegetarians who avoid animal products altogether rarely develop obvious deficiencies.[92] However B_{12} deficiencies do occur in people who can't absorb it—for example folks who have stomach surgery and those who simply don't produce the body chemical (called gastric intrinsic factor) which is crucial for absorbing appropriate amounts. Such people need to have injections of vitamin B_{12} every two to four weeks for as long as they live.[93]

Just how common these people may be is not quite clear. There has been a lot of hoopla in medical journals lately about the development of B_{12} deficiency in babies breast-fed by their vegetarian mothers,[94] and some case reports of infants admitted to the hospital extremely ill with a deficiency have been published. On the other hand, some medics argue that most vegetarians do not develop B_{12} deficiency and that breast-feeding by any mother shouldn't be discouraged. In our opinion all this discussion represents more smoke than fire. Increased demand for B_{12} during pregnancy may deplete body stores. Since the vitamin is available in tablet form and is chemically produced rather than derived from animal sources it would seem prudent for pregnant and lactating vegetarians to take a vitamin B_{12} supplement for insurance sake just to keep their babies from becoming another case history in the doctors' magazine battle. Since high doses of vitamin C can destroy some of the B_{12} in food,[95] it would also be wise for anyone whose diet is low in this vitamin to avoid vitamin-C supplements at mealtime.

So far vitamin B_{12} sounds boring as the dickens. But it has gained a certain popular notoriety as an "energy booster." Some public figures have claimed that their B_{12} injections give them the extra energy they need to cope with their hectic lives. Naturally, others who feel they could use more dynamism in their lives are interested. But sad to say, for anyone who is not actually B_{12}-deficient, the injections are no more than a placebo—like a sugar pill—and an expensive one at that.

THE RUSSIANS ARE COMING: VITAMIN B_{15}

From B_{12} to B_{15} may not seem a big jump numerically, but it is a giant leap in terms of orthodoxy and credibility. Vitamin B_{15}, otherwise known as pangamic acid, has been at the center of a firestorm lately. Russian researchers claim that the substance is a cure-all for such conditions as aging, senility, mental illness (including autism), alcoholism, drug addiction, and allergies. As one skeptical physician cracked, "It does everything but raise the dead."[96] Critics in this country are not convinced that pangamic acid is even a vitamin because it is not clear if it is essential to human nutrition, but international research does suggest that the chemical is extremely widespread in foods and that it probably has some important biochemical actions in the body.[97] The FDA, as usual, has been very upset about the extravagant claims made for B_{15}, and has even seized a few shipments of the substance.[98] Naturally, that hasn't stopped the enthusiasts from popping the pills whenever they can get them, even tripling the 50-mg dose recommended by the Russians.[99] Although there are some suggestive reports that pangamic acid may have beneficial effects on "impaired cerebral, cardiac or cutaneous oxygenation," one expert, Peter Stacpoole, states that "definitive studies, involving large, carefully matched treated and control populations and long-term follow-up surveys, are lacking."[100] The final chapter on B_{15} is far from in. It's a sure-fire bet that many of the excessive claims now being made will be debunked. After all, nothing cures everything, and even vitamins, as wonderful as they are, aren't miracle drugs.

Other disputed members of the B-complex have included biotin, bioflavonoids, choline, and inositol. Only biotin has been accepted by the nutrition establishment as a vitamin. Part of the delay in accepting any of these compounds is the difficulty in demonstrating that deficiency creates disease. Which brings us right back to where we started. Are vitamins necessary for providing optimum health or preventing disease? Clearly, modern-day "medicine shows" like the ones which insist they can "wake up 'sleeping' hair" are baloney. But just because you don't develop some dreadful deficiency disease if your diet lacks one of these nutrients does not mean that it isn't important for good health.

C IS FOR CHOLESTEROL, CANCER, AND COLDS

The history of ascorbic acid, or vitamin C, has been filled with romance and controversy. Although Dr. James Lind conclusively established in 1747 that citrus fruits could prevent and cure the dreaded scourge of scurvy, the British Navy waited nearly fifty years to adopt the citrus and gain the epithet "limeys."[101] Although it took the "establishment" a long time to recognize the value of vitamin C it is likely that the eventual establishment of this policy made it possible for Britannia to rule the waves for many years to come. The French and Spanish crews, their main competition, were regularly debilitated and decimated by scurvy.

So much for history. Nowadays, scurvy sounds like an exotic disease, although subclinical scurvy is not uncommon among heavy drinkers.[102] Even more serious, the Ten-State Nutrition survey of the late sixties demonstrated that one in every twenty-five Americans had actual symptoms of scurvy, and 12 to 16 percent of those surveyed had abnormally low levels of vitamin C. [103] Most of the controversy about vitamin C, though, has centered on its pharmacological properties: should the recommended intake be boosted or should we stick to the minimum dose necessary to prevent scurvy (10 to 60 mg)?[104] And are the reported benefits of large doses real, or just so much hype? These are the questions that have more than any others raised the Great Vitamin War to the extraordinary levels we mentioned at the very beginning of this chapter.

You don't have to be a counter-establishment vitamin enthusiast to recognize that ascorbic acid has many vital functions in the body. Two doctors in the Department of Pediatrics at Vanderbilt University School of Medicine point out that "in biochemical terms, the ascorbic acid molecule possesses considerable versatility."[105] It is essential for the proper formation of collagen, the "cement" that keeps our bodies together. It participates in a number of very important biochemical reactions, and stops many substances from deteriorating. In fact, these "anti-oxidant" properties are so potent that the steel industry is considering using vitamin C in rust-proofing (remember iron oxide?) instead of the toxic chemicals now in use.[106] Perhaps because of this anti-oxidant property, vitamin C has a sparing effect on other vitamins, especially A, E, and B-complex, which means that requirements for other vitamins are lower when vitamin C is in good supply.

A good many research reports have accumulated in recent years that demonstrate ascorbic acid is capable of lowering cholesterol and certain other fats in the bloodstream. Guinea pigs are handy critters if you want to study arteriosclerosis because they develop this human problem readily when fed a high-cholesterol diet. And like people, guinea pigs die of scurvy when their diets are deficient in vitamin C. Guinea pig studies have repeatedly shown that in sufficient doses ascorbic acid protects against the arteriosclerosis they get from eating cholesterol. Conversely, guinea pigs with long-term deficiencies in vitamin C, but without the excess cholesterol in their diets, still end up with more fat deposited in their arteries.[107-109] There is some tantalizing evidence that human beings may react in pretty much the same way.[110-112]

There are three ideas that are floating around to explain how vitamin C could help protect against heart disease: (1) ascorbic acid seems to promote the conversion of cholesterol to bile acids, which speeds extra cholesterol out of the body;[113, 114] (2) vitamin C may protect against deterioration and damage to the walls of the blood vessels themselves, because of its important role in collagen manufacture and maintenance (remember the cement);[115] and/or (3) vitamin C may increase fibrinolytic (anticoagulant) activity of the blood serum, helping to prevent the tiny blood clots we think may be important in the early development of arteriosclerosis.[116] Whether or not cholesterol is the true villain in hardening of the arteries and heart disease, it would be well worth the effort to conduct a good study in order to determine whether vitamin C has a protective effect on blood vessels and the heart, and if so, at what levels. An eminent researcher in this field, Dr. Emil Ginter of the Institute for Human Nutrition Research in Czechoslovakia, has made a plea for just such a study:

> **The only way to obtain a full answer to this question [does vitamin C help prevent atherosclerosis in humans?] would be to conduct an extensive field investigation among a large number of subjects given ascorbic acid over a long period, carrying out a longitudinal study of their blood lipid levels, signs of atherosclerosis and total mortality, which is a more meaningful end point when assessing the health of a whole community . . .[117]**

Unfortunately, the nutrition establishment and the medical community appear reluctant to undertake this sort of in-depth study, preferring instead to evaluate expensive cholesterol-lowering drugs like ATROMID-S (clofibrate). Turn to page 134 for the full story on how this drug apparently was killing patients faster than their elevated cholesterol levels.

Pleas for careful studies of vitamin C and its pharmacological effects are now being made on other fronts as well. In 1978 Linus Pauling and his Scottish associate, Dr. Ewan Cameron, published a reevaluation of their 1976 study of terminal cancer patients; the cancer patients who were given whopping doses of vitamin C survived nearly a year longer, on the average, than patients with similar cancers who did not receive the vitamin.[118,119] Although many cancer researchers wrinkled their noses at the research done in Loch Lomondside because the procedures left room for error, the results were still exciting. Dr. Paul Chretien, chief of tumor immunology in the National Cancer Institute, expressed his duly cautious response:

> **This study should prompt a repeat study of an identical nature that is controlled by a statistician ... There would be no question about the results if it had been done by random patient selection as a double-blind test in which neither doctors nor patients knew what medication was being given.** [120]

Such a study has, in fact, been conducted at the prestigious Mayo Clinic. And unfortunately, for terminal cancer patients and their families, the results do not support Cameron's and Pauling's findings.[121] The doctors found no difference in survival time or quality of life between the terminal patients treated with ascorbic acid and those who received placebos. The fight is not over yet, however, because Dr. Pauling claims that the potent chemotherapy that the Mayo patients had undergone wiped out their natural immune responses.[122] Without further studies, this argument could go on for a long time.

If we turn our attention now to the potential of ascorbic acid for *preventing* cancer in certain situations, we find a whole new cast of characters—and a good deal more consensus. If you eat foods containing sodium nitrite (a common preservative in everything from hot dogs and bacon to salami and pepperoni), you should be concerned about a chemical reaction that takes place in your stomach with compounds called amines. The combination of nitrites and amines can lead to the formation of potent cancer-causing substances called, logically enough, nitrosamines. There is, however, some pretty solid evidence that vitamin C taken at the same time prevents this interaction, thus saving your system from one more cancer-provoking exposure.[123,124] But that's not all. Some Swiss scientists have found that vitamin C "protects against or reverses abnormal growth and malignant transformation occurring (in cell cultures) ... after repeated exposure to smoke from tobacco or marijuana cigarettes."[125] And some researchers in Dublin found that cells treated with vitamin C resisted the toxic effects of radiation better than untreated cells.[126] Dr. Linus Pauling's own sophisticated research on the ability of vitamin C to protect a special breed of mice from getting skin cancer after exposure to ultraviolet light also looks impressive as the dickens.[127] Now it is a big jump from cell cultures and hairless mice to human beings, we grant you. Even the scientists trying to make that leap express some reservations; another group of Irish researchers gave 6,000 mg of ascorbic acid to skin cancer patients every day for a week before their tumors were surgically removed. Their work led them to theorize that large doses of vitamin C may serve a protective function for normal cells during radiation therapy.[128] Another researcher, Dr. J. U. Schlegel at Tulane University School of Medicine, is investigating the possible use of vitamin C in bladder cancer. He believes some tentative evidence supports the view that the antioxidant action of ascorbic acid may counteract the carcinogenic effect of a bladder carcinogen and may possibly help prevent bladder cancer.[129] Now none of this is what you'd call conclusive scientific proof. Still, there is more than a hint that ascorbic acid may be of some value in helping the body sidestep those toxic chemicals to start with, or in mustering the natural immune response against a developing cancer. This line of research deserves a lot more attention—from scientists and the public alike.

And now, dear friend, strap on your helmet and bulletproof vest, because we're about to venture into the real battle zone. Can vitamin C prevent the common cold? Our friend, Pauling, of course boldly initiated the fray, with a resounding *YES!*[130] Others, however, aren't so sure. A group of scientists at the "Common Cold Research Unit" of Britain's Medical Research Council found that, although the men who took ascorbic acid rather than a placebo had fewer colds, this did not hold for the women, and consequently results for the entire sample were not statistically significant. They conclude that the "preventive effect of vitamin C, if any, is not such as to justify advising its general use as a prophylactic measure."[131]

A noted Irish researcher, on the other hand, found that 550 mg of vitamin C daily would protect from 30 to 40 percent of the schoolgirls he studied against the common cold, but had little effect on the boys.[132] After reviewing a number of other relevant studies, he concluded, "Significant benefit was produced by vitamin C therapy in the naturally produced colds, whereas it was ineffective in the smaller number of subjects who were subjected to nasally instilled viral infection."[133]

Insofar as there is any agreement in this hotly disputed arena, it seems to be that ascorbic acid reduces the disability resulting from cold symptoms and has a positive effect on the general feeling of well-being.[134,135] Which is a heck of a lot more than you can say about the vast majority of over-the-counter cold remedies on the market. Vitamin C has been put under the microscope and examined with extraordinary critical care, something that has never been done with the expensive drug-company products. One can only marvel that doctors manage to get themselves so exercised over a simple vitamin but can't muster enough energy to let out a peep over some of the potentially hazardous medications that offer doubtful benefit. Perhaps the most beneficial effect of the entire brouhaha is the interest it has sparked on precisely how vitamin C works to enhance the immune process.[136,137] A better understanding of the functions of ascorbic acid in the immune system will go far in helping to determine its usefulness in warding off common infections like the cold or flu as well as battling those less common diseases we call cancer.

Now what about the claim that ascorbic acid can extend the life span and help us all reach a vigorous old age?[138] There is, unfortunately, little evidence to support this hypothesis. In fact, one of the few direct studies of the effects of vitamin C on life span (of guinea pigs, not people) found no protective effect of large doses of vitamin C.[139] But the news isn't all so pessimistic. There are some clues that ascorbic acid can improve the later years. One double-blind study in a British "long-stay" hospital found more improvement in outlook and less psychological deterioration in the patients given 1 gram of vitamin C daily for a month than in those who received a placebo, even though tissue levels of the vitamin never rose to normal.[140] Vitamin-C blood and tissue levels are frequently lower than they should be in older people, a fact which is often attributed to changes in diet but may also be related to hormonal changes associated with aging.[141]

Some degenerations of tongue and mouth tissue which were once considered to be a "natural" consequence of aging are not present to the same degree in elderly life-long vegetarians. This suggests that some of the aging degenerations we take for granted might be staved off with higher intakes of ascorbic acid.[142] Drs. T. P. Eddy and G. F. Taylor who did this research at the London School of Hygiene and Tropical Medicine propose "that previous, perhaps recurrent, vitamin deficiencies may lead to irreversible changes in the elderly that cannot subsequently be changed by vitamin-therapy."[143] The suggestion has even been made that the low levels of cholesterol and fats found in the blood of vegetarians may be partially due to their generally higher intake of ascorbic acid.[144] It would certainly be of interest to see if people whose vitamin-C intake is high their entire lives make it to a riper, older age more often than the rest of the population.

All right already, what about your basic question—should you be taking vitamin C every day? Well, that is a personal matter that only you can answer for yourself. To be honest, we are impressed enough with the early glimmerings to gorp down vitamin-C supplements on a daily basis, but we have a weak spot in our heart for Linus Pauling. What if you drink a glass of orange juice every morning, won't that do the trick? Unfortunately not. *Consumer Reports* did an excellent comparison of different brands of orange juice a few years back and discovered some extraordinary facts:

> **People think of fresh orange juice as excellent in nutrition, a nationwide survey revealed some years back ... Except for its vitamin C and potassium content, orange juice—fresh or processed—has little nutritional importance.**
>
> **Orange juice is, to be sure, one of the few good natural sources of vitamin C. But it's a less reliable source than you might expect.**
>
> **Unfortunately, few of the frozen juices could be relied on to deliver enough vitamin C to meet the recommendation for adults (45 mg) if served in the common 3½ ounce portion. A few, indeed, wouldn't even meet the recommendation for infants (35 mg).**
>
> **Moral: You can't rely on a small glass of frozen orange juice to meet your day's needs.**[145]

Now that's distressing, especially when you keep in mind that the medical experts for Consumers Union are a pretty conservative bunch. They have taken a traditional view of the vitamin-C issue. Although they have slowly increased their recommendations over the years, they are not convinced that megadoses are beneficial. In their large sampling they found that 3½ ounces of most brands of orange juice only contained between 20 and 40 mg of ascorbic acid (with quite a few familiar brands weighing in at less than 25 mg: SNOW CROP, SHURFINE, SUNNY SEVEN, SUNKIST, and SUNSHINE STATE). There were surprisingly large variations in C content depending upon the time of year. For example, their first test of SNOW CROP only had 22 mg but a later measurement on a different batch produced 51 mg.[146]

Well, what foods are really high in vitamin C? If orange juice isn't so great, is anything else any better? Here's a list of the big winners:

FOODS HIGH IN VITAMIN C

FOOD	SERVING SIZE	VITAMIN C (MG)
Brussels sprouts	½ cup	68
Strawberries	¾ cup	66
Orange	1	66
Orange juice (fresh)	½ cup	60
Broccoli	½ cup	52
Grapefruit juice	½ cup	48
White grapefruit	½	44
Pink grapefruit	½	44
Collard greens	½ cup	44
Mustard greens	½ cup	34
Cauliflower	½ cup	33
Cantaloupe	¼	32
Tangerine	1	27
Cabbage	½ cup	24
Beef liver	3 oz.	23
Cooked tomatoes	½ cup	21
Tomato juice	½ cup	20

Source: Whitney, Eleanor, and Hamilton, Eva May. *Understanding Nutrition.* St. Paul: West, 1977, pp. 318–319.

"FOODS HIGH IN VITAMIN C"

If we've still got your attention, you'll notice quickly that the batting averages are pretty puny. You'd have to eat a bushel of Brussels sprouts to get close to Linus Pauling's recommended dose.

So how much vitamin C do you need? That is a zillion-dollar question. Quite clearly there is no one single answer that is right for everyone. In fact, there is even less agreement on the *levels* of vitamin C which might protect against certain cancers or arteriosclerosis than there is on whether or not the vitamin may really be useful for such prevention in the first place. People under certain life stresses clearly need more vitamin C than the average government bureaucrat. Pregnancy and lactation both increase the need for vitamin C, but megadoses may not be a good idea because an infant accustomed to such a high level in the womb may develop scurvy after birth, when it can no longer obtain such amounts.[147] Smokers, boozers and people with unbalanced diets would be wise to goose their vitamin-C levels on a regular basis. And if you are unlucky enough to be exposed to toxic chemicals (or you just can't give up nitrite-preserved meat like hot dogs, bologna, salami, pepperoni, etc.) extra vitamin C may be a good insurance policy.

There are, of course, a few dangers associated with the use of vitamin C as a drug. Naturally the "experts" differ about the significance of these effects. People with a relatively rare genetic abnormality of the blood called glucose- 6- phosphate dehydrogenase deficiency (now there's a tongue twister for you) and people with sickle- cell anemia would probably be smart to avoid big doses (over 1 or 2 grams per day).[148,149] But these conditions are not common.

There is a good bit of controversy as to whether and in what doses ascorbic acid might lead to the formation of kidney stones in susceptible individuals. Given the fact that most doctors are gunning for any adverse reaction they can find there has been a surprising paucity of case reports in the medical literature. But if you have ever had a kidney stone, you know you're susceptible, and you sure as shooting do not want to repeat the experience. You'd be smart to keep your vitamin- C intake below the daily 4 g (4,000 mg) which have been implicated in causing oxalate stones.[150,151] Diabetics who must rely on urine tests to insure that their blood sugar is in line will get false results on high doses of ascorbic acid.[152] And people who have become accustomed to megadoses of C and then suddenly stop taking it may get into trouble—a case of scurvy.[153] This "rebound" effect is probably not terribly relevant to most people.

But enough beating around the bush. Assuming that there is no health reason to avoid megadoses of vitamin C how much should the average person take? What's the bottom line? Well, we keep repeating that there is no one perfect dose for everyone. Linus Pauling concludes from analysis of how much animals manufacture, the "optimum intake of vitamin C by man probably also lies in the range of 1.75 g to 3.50 g per day."[154] He suggests that under stressful situations (such as during a cold) higher amounts are helpful. In general, Dr. Pauling suggests that depending upon your own particular body makeup an adequate dose of vitamin C should range from 250 mg up to 10,000 mg per day. We refuse to give you any more specific answer than that because, quite honestly, there are just too many variables to be dogmatic. Is vitamin C important? Absolutely. How important, we may have to wait to find out.

DAZZLING D—THE SUNSHINE VITAMIN

If ever there was a confusing name for a vitamin, this one from the old- time nutrition books has to be it. How could a vitamin which we need to get from our food to maintain good health have anything to do with sunshine? The answer: vitamin D is very peculiar indeed. It is the only substance known which is classified as both a vitamin and a hormone. You heard right—vitamin D acts as a hormone in the body, and what's more, your body even makes some itself when ultraviolet rays from the sun strike your naked skin. So if you spend a lot of time outdoors in a sunny climate, you need never take any vitamin D, which like vitamin A, is stored in the liver. Your normal stores can carry you through a few cloudy days.

If, on the other hand, you're living in a big city where the sun doesn't shine that often, you must get vitamin D from your food. This was a major medical breakthrough in the 1920s when researchers discovered that cod liver oil kept New York City youngsters from getting rickets. Since then, fortification of milk with vitamin D has made both cod liver oil and rickets almost obsolete in this country.

Now, if you've guessed that body storage of this vitamin may lead to some of the same kinds of potential overdose problems we discussed with vitamin A, you are right. The recommended daily intake of 400 IU for both children and adults is probably ample to insure proper mineral metabolism and bone growth in youngsters. Daily intakes of 1,000 IU are considered potentially dangerous, and poisoning has occurred at levels of 50,000 IU and more. Symptoms of vitamin D toxicity range from nausea, diarrhea, and weight loss up to the most serious—irreversible kidney damage. On the whole, it would be a lot smarter not to take the risk of overdosing on D.

The principal action of vitamin D is regulation of calcium in the body, but there is an enormous number of variables influencing this action. The parathyroid and thyroid glands both produce substances which work with vitamin D (remember its hormone status?) in maintaining mineral balance. Dietary levels of minerals, not only calcium, but also phosphorus and magnesium, are also important. In fact, the whole juggling act is much too complicated to go into here without a raft of diagrams and flow charts. Vitamin D or some of its more potent variants are sometimes prescribed for diseases involving the parathyroid gland, chronic renal failure, and abnormal bone metabolism. For the most exciting news we've had recently on the use of vitamin D in conjunction with calcium to prevent and treat osteoporosis, turn to page 249, in the chapter "For Women Only."

A few drugs interfere with vitamin D's action in the body. The anticonvulsants used for epilepsy and DORIDEN (glutethimide), a sleeping pill, can all deplete vitamin D levels and interfere with mineral metabolism. Mineral oil and a medication called cholestryramine (QUESTRAN) when taken with food keep it from being absorbed into the body at all. In addition, over-the-counter laxatives containing phosphates can throw a real monkey wrench in the works if you depend on them regularly. For more details, check the chart on page 226.

ENIGMATIC E

Few vitamins have incited such emotion and controversy right from the moment of their discovery as vitamin E. Because the Berkeley chemists who isolated the compound in 1922 had found that laboratory animals on a vitamin-E-deficient diet did not reproduce normally, the word soon spread to all and sundry that vitamin E would pep up sex life. (There is, we hasten to add, a big difference between white rats and human beings in this regard, since humans don't appear to gain any sort of reproductive or sexual benefit that has ever been documented.) Since then the "enthusiasts" have been dreaming up new therapeutic uses for vitamin E, while the establishment long maintained a skepticism that vitamin E was even essential to human nutrition. To compound the confusion, there are few foods which are naturally rich in this vitamin. The best sources are the oils, but even these are hardly loaded: one tablespoon of safflower oil contains 12.6 mg, olive oil supplies 9.4 mg in a tablespoon, and peanut and cottonseed oil check in at 8.5 mg per tablespoon.

Although the controversy still rages, by now even the old-establishment types have embraced the tocopherols, as the E vitamins are known, for several "pharmacologic" uses. A majority of these are focused on premature infants, who are demonstrably deficient in vitamin E.[155] These babies commonly develop anemia due to the rapid destruction of their red blood cells; administering vitamin E protects them from this problem.[156] Vitamin E may also help protect them from some of the adverse effects of the concentrated oxygen that they sometimes require. Oxygen damage to the retina of the eye and to the lungs appears to be minimized when "preemies" are treated with E.[157–159]

Another establishment-approved use of vitamin E is in the treatment of people who do not absorb fats normally, especially children with cystic fibrosis.[160,161] The medical establishment also approved one other use for vitamin E in relatively high doses: daily doses of 300 or 400 mg taken over a fairly long time—at least three to six months—are effective in combating disconcerting cramps in the calf muscle while walking (given the high-falutin' term "intermittent claudication").[162–164] And that's it. As far as the doctors know, we're on our own and strictly out in left field when it comes to any other uses of vitamin E.

Luckily, there are some researchers out there with us. In several studies, rats and mice given about as much tocopherol for their size as the average American gets in his diet were subjected to polluted air. These poor critters developed lung damage strikingly similar to human emphysema, while their buddies treated with high doses of vitamin E were largely protected.[165,166] The respected journal *Nutrition Reviews* went so far as to conclude that the antioxidant properties of vitamin E "and the related protective systems now appear to be among the most important defensive systems against oxidant insult to lungs from air pollution."[167] None of these researchers is willing to go out on a limb and actually recommend higher doses of the vitamin for city dwellers, because it will probably be some time before definitive studies on human populations are published. You might want to draw your own conclusions before then.

Now we get into the murky middle earth. The women's underground has long suggested that vitamin E might be of use in combating the symptoms of menopause, and in fact some physicians did clinical tests, with positive effects, back in the 1940s.[168] Of course, research done that long ago is not always up to "snuff" by today's standards; but practicing gynecologists these days have not followed up on this early lead, sticking instead to their now conventional use of replacement estrogens. Of course, we really don't have any good explanation of how vitamin E might help alleviate menopausal discomfort; but the fact that it's apparently a lot less toxic than artifical estrogens should surely get someone interested enough to give it a whirl. We doubt that improvement will be dramatic but any little bit could help.

One isolated study done in Israel points to another tantalizing suggestion. The scientists at the Rheumatology Clinic of Hasharon Hospital found that tocopherol in a dose of 600 mg per day significantly lessened the pain reported by the osteoarthritis patients they studied.[169] Now this study alone is not enough to lead to any conclusions, but if future investigations support these results, it may be because vitamin E has a dampening effect on prostaglandins.[170] "Prosta" who? Well, it's interesting that this family of chemicals which is found throughout the body is "inhibited" by almost all arthritis drugs—from aspirin to INDOCIN, NAPROSYN, and MOTRIN. It is just barely possible that vitamin E may be doing much the same thing as these drugs, at least on a small scale.

How about vitamin E and the heart? Even though we now know that vitamin E can be metabolized in the body to a substance called tocopheryl hydroquinone, which works as an anticoagulant,[171] most evidence suggests that vitamin E is not effective against heart disease.[172,173] This fancy byproduct of vitamin E may boost the power of anticoagulant medication, and so if you are taking a drug like COUMADIN (warfarin), watch out. If you aren't careful to check in with your doctor and have your blood tested you could check out with a horrendous hemorrhage. With some subtle adjustments in the drug dose your doctor should be able to keep you out of trouble.[174]

Oh yes, mustn't forget side effects. Will large doses get you into trouble? Even though vitamin E is a fat-soluble vitamin the good news is that even in relatively high doses (750 mg/IU) per day, there haven't been any blatant examples of toxicity. The research that investigated this question was carried out for only a few months, however.[175,176] Although we haven't managed to locate any reports of studies on the safety of large doses over longer periods of time, there have also been no warnings of hazards.[177] Since people have been loading up on the stuff for years, it seems fair to guess that any really dreadful danger would probably have been trumpeted to the world by docs who disapprove of folks taking pills into their own hands.

COAGULATION WITH K

Now here is a vitamin that is about as straightforward as you can get. It was discovered to be the mysterious factor whose deficiency caused chickens to bleed to death, and named vitamin K for "koagulation." (Vitamin C had already been named, and besides, the scientist didn't speak English.) As would be expected, in humans too vitamin K is essential for proper blood clotting. About half the vitamin K you need comes from your diet, especially green vegetables like collard or turnip greens, broccoli, cabbage, lettuce, or spinach; the other half is manufactured by the friendly bacteria which live in your intestine. Consequently, vitamin-K deficiency is pretty uncommon, and the vitamin is available only as injections, with a doctor's prescription. Because of its influence on blood-clotting time, maintaining a steady vitamin K intake, without big fluctuations, is important for people on anticoagulant medications (see pp. 81-82, 101 in the drug-interaction chapter).

SHALL WE DECLARE A TRUCE?

Well, dear reader, we have come to the end of the line. There is much we haven't covered because there is just *so* much to talk about when it comes to vitamins. And who, you ask, will win The Great Vitamin War? We leave that question to you to resolve within your own beating breast. We confess that we do take some vitamins each day, (won't get any more specific than that, though) but we tried very hard not to let our personal lives influence what's included in this chapter. We truly believe that there are a lot of inflated claims and altogether too much hot air when it comes to some purported vitamin "treatments." But we also believe that the medical/nutrition establishment has been entirely too close-minded. The FDA almost seems vindictive in some of its pronouncements. They seem to be saying, if you don't like our artificial flavors and colors, emulsifiers, texturizers, and preservatives, then we won't like your vitamins.

The establishment experts put a lot of stock in a "well-balanced diet" without really bothering to get very specific. If you've been paying any attention to the tables in this chapter you discovered that some of the most nutritious foods aren't all that popular. If you aren't regularly eating **liver, greens, broccoli, spinach, sweet potatoes, cantaloupe,** and **Brussels sprouts** you may not be as well off as the bureaucrats imply. But does that mean you need high-potency supplements? Well, if your thing is tea and toast for breakfast, a "plastic" burger or a carton of yogurt for lunch, and a steak and mashed potatoes for supper, you may want to refer back to our suggested vitamin formulations on page 187.

There is little doubt that the Vitamin War will be with us for many years to come. Use your own common sense and you shouldn't get wounded. If we had our druthers we would declare a truce. It's time for more research and less arguing. If everyone started working together we might find out if vitamins really can live up to some of the hopes and claims.

INTERACTIONS OF VITAMINS AND DRUGS

THIS VITAMIN:	INTERACTS WITH:	SO THAT:
VITAMIN A	Mineral oil	the vitamin is not absorbed well. If you feel compelled to use this kind of laxative, take it at bedtime on an empty stomach.
VITAMIN A	Cholestyramine Questran	less vitamin A is absorbed. If this cholesterol-lowering drug has to be taken for a long time better play it safe and go with a vitamin supplement.
THIAMINE (vitamin B_1)	Tea	if you're an iced-tea lover or just like it hot you could run the risk of developing a thiamine deficiency. If you're into tea, better keep the thiamine flowing.
THIAMINE	Antacids	thiamine is destroyed when antacids are taken at meal time. Even if you opt for some vitamin "insurance," antacids may obliterate the benefits if taken at the same time.
THIAMINE	Alcohol	boozers get busted! Alcohol increases the body's need for thiamine. If an extra effort isn't made to improve the diet or take a strong supplement, dangerous nerve damage may result.
RIBOFLAVIN (vitamin B_2)	Methotrexate	the action of this anticancer drug may be sandbagged if too much riboflavin is taken. Here is a case where a vitamin may reduce the effectiveness of an important therapeutic agent.
VITAMIN B_6 (pyridoxine)	Levodopa Bio/Dopa Dopar Larodopa Parda	the drug becomes much less effective because vitamin B_6 speeds the breakdown of levodopa. If you want this anti-Parkinsonism drug to work, either reduce B_6 intake or switch to a medication called SINEMET which prevents the drug/vitamin interaction.

INTERACTIONS OF VITAMINS AND DRUGS

THIS VITAMIN:	INTERACTS WITH:	SO THAT:
VITAMIN B$_6$	*Isoniazid* INH Laniazid Niconyl Nydrazid Rifamate *Cycloserine* Seromycin	vitamin B$_6$ deficiency can develop during tuberculosis treatment with these drugs; seizures and nerve damage may result. This is a "double whammy," though, since vigorous supplementation may reverse the anti-TB effect. Check with a doctor for appropriate vitamin B$_6$ dosage.
VITAMIN B$_6$	*Anti-depressants* Adapin Aventyl Elavil Limbitrol Norpramin Pertofrane Presamine Sinequan Triavil Tofranil	25 mg of vitamin B$_6$ (2 to 4 times a day) may help reduce the nasty dry mouth and urination difficulties often caused by these tricyclic anti-depressants. We don't guarantee this one, but if it works, zounds! It would be a big break for a great many dry-mouthed depressed people.
VITAMIN B$_6$	*Penicillamine* Cuprimine	vitamin B$_6$ deficiency can develop during arthritis treatment with **CUPRIMINE**. A daily dose of pyridoxine should be a must. But skip the mineral supplements—they can block the effectiveness of the drug. If you have to take iron, take it for short periods of time and space the dose at least 2 hours from the arthritis medication.
VITAMIN B$_6$	*ESTROGENS* Oral Contraceptives Brevicon Demulen Enovid Loestrin Modicon Norinyl Norlestrin Ortho-Novum Ovcon Ovral Ovulen	the need for vitamin B$_6$ is increased. Here is where a little vitamin insurance might come in handy. A supplement of about 20 mg per day is often recommended.

INTERACTIONS OF VITAMINS AND DRUGS

THIS VITAMIN:	INTERACTS WITH:	SO THAT:
VITAMIN B$_6$	*Post-menopausal* Estinyl Estrace Menrium Milprem Ogen Premarin	the need for vitamin B$_6$ is increased. Here is where a little vitamin insurance might come in handy. A supplement of about 20 mg per day is often recommended.
VITAMIN B$_6$	*Hydralazine* Apresazide Apresoline Dralzine Ser-Ap-Es Unipres	the body is depleted of vitamin B$_6$. Signs and symptoms of a serious deficiency include numbness and tingling in extremities. It might not hurt to try to prevent nerve damage by starting with adequate B$_6$ levels and then maintaining them.
FOLIC ACID	*Phenytoin* Dilantin Di-Phen Diphenylan Ekko	all hell breaks loose on this one. Pay attention, this gets sticky! The anticonvulsant drug **phenytoin** depletes the body of folic acid. If you attempt to replace it, however, the drug won't work very well and seizures may result. It takes a special effort to stay on this tightrope. If anemia develops or a woman becomes pregnant most doctors add a folic-acid supplement. Up to 1 mg may be prescribed per day. Careful monitoring is a must!
FOLIC ACID	*Oral Contraceptives* See list under B$_6$.	the need for folates is increased. If you don't eat a lot of green leafy vegetables (spinach, collards, kale, Swiss chard, etc.) better take a dietary supplement.
FOLIC ACID	*Trimethoprim* Bactrim Septra *Pyrimethamine* Daraprim *Methotrexate*	these drugs and the vitamin "fight" each other in the body. If a deficiency develops (anemia), it should probably be treated with folinic acid injections (**LEUCOVORIN**), which will not counteract the drugs' effectiveness.

INTERACTIONS OF VITAMINS AND DRUGS

THIS VITAMIN:	INTERACTS WITH:	SO THAT:
FOLIC ACID	Alcohol	unless the diet is super-fine and high in those yucky greens, megaloblastic anemia is likely because of folic-acid deficiency.
FOLIC ACID	Aspirin (in high doses over a long period of time)	folic-acid anemia (macrocytic) may result in some people.
VITAMIN B_{12} (cyanocobalamin)	Alcohol	you can bet your booties that if you're a boozer you'll be short on B_{12}. Better supplement or eat well.
VITAMIN B_{12}	Colchicine ColBENEMID	vitamin B_{12} absorption is fouled up. If long-term use of the gout medicine is necessary, monitor for a deficiency state.
VITAMIN B_{12}	Clofibrate Atromid-S	the possibility exists that vitamin B_{12} absorption will be reduced.
VITAMIN B_{12}	p-Aminosalicylic Acid P.A.S.	vitamin B_{12} is not absorbed. People taking this anti-tuberculosis drug may develop a deficiency.
VITAMIN B_{12}	Potassium Chloride K-Lor Kaochlor Kaon-Cl Slow-K	once again we see poor vitamin B_{12} absorption in combination with potassium supplements. Check on it with your doctor.
VITAMIN B_{12}	Vitamin C	Vitamin B_{12} could get zapped. 500 mg of vitamin C can destroy vitamin B_{12} in food or in a supplement. To be on the safe side take your vitamin C at least two hours before or after meals.
VITAMIN C (ascorbic acid)	Anti-coagulants Coumadin Dicumarol Panwarfin	the blood-thinning effect may be altered. This is somewhat controversial. Play it safe, have blood levels checked if you start or stop large doses of vitamin C.
VITAMIN C	Aspirin	the aspirin lasts longer and provides more zip for the zap. High doses could lead to aspirin tox-

INTERACTIONS OF VITAMINS AND DRUGS

THIS VITAMIN:	INTERACTS WITH:	SO THAT:
		icity. Conversely, aspirin prevents vitamin C from getting into cells and reduces its effectiveness.
VITAMIN C	*Fluphenazine* Permitil Prolixin	ascorbic acid in high doses reduces the levels and effectiveness of this anti-psychotic medication.
VITAMIN C	*Iron*	absorption of the iron is significantly improved if 200 mg or more of vitamin C is taken at the same time.
VITAMIN C	*Oral Contraceptives*	birth control pills deplete the body of vitamin C. Regular daily supplements are essential.
VITAMIN C	*Methenamine* Mandelamine Methavin Prosed Trac Thiacid Uroqid Urex	the effectiveness of these drugs in the urinary tract is significantly improved. Very large doses of vitamin C are often recommended.
VITAMIN C	*Nitrites (in food)* Hot dogs Bacon Bologna Salami Etc.	the formation of cancer-causing **nitrosamines** from the nitrites is prevented. The regular intake of vitamin C appears to be a dynamite prophylactic agent if you dig these preserved meat products.
VITAMIN C	*Sulfa Drugs* Azo Gantanol Thiosulfil Gantrisin SK-Soxazole Soxomide	kidney stones could develop. Many doctors fail to mention that vitamin C makes the urine more acidic and this in turn makes many sulfa drugs dangerous.
VITAMIN C	*Tobacco smoke*	the body's need for ascorbic acid is increased by about 40 percent. Smokers—make sure you take extra vitamin C to make your body a little healthier.

INTERACTIONS OF VITAMINS AND DRUGS

THIS VITAMIN:	INTERACTS WITH:	SO THAT:
VITAMIN C	Vitamin E Vitamin A	these vitamins are "protected" from early destruction. By combining vitamin C with E and A their effects are stronger and longer-lasting.
VITAMIN C	Urine Glucose Tests 　Tes-Tape 　Clinistix	these tests may give false-negative results when large doses of vitamin C are taken.
VITAMIN C	Urine Glucose Tests 　Clinitest 　Benedict's 　Solution	these tests may give false-positive results if large doses of vitamin C are taken.
VITAMIN D	ANTICONVUL-SANTS Phenobarbital Phenytoin 　Dilantin 　Di-Phen 　Diphenylan 　Ekko Primidone 　Mysoline	vitamin D may become depleted which in turn may interfere with calcium and phosphate metabolism. The result: bones can be weakened. Vitamin-D intake should probably be increased during treatment.
VITAMIN D	Cholestyramine 　Questran	less of the vitamin is absorbed.
VITAMIN D	Glutethimide 　Doriden	long-term use of this sleeping pill may deplete vitamin-D levels. This may foul up calcium and phosphorus metabolism.
VITAMIN D	Laxatives containing phosphates	regular use can deplete body calcium and interfere with vitamin-D utilization. Over the long term a negative effect on bone can occur.
VITAMIN D	Mineral Oil	vitamin D is not well absorbed. If you feel compelled to take this kind of laxative use it at bedtime on an empty stomach.

INTERACTIONS OF VITAMINS AND DRUGS

THIS VITAMIN:	INTERACTS WITH:	SO THAT:

VITAMIN E (tocopherol)	Anticoagulants
	  Coumadin
	  Dicumarol
	  Panwarfin
		there is fear the blood-thinning action of these drugs will be strengthened. Better have regular blood tests or avoid vitamin E if you want to keep the anticoagulant effect stable.

VITAMIN E	Iron	the effectiveness of vitamin E is diminished if iron is taken simultaneously. If you are one of those people who gorps down all your vitamins and minerals at breakfast, better think again.
VITAMIN E	Mineral Oil	vitamin E is not well absorbed. If you feel compelled to use this kind of laxative, take it at bedtime on an empty stomach.

VITAMIN E	Oral Contraceptives
	  Brevicon
	  Demulen
	  Enovid
	  Loestrin
	  Modicon
	  Norinyl
	  Norlestrin
	  Ortho-Novum
	  Ovcon
	  Ovral
	  Ovulen
		blood levels of vitamin E may drop. Women on the Pill may need more vitamin E than other people.

VITAMIN E	Vitamin A Retinoids	retinoids become more effective if a person also takes vitamin E. In high doses retinoids also can be more toxic in the presence of vitamin E.

VITAMIN K	Antibiotics
	  Broad spectrum
	  (long-term)
	  Tetracycline
	  Ampicillin
		a vitamin-K deficiency may result. This can be terribly important, so pay heed. The normal "good" bacteria in your gut make a significant amount of vitamin K. Antibiotics wipe the buggers out and needless to say their productivity declines correspondingly. Without vitamin K

INTERACTIONS OF VITAMINS AND DRUGS

THIS VITAMIN:	INTERACTS WITH:	SO THAT:
		your body is more susceptible to bleeding, especially if you are on an anticoagulant. Be very careful!
VITAMIN K	Anticoagulants Coumadin Dicumarol Panwarfin	the blood-thinning action of these drugs is diminished. Watch out! Too many green leafy vegetables that contain lots of vitamin K (spinach, kale, cabbage, cauliflower, etc.) can reverse the anticoagulant effect.
VITAMIN K	Mineral Oil	the vitamin is not absorbed well. If you feel compelled to use this kind of laxative, take it at bedtime on an empty stomach.

Knowledge about the effects of drugs on nutrition is still crude at best. We do know that alcohol, anticonvulsants, oral contraceptives, and **DORIDEN** can cause deficiencies of several different vitamins simultaneously. Mineral oil does a nasty job on all fat-soluble vitamins and other laxatives that contain the ingredient phenolphthalein (**AGORAL**, **ALOPHEN**, **AMLAX**, **EVAC-Q-KIT**, **EX-LAX**, **FEEN-A-MINT**, **PHENOLAX**, etc.) can cause nutritional deficiencies by interfering with adequate absorption. Vitamins can also interfere with the appropriate action of many drugs. This whole area has been neglected for too long and requires much closer examination. You may know more than your doctor when you finish digesting this chapter.

TABLE REFERENCES

1. DiPalma, Joseph R. "Vitamin Toxicity." *American Family Physician* 18:106—109, 1978.

2. DiPalma, Joseph R., and Ritchie, David M. "Vitamin Toxicity." *Ann. Rev. Pharmacol. Toxicol.* 17:133—148, 1977.

3. Haithcock, John N. "Nutrition: Toxicology and Pharmacology." *Nutrition Reviews* 34:65—69, 1976.

4. Ivey, Marianne. "Nutritional Supplement, Mineral and Vitamin Products." In *Handbook of Non-Prescription Drugs,* (5th edition), Washington, D. C., American Pharmaceutical Association, 1977, pp. 135—165.

5. Lambeth, Martin L. "Drug and Diet Interactions." *American Journal of Nursing* 75:402—406, 1975.

6. Lehmann, Phyllis. "Food and Drug Interactions." *FDA Consumer* March, 1978.

7. Martin, Eric W. *Drug Interactions Index,* Philadelphia: J. B. Lippincott, 1978.

8. Reiss, Barry S., and McLean, Ronald W. "Drug-Induced Vitamin Deficiencies." *Pharmacy Times* February: 68—69, 1979.

9. Roe, Daphne A. "Nutritional Side Effects of Drugs." *Food and Nutrition News* 45(1):1, 4, 1973.

10. Rosenberg, Jack M. "Vitamins: The Hazards are Subtle." *Current Prescribing* July:123—128, 1978.

REFERENCES

1. Pauling, Linus. *Vitamin C, the Common Cold and the Flu,* San Francisco: W. F. Freeman, 1976, p. 33.

2. Morton, R. A. "Vitamins in Western Diets: Symposium on Some Aspects of Diet and Health." *Proceedings of the Nutrition Society* 35:23—29, 1976.

3. Davis, Adelle. *Let's Get Well.* pp. 40—41.

4. Taylor, Keith B. "Uses and Abuses of Vitamin Therapy." *Rational Drug Therapy* 9(10):1—6, 1975.

5. Rodale, Robert. "Why Some Crazy Diets Work" (editorial). *Prevention* 30(2):25—30, 1978.

6. Disler, P. B., et al. "The Effect of Tea on Iron Absorption" *Gut* 16:193—200, 1975.

7. Williams, Roger J. "Nutritional Individuality." *Human Nature* 1(6): 46—53, 1978.

8. Ibid., p. 50.

9. Truswell, A. S. "A Comparative Look at Recommended Nutrient Intakes. Symposium on 'Some Aspects of Diet and Health.' " *Proc. Nutr. Soc.* 35:1—14.

10. Benowicz, Robert J. *Vitamins and You,* New York: Grosset and Dunlap, 1979, p. 52.

11. "How Nutritious are Fast-Food Meals?" *Consumer Reports* 40(5):278—281, 1975.

12. Ibid., p. 280.

13. Krupp, Marcus, and Chatton, Milton, eds. *Current Medical Diagnosis and Treatment,* Los Altos, Calif. Lange, 1978, p. 803.

14. Sabry, Zak. "Take a Sensible Stand on Vitamin Pills." *Nutrition and the M.D.* 4(1):1—2, 1977.

15. Ibid., pp. 1—2.

16. Williams, Roger J. "Nutritional Individuality." *Human Nature* 1(6): 46—53, 1978.

17. Ibid., p. 53.

18. Robinson, Corinne H., and Lauler, Marilyn R. *Normal and Therapeutic Nutrition,* 15th ed. New York: Macmillan, 1977, pp. 184—185.

19. Hecht, Annabel. "Vitamins Over the Counter: Take Only When Needed." *FDA Consumer* April 1979:17—19.

20. Sporn, Michael B.; Dunlop, Nancy M.; Newton, Dianne L.; and Smith, Joseph M. "Prevention of Chemical Carcinogenesis by Vitamin A and Its Synthetic Analogs (Retinoids)." *Federation Proceedings* 35:1332—1338, 1976.

21. Babb, Richard R., and Keraldo, John H. "Cirrhosis Due to Hyper-vitaminosis A." *Western J. Medicine* 128:244—246, 1978.

22. Krupp, Marcus A., and Chatton, Michael J. "Nutrition and Metabolic Disorders." In *Current Medical Diagnosis and Treatment,* rev. ed. Los Altos, Calif. Lange, 1978, p. 799.

23. Roels, Oswald A., and Lui, Nan S. T. "The Vitamins: Vitamin A and Carotene." In *Modern Nutrition in Health and Disease: Dietotherapy,* 5th ed. R. S. Goodhart and M. S. Shils, eds. Philadelphia: Lea and Febiger, 1973, p. 152.

24. Shaywitz, Bennett A.; Siegel, Norman J.; and Pearson, Howard A. "Megavitamins for Minimal Brain Dysfunction: A Potentially Dangerous Therapy." *JAMA* 238:1749—1750, 1977.

25. Morriss, Gillian M. "Vitamin A and Congenital Malformations." *Inter. J. Vit. Nutr. Res.* 46:220—222, 1976.

26. Cheraskin, E.; Ringsdorf, W. M., Jr.; and Medford, F. H. "The 'Ideal' Daily Vitamin A Intake." *Inter. J. Vit. Nutr. Res.* 46:11—13, 1976.

27. Wolf, George. "Vitamin A—Not Too Little, Not Too Much." *Nutrition and the M.D.* 4(12):1—2, 1978.

28. Agricultural Research Service. "Nutritive Value of Foods." Home and Garden Bulletin No. 72, 1970.

29. Guilhou, J. J., et al. "Traitement Oral des Psoriasis Graves par un Nouveau Retinoide Aromatique (Ro 10-9359)." *Ann. Dermatol. Venereol. (Paris)* 105:813—818, 1978.

30. Pekamberger, H., et al. "Oral Treatment of Ichthyosis With an Aromatic Retinoid." *Br. J. Dermatol.* 99:319—324, 1978.

31. Schuppli, R. "The Efficacy of a New Retinoid (Ro 10-9359) in Lichen Planus." *Dermatologica* 157 (Suppl. 1): 60—63, 1978.

32. Peck, G. L., et al. "Treatment of Darier's Disease, Lamellar Ichthyosis, Pityriasis Rubra Pilaris, Cystic Acne and Basal Cell Carcinoma with Oral 13-cis-Retinoic Acid." *Dermatologica* 157 (Suppl. 1): 11−12, 1978.

33. Orfanos, Constatin E., et al. "Oral Treatment of Keratosis Follicularis with a New Aromatic Retinoid." *Arch. Dermatol.* 114:1211−1214, 1978.

34. Dominguez-Soto, Luciano, and Hojoyo-Tomoka, Maria Teresa. "Aromatic Retinoid (Ro 10-9359) on the Treatment of Psoriasis." *Cutis* 22:376−379, 1978.

35. Fredriksson, T., and Pettersson, U. "Severe Psoriasis−Oral Therapy with a New Retinoid." *Dermatologica* 157 (Suppl. 1): 238−244, 1978.

36. Viglioglia, P. A., and Barclay, A. "Oral Retinoids and Psoriasis." *Dermatologica* 157 (Suppl. 1):32−37, 1978.

37. Goerz, G., and Orfanos, C. E. "Systemic Treatment of Psoriasis with a New Aromatic Retinoid." *Dermatologica* 157 (Suppl. 1):38−44, 1978.

38. Bjelke, E. "Dietary Vitamin A and Human Lung Cancer." *Int. J. Cancer* 15:561−565, 1975.

39. Cohen, Martin H., et al. "Vitamin A Serum Levels and Dietary Vitamin A Intake in Lung Cancer Patients." *Cancer Letters* 4:51−54, 1977.

40. Smith, P. G., and Jick, Hershel. "Cancers Among Users of Preparations Containing Vitamin A: A Case-Control Investigation." *Cancer* 42:808−811, 1978.

41. Sporn, Michael B. "Retinoids and Carcinogenesis." *Nutrition Reviews* 35(4): 65−69, 1977.

42. Ibid., p. 66.

43. Crocker, T. Timothy, and Sanders, Lora L. "Influence of Vitamin A and 3,7-Dimethyl-2,6-Octadienal (Citral) on the Effect of Benzo(a)pyrene on Hamster Trachea in Organ Culture." *Cancer Research* 30:1312−1318, 1970.

44. Lasnitzki, Ise, and Goodman, Dewitt S. "Inhibition of the Effects of Methylcholanthrene on Mouse Prostrate in Organ Culture by Vitamin A and its Analogs." *Cancer Research* 34:1564−1571, 1974.

45. Nettesheim, P., et al. "The Influence of Retinyl Acetate On the Potentiation Phase of Preneoplastic Lung Nodules in Rats." *Cancer Research* 36:996−1002, 1976.

46. Sporn, Michael B., et al. "13-Cis-Retinoic Acid: Inhibition of Bladder Carcinogenesis in the Rat." *Science* 198:487−489, 1977.

47. Grubbs, Clinton J., et al. "13-Cis-Retinoic Acid: Inhibition of Bladder Carcinogenesis Induced in Rats by N-Butyl-n-(4-Hydroxybutyl) Nitrosamine." *Science* 198:743−744, 1977.

48. Felix, Edward L., et al. "Inhibition of the Growth and Development of a Transplantable Murine Melanoma by Vitamin A." *Science* 189:886−887, 1975.

49. Becci, Peter J., et al. "Inhibitory Effect of 13-Cis-Retinoic Acid on Urinary Bladder Carcinogenesis Induced in C57BL/6 Mice by N-Butyl-N-(4-Hydroxybutyl) Nitrosamine." *Cancer Research* 38:4463—4466, 1978.

50. Bollag, Werner, "Prophylaxis of Chemically Induced Benign and Malignant Epithelial Tumors by Vitamin A Acid (Retinoic Acid)." *Europ. J. Cancer* 8:689—693, 1972.

51. Ibid.

52. Sporn, Michael B., et al., 1976, op. cit.

53. Rettuva, Giuseppe, et al. "Antitumor Action of Vitamin A in Mice Inoculated with Adenocarcinoma Cells." *J. National Cancer Institute* 54:1489—1491, 1975.

54. Lotan, Reuben, et al. "Characterization of the Inhibitory Effects of Retinoids on the In Vitro Growth of Two Malignant Murine Melanoma." *J. National Cancer Institute* 60:1035—1041, 1978.

55. Bollag, Werner. "Therapeutic Effects of an Aromatic Retinoic Acid Analog on Chemically Induced Skin Papillomas and Carcinomas of Mice." *Europ. J. Cancer* 10:731—737, 1974.

56. Lapis, K., et al. "The Effect of Retinoic Acid on Lewis Lung Carcinoma Model in Mice." *Dermatologica (Suppl. 1)* 157:52—53, 1978.

57. Crocker, T. Timothy, and Sanders, Lora L., op. cit.

58. Lasnitzki, Ise, et al., op. cit.

59. Sporn, Michael B. "Vitamin A and its Analogs (Retinoids) in Cancer Prevention." in *Nutrition and Cancer,* ed. M. J. Winick, New York: Wiley Interscience, 1977.

60. Sporn, Michael B., et al., 1976, op. cit.

61. Todaro, George J., et al. "Retinoids Block Phenotypic Cell Transformation Produced by Sarcoma Growth Factor." *Nature* 276:272—274, 1978.

62. Seifter, Eli. "Of Stress, Vitamin A, and Tumors (letter)." *Science* 193:74—75, 1976.

63. Michsche, M., et al. "Stimulation of Immune Response in Lung Cancer Patients by Vitamin A Therapy." *Oncology* 34:234—238, 1977.

64. Kurata, T., and Micksche, M. "Suppressed Tumor Growth and Metastasis by Vitamin A and BCG in Lewis Lung Tumor Bearing Mice." *Oncology* 34:212—215, 1977.

65. Allen, Norman, et al. "Effect of Vitamin A on Radiation Enhancement and Survival in Experimental Rat Gliomas." *Trans. Am. Neurol. Assn.* 102:160—163, 1977.

66. Dennert, G., and Lotan, R. "Effects of Retinoic Acid on the Immune System: Stimulation of T Killer Cell Induction." *Eur. J. Immunol.* 8:23—29, 1978.

67. Sporn, Michael B., op. cit., 1977.

68. Sporn, Michael B., op. cit., 1976.

69. Koch, Herbert F. "Biochemical Treatment of Precancerous Oral Lesions: The Effectiveness of Various Analogues of Retinoic Acid." *J. Maxillo-Facial Surg.* 6:59−63, 1978.

70. Gunby, Phil. "Retinoid Chemoprevention Trial Begins Against Bladder Cancer." (Medical News) *JAMA* 240:609−614, 1978.

71. Sporn, Michael B., et al., op. cit., 1976.

72. Sporn, Michael B., op. cit., 1977.

73. Greene, Harry L. "The B Vitamins." *Nutrition and the M.D.* 4(8):1−2, 1978.

74. Ivey, Marianne. "Nutritional Supplement, Mineral and Vitamin Products." In *Handbook of Non-Prescription Drugs.* Washington, D. C.: American Pharmaceutical Association, 1977.

75. "Morsels and Tidbits." *Nutrition and the M.D.* 4(5):4, 1978.

76. Charaskin, E., et al., "The 'Ideal' Daily Niacin Intake." *Inter. J. Vit. Nutr. Res.* 46:58−60, 1976.

77. Greene, Harry L., op. cit.

78. "Morsels and Tidbits," op. cit.

79. Moran, J. Roberto, and Greene, Harry L. "The B Vitamins and Vitamin C in Human Nutrition." *Am. J. Dis. Child.* 133:308−314, 1979.

80. Pfeiffer, Carl C. *Mental and Elemental Nutrition.* "Niacin and Megavitamin Therapy." New Canaan, Conn.: Keats, 1975, p. 118.

81. Ivey, Marianne, op. cit.

82. Pollitt, Norman T., and Salkeld, Richard M. "Vitamin B Status of Geriatric Patients." *Nutr. Metabl.* 21(Suppl. l): 24−27, 1977.

83. Thornton, William E., and Thornton, Bonnie Pray. "Folic Acid, Mental Function and Dietary Habits." *J. Clin. Psychiatry.* April 1978:315−320, 1978.

84. Ivey, Marianne, op. cit.

85. Underwood, Barbara A.; del Pozo, E.; and Brun del Re, R. "Vitamin B6 in Nursing Mothers." (letters) *New Engl. J. Med.* 301:107, 1979.

86. Ivey, Marianne, op. cit.

87. "Infertile Women Conceive After Vitamin B6 Therapy." *Medical World News,* March 19, 1979, p. 43.

88. "Vitamin B6 Effectively Treats Bladder Cancer." (News) *Am. Fam. Physician* 17:290−293, 1978.

89. Smith, Tom. "Vitamin B_6 Can Prevent Heart Attacks." *National Enquirer,* July 31, 1979, p. 52; and Raymond, Stephen A., and Gruberg, Edward R. *Atlantic Monthly,* 1979, and Personal Communication.

90. Gruberg, Edward R., Personal Communication, 1979.

91. Herbert, Victor. "Folic Acid and Vitamin B_{12}." In *Modern Nutrition in Health and Disease: Dietotherapy,* 5th ed., eds. R. S. Goodhart and M. E. Shils, Philadelphia: Lea and Febiger, 1973, p. 234.

92. Carmel, Ralph. "Nutritional Vitamin-B_{12} Deficiency: Possible Contributory Role of Subtle Vitamin-B_{12} Malabsorption. *Ann. Intern. Med.* 88:647−649, 1978.

93. McCurdy, Paul R. "B_{12} Shots: Flip Side." *JAMA* 231:289−290, 1975, and "The Nutritional Anemias." *Nutrition and the M.D.* 5(5):4, 1979.

94. Higginbottom, Marilyn C., et al. "A Syndrome of Methylmalonic Aciduria, Homocystinuria, Megaloblastic Anemia and Neurologic Abnormalities in a Vitamin B_{12}-Deficient Breast-Fed Infant of a Strict Vegetarian." *New Engl. J. Med.* 299:371−323, 1978.

95. Herbert, V., and Jacob, E. "Destruction of Vitamin B_{12} by Ascorbic Acid." *JAMA* 230:241−242, 1974.

96. Cooney, John E. "B_{15} Is Taking Off: It's a Bird! It's a Plane! It's Superpill! Maybe." *Wall Street Journal,* April 24, 1978.

97. Stacpoole, Peter W. "Pangamic Acid ('Vitamin B_{15}'): A Review." *World Review of Nutrition and Dietetics* 27:145−163, 1977.

98. Cooney, John E., op. cit.

99. Nobile, Philip. "Will Vitamin B-15 Cure What Ails You?" *New York,* March 13, 1978.

100. Stacpoole, Peter W., op. cit.

101. Hodges, Robert E., and Baker, Eugene M. "Ascorbic Acid." In *Modern Nutrition in Health and Disease: Dietotherapy,* 5th ed., eds, R. S. Goodhart and M. E. Shils, Philadelphia: Lea and Febiger, 1973, pp. 245−255.

102. Sprince, H. "Influence of Smoking and Drinking on Vitamin C." *Inter. J. Vit. Nutr. Res.* Supplement 16: 185−218, 1977.

103. Robinson, Corinne H., and Lawler, Marilyn R. *Normal and Therapeutic Nutrition,* 15th ed., New York: MacMillan, 1977, p. 16.

104. Harper, Alfred E. "The Recommended Dietary Allowances for Ascorbic Acid." *Ann. N.Y. Acad. Sciences* 258:491−496, 1979.

105. Moran, J. Roberto, and Greene, Harry L. "The B Vitamins and Vitamin C in Human Nutrition." *Am. J. Dis. Child.* 133:308−314, 1979.

106. Horwitz, Nathan. "Vitamin C Gives Proof of Metal as Ca Fighter." *Medical Tribune* 19(35): 1,7, (Nov. 1, 1978).

107. Weiser, H.; Hanck, A.; and Hornig, D. "Ascorbic Acid and Cholesterol Interaction in Guinea Pigs." *Nutr. Metab.* 21(Suppl. 1):240–244, 1977.

108. Hayashi, Eiichi, et al. "Fundamental Studies on Physiological and Pharmacological Actions of L-Ascorbate 2-Sulfate. VI. Effects of L-Ascorbate 2-Sulfate on Lipid Metabolism in Guinea Pigs." *Japan J. Pharmacol.* 28:133–143, 1978.

109. Ginter, Emil. "Marginal Vitamin C Deficiency, Lipid Metabolism, and Atherogenesis." *Advances in Lipid Res.* 16:167–220, 1978.

110. Ginter, E., et al. "Hypocholesterolemic Effect of Ascorbic Acid in Maturity-Onset Diabetes Mellitus." *International J. Vit. Nutr. Res.* 48:368–373, 1978.

111. Cerna, O., and Ginter, E. "Blood Lipids and Vitamin-C Status." *The Lancet* 1:1055–1056, 1978.

112. Ginter, Emil. "Vitamin C and Plasma Lipids." (letter) *New Engl. J. Med.* 294:559–560, 1978.

113. Weiser, H., op. cit.

114. Ginter, E., et al., op. cit., 1978. [refers to ref. 109]

115. Ibid.

116. Bordia, Arun, et al. "Acute Effect of Ascorbic Acid on Fibrinolytic Activity." *Atherosclerosis* 30:351–354, 1978.

117. Ginter, Emil, op. cit., 1978 [refers to ref. 112].

118. Cameron, Ewan, and Pauling, Linus. "Supplemental Ascorbate in ᵗᵉ Supportive Treatment of Cancer: Prolongation of Survival Times in ᵗᵐinal Human Cancer." *Proc. Natl. Acad. Sci. USA.* 73:3685–3689, 1976.

119. Cameron, Ewan, and Pauling, Linus. "Supplemental Ascorbate in the Supportive Treatment of Cancer: Reevaluation of Prolongation of Survival Times in Terminal Human Cancer." *Proc. Natl. Acad. Sci.* 75:4538–4542, 1978.

120. Leary, Warren E. "Vitamin C Gives Cancer Patients Longer Life, Nobel Winner Finds." *Durham Sun,* October 26, 1976, p. 4-B.

121. "No Vitamin-C Benefit Found in Ca Trial." *Medical World News* June 25, 1979, p. 19.

122. Ibid.

123. Kamm, Jerome J., et al. "Effect of Ascorbic Acid on Amine-Nitrite Toxicity." *Ann. N.Y. Acad. Sci.* 258:169–174, 1978.

124. "Can Vitamin C Stop Cancer?" (News) *Drug Topics,* July 2, 1979, p. 12.

125. Leuchtenberger, C., and Leuchtenberger, R. "Protection of Hamster

Lung Cultures by L-Cysteine or Vitamin C Against Carcinogenic Effects of Fresh Smoke from Tobacco or Marihuana Cigarette." *Br. J. of Exp. Pathol.* 58:625—634, 1977.

126. O'Connor, M. K., et al. "A Radioprotective Effect of Vitamin C Observed in Chinese Hamster Ovary Cells." *Br. J. of Radiology* 50:587—591, 1977.

127. Pauling, Linus, Personal Communication, 1978.

128. Moriarty, M., et al. "Some Effects of Administration of Large Doses of Vitamin C in Patients with Skin Carcinoma." *Irish J. of Med. Sci.* 147:166—170, 1978.

129. Schlegel, J. U. "Proposed Uses of Ascorbic Acid in Prevention of Bladder Carcinoma." *Ann. N. Y. Acad. Sci.* 258:432—437, 1978.

130. Pauling, Linus. *Vitamin C, the Common Cold and the Flu.* San Francisco: W. H. Freeman, 1976.

131. Tyrrell, A. J., et al. "A Trial of Ascorbic Acid in the Treatment of the Common Cold." *Br. J. of Prevent. and Soc. Med.* 31:189—191, 1977.

132. Wilson, C. W. M. "Ascorbic Acid Function and Metabolism During Colds." *Ann. N. Y. Acad. Sci.* 258:529—539, 1978.

133. Ibid.

134. Editorial. "Vitamin C and the Common Cold." *Br. Med. J.* March 13, 1976, p. 606—607.

135. Kent, Saul. "Vitamin C Therapy: Colds, Cancer and Cardiovascular Disease." *Geriatrics* 33(10):91—99, 1978.

136. Thomas, W. R., and Holt, P. G. "Vitamin C and Immunity: an Assessment of the Evidence." *Clin. Exp. Immunol.* 32:370—379, 1978.

137. Leibovitz, Brian, and Siegel, Benjamin V. "Ascorbic Acid Neutrophil Function, and the Immune Response." *International J. Vit. Nutr. Res.* 48:159—164, 1978.

138. Pauling, Linus, op. cit., 1976.

139. Davies, J. E. W., et al. "Dietary Ascorbic Acid and Life Span of Guinea Pigs." *Exp. Gerontol.* 12:215—216, 1977.

140. "On Psyche of Geriatric Patients." *The Lancet* 1:403, 1979.

141. Sokoloff, Boris, et al. "Aging, Atherosclerosis and Ascorbic Acid Metabolism." *J. of the Amer. Geriat. Soc.* 14:1239—1257, 1966.

142. Eddy, T. P., and Taylor, G. F. "Sublingual Varicosities and Vitamin C in Elderly Vegetarians." *Age and Ageing* 6:6—13, 1977.

143. Ibid.

144. Ginter, Emil, op. cit., 1978 [refers to ref. 112].

145. "Orange Juice: Frozen, Canned, Bottled, Cartoned, Fresh." *Consumer Reports* 41(8):435—442, 1976.

146. Ibid.

147. Hughes, R. E. "Use and Abuse of Ascorbic Acid—A Review." *Food Chemistry* 2:119—133, 1977.

148. Ibid.

149. Campbell, G., et al. "Ascorbic Acid-induced Hemolysis in G-6-PD Deficiency." (Letter) *Ann. Int. Med.* 82:810, 1975.

150. Herbert, Victor, and Smith, Lynwood H. "Risk of Oxalate Stones From Large Doses Vitamin C." (Letters) *New Engl. J. Med.* 298:856, 1978.

151. Siest, G., et al. "Drug Interferences in Clinical Chemistry: Studies on Ascorbic Acid." *J. Clin. Chem. Clin. Biochem.* 16:103—110, 1978.

152. Ibid.

153. Hughes, R. E., op. cit., 1977.

154. Pauling, Linus, op. cit., p. 83.

155. Bieri, John G., and Farrell, Philip M. "Vitamin E." *Vitamins and Hormones* 34:47, 1976.

156. Editorial. "Vitamin E for Babies." *The Lancet,* Dec. 17, 1977, 1268—1269.

157. Bieri, John G., and Farrell, Philip M., op. cit., p. 50.

158. Ehrenkranz, Richard A., et al. "Amelioration of Bronchopulmonary Dysplasia After Vitamin E Administration: A Preliminary Report." *New Engl. J. Med.* 299:564—601, 1978.

159. Oski, Frank A. "Metabolism and Physiologic Roles in Vitamin E." *Hosp. Prac.* 12:79—85, 1977.

160. "Vitamin E." *Nutrition Reviews* 35:58, 1977.

161. Winick, Myron. "Setting the Facts Straight on Vitamins E and K." *Mod. Med.* Oct. 15—Oct. 30, 1978, pp. 103—108.

162. Oski, Frank A., op. cit., p. 84

163. "Vitamin E," op. cit., p. 58.

164. Horwitt, M. K. "Vitamin E: A Reexamination." *Amer. J. Clin. Nutr.* 29:569—578, 1976.

165. News. "Vitamin E Found to Protect Mouse Lung in Polluted Air." *Medical Trib.,* May 3, 1978:1.

166. Horwitt, M. K., op. cit., p. 573—574.

167. "Vitamin E," op. cit., p. 61.

168. Seaman, Barbara, and Seaman, Gideon. "Vitamin E and Other Helps for Menopause." Chapter 32. *Women and the Crisis in Sex Hormones.* New York: Rawson Assoc., 1977, pp. 363—367.

169. Machtey, I., and Ouaknine, L. "Tocopherol in Osteoarthritis: A Controlled Pilot Study." *J. Am. Geriat. Soc.* 27:328—330, 1978.

170. Hope, W. C., et al. "Influence of Dietary Vitamin E on Prostaglandin Biosynthesis in Rat Blood." *Prostaglandins* 10:557—570, 1975.

171. Horwitt, M. K., op. cit., pp. 574—575.

172. "Vitamin E," op. cit., p. 59.

173. Bieri, John G., and Farrell, Philip M., op. cit., p. 66.

174. Horwitt, M. K., op. cit., p. 576.

175. Tsai, Alan C., et al. "Study on the Effect of Megavitamin E Supplementation in Man." *Am. J. Clin. Nutr.* 31:831—837, 1978.

176. Horwitt, M. K., op. cit., p. 576.

177. "Vitamin E," op. cit., p. 61.

For Women Only

Shafted by the system: Discrimination by doctors and prejudices in prescribing • Sex differences that count • Menstrual cramps are **NOT** in your head: Drugs that really help—PONSTEL, MOTRIN, and NAPROSYN • Periodic puffiness—Dubious diuretics. Calcium and magnesium: some hope for help • Feminine hygiene is unhygienic: Dangerous douches • Yeast infections: Causes and cures—MY-COSTATIN, MONISTAT 7, and GYNE-LATRIMIN. Vaginitis and FLAGYL: The controversy rages on. Nonspecific bugs: vinegar, yogurt or . . . ? • Horr le Herpes—Help is on the way: **2-deoxy-D-glucose** or ACYCLO-VIR • Cystitis: Home lab tests are in. Successful treatment means goodbye to **UTI** • Menopause and estrogen therapy—the fight goes on • Calcium and exercise: Better ways to fight osteoporosis.

Women are getting shafted by the medical system! Now we know that may sound either harsh and emotional or like yesterday's news depending upon your perspective. However, let us assure you, we do not go around looking for sexists under every bed or stethoscope. But we have it straight from the dragon's den (*Journal of the American Medical Association,* May 18, 1979) that what we have suspected for a long time is indeed true—male doctors don't take their women patients as seriously as they do their men patients. The physicians who undertook this research set out to investigate how their California colleagues would respond to five common complaints: back pain, headache, dizziness, chest pain, and fatigue. The results of their work are shocking!

> **Because we were curious about the degree to which sexism might affect general medical care, we undertook such a study . . . The only variable that correlated with the extent of workup was the sex of the patient. For the total group of complaints, back pain, headache, dizziness,**

chest pain, and fatigue, the physician workups
were significantly more extensive for the men.
Finally and most controversially, the data may
bear out what many critics already claim:
namely, that the physicians—who in this study
were all male—tend to take illness more
seriously in men than in women.[1]

OVERPRESCRIPTION TO WOMEN

So what else is new? Well it is new! As far as we can tell, this is the
first scientific study which substantiates the claims of the women's
health movement and it has implications far beyond the damage that
has been done to women's self-respect. Not only does this practice
influence the diagnostic process, it also has a major impact on the
kind of drugs that are prescribed. In 1978 the House Select
Committee on Narcotics Abuse and Control held hearings in order to
find out "why so many women are taking mood-altering drugs." The
testimony produced some frightening statistics:

> Thirty-two million (42%) women compared to
> 19 million (26%) men have used tranquilizers
> prescribed by a doctor. Sixteen million (21%)
> women as compared to 12 million(17%) men
> have used physician prescribed sedatives and 12
> million (17%) women as compared to 5 million
> (8%) men have used amphetamines ordered by a
> doctor. In 1977 8½ million women used tran-
> quilizers, 3 million women used sedatives and 1
> million women took their first stimulants
> prescribed by a doctor.[2]

Now that represents an awful lot of VALIUM, LIBRIUM, PHENOBAR-
BITAL, TRANXENE, DEXEDRINE, and DALMANE, not to mention antidepressants like ELAVIL, MELLARIL and TRIAVIL. Men probably have
to face as much stress as women. And there is little evidence that
they are coping with it any better. So why do women receive so much
more heavy head medicine than men? It is tempting to speculate that
doctors see men as stoics and women as hypochondriacs. Another
reason may be that drug companies work very hard at creating an
image of the nervous, uptight woman when they pitch their drugs to
doctors. Dr. Jere Goyan, the Commissioner of the Food and Drug
Administration, showed surprising sensitivity when he said:

> I have a lot of concerns about these minor
> tranquilizers. One of the things that bothers me

**about them is that the advertising for them—
which is aimed not at the patient, but at the
physician and the pharmacy—is basically sexist. I'll bet 80% of the ads—that are aimed at the
minor tranquilizer market—show a woman
anxious. Now I would contend that lots of men
are anxious from time to time, too.**[3]

That's pretty strong stuff coming from the top-dog at the FDA.
Another possible reason for the frequent prescribing of tranquilizers
is that it may be easier to give a drug than to help a patient resolve
conflict and anxiety that stem from real-life problems, especially if
those problems have deep roots in social institutions.

Whatever the reasons for these prescribing patterns we find them
deplorable. It is past time for women to insist on fair treatment.
Condescending attitudes have got to go! If your doctor makes you
feel uncomfortable, tense, self-conscious, apprehensive, or just plain
mad, maybe it's time to change doctors. A pat on the back and a
prescription aren't acceptable. If your doctor makes you cool your
heels for an hour in the waiting room and then makes you feel as if
you're on a conveyor belt once you do get to see him, let the fink
know that you are dissatisfied. And if his solution to your problems is
always VALIUM find another doctor. There are many really fine
physicians out there who DO NOT perform this way. Conscientious
doctors will not be ready to reach for the prescription pad at the drop
of a hat.

"VIVE LA DIFFERENCE"

From what you have read so far you may have gotten the idea that
we believe men and women should be treated alike by doctors. For
most things, yes. But when it comes to drugs, men and women are
not equals and they shouldn't be treated as if they are. Unfortunately,
this is one instance when doctors don't discriminate enough. For one
thing, women tend to weigh less than men, sometimes a lot less. Take
Fred and Jennifer for example. Fred is six feet tall and weighs 194
pounds. Jennifer is only five feet four inches and weighs 105 pounds.
They both have high blood pressure and are taking DYAZIDE. The
drug company only makes one dose of this medication and the doctor
followed a standard recommendation—one capsule twice a day. That
was fine for Fred, but Jennifer experienced a whole host of side
effects including dizziness, headache, dry mouth, nausea, and
diarrhea. Because she was small, with less fat and muscle, Jennifer
was receiving, on a milligram per kilogram basis, almost twice the

dose that Fred got. Even one capsule a day might have been too much for her. But the doctor didn't take weight differences into account.

Body size is only the most obvious difference between men and women. Other sex-related factors that can profoundly affect the ways in which drugs are handled in the body include basic metabolism and levels of circulating hormones.[4] For example, women tend to metabolize some anticonvulsant drugs more rapidly than men. As a result, drugs like DILANTIN (phenytoin) and MYSOLINE (primidone) may never reach the anticipated level in the bloodstream and therefore may not be as effective in preventing seizures. On the other hand, women may be more vulnerable to adverse reactions than men. Anesthetics like NITROUS OXIDE (laughing gas) or HALOTHANE are more likely to cause nausea and vomiting in women, who are also more susceptible to increased bleeding from HEPARIN (an anticoagulant frequently given after strokes and heart attacks).[5] The moral of this tale is that doctors must take women's illnesses as seriously as they do men's illnesses. But they must also take sex differences into account when they prescribe drugs since women may be more *or* less sensitive to some medications than men.

MENSTRUAL CRAMPS—CURSE THE DOCTOR

Women have suffered far too long with misinformed, insensitive doctors when it comes to the treatment of cramps. It has often been suggested that the pain, headache, backache, nausea, and vomiting that some experience during menstruation were due to some amorphous psychological factors. Many doctors minimized the problem as "psychosomatic," implying that the woman was imagining things, and recommended a hot water bottle or a "muscle-relaxant" (read VALIUM) to reduce anxiety. This attitude led women to believe that they weren't supposed to feel bad, which in turn often made them feel guilty, which only made matters worse. Other physicians overreacted by prescribing heavy-duty pain relievers (including narcotics) or birth control pills. A few women finally gave up and resorted to a hysterectomy to obtain relief. Drastic measures? You bet! But if you don't believe us, here are some actual letters from readers of *The People's Pharmacy* newspaper column that tell a sad story:

> I wish I had $20 for every doctor who told me my cramps were psychosomatic; $10 for every sadist who suggested I do exercises and they'll go away and "We wouldn't be women without our periods" (indeed! my foot); $5 for every well-

meaning but non-suffering friend or relative who suggested that I should ignore them and make the best of it; and $1 for every pill, tablet, capsule, shot of scotch and bottle of wine I consumed to kill the pain.

Finally, I found a good sympathetic doctor, padded the cancer and abnormal uterus cases in my family, borrowing incidents that suited my purpose from families or friends, I confess. He consented to a vaginal hysterectomy.

The surgeon ended what h'ad been for me twenty years (from the time I was 12) of spending at least one day a month curled around a hot water bottle or heating pad. He ended at least one day a month of missing school or work, or half a day (or more) of living. He ended that one day each month that I would be bombed out so I could sleep long enough for the pain to go away, or walking around with my mind at least twenty miles away because I was wasted on codeine.

Granted, the hysterectomy sounds drastic, but it was the only thing that ever brought relief.

Mrs. C.S., St. Petersburg, Fla.

I suffer from debilitating cramps for 2 days every 26 days. I can barely stand for the pain. My lower back and legs ache horribly and I'm nauseous. I still try to go to work (I'm a teacher) but after taking muscle relaxers, which help only a little, I'm certainly not doing anyone much good. I feel perfectly worthless during this time. I've been told by doctors that I am imagining things and at age 18 I was given a prescription for strong tranquilizers to keep me from worrying. (That never was my problem, and after taking a few of them, I threw the rest away.) Even being self-assured enough to know the cramps weren't all in my head, I often wondered if there might be something wrong with me.

L.F., Seattle, Wash.

> I am one of the millions of women who suffer
> from menstrual cramps. My family doctor
> pushes me aside with barbiturates and tells me
> it is psychological. I have been suffering since I
> was a teenager. Each year it seems to get worse.
> The pain spreads to my back, the headaches are
> unbearable and my joints ache. I am tired of
> suffering and need help now!
>
> **I.H., Philadelphia, Pa.**

Are you angry? You have every right to be. And so do the women
who wrote those letters. Painful menstrual cramps (dysmenorrhea)
sure as heck aren't "all in your head." The backache, headache,
nausea, vomiting, and diarrhea are all too real and these symptoms
have very little to do with the state of your psyche. New research has
conclusively demonstrated that women who suffer persistent and
debilitating menstrual cramps are biologically different from those
who don't. It would appear that many of the women who suffer most
are more likely to have high levels of substances called prostaglandins
which can trigger uterine contractions as well as headache, fatigue,
nervousness, nausea, vomiting, and diarrhea.[6,7]

Prostaglandins are hormone-like chemical messengers that play an
important role in a wide variety of life processes. They help regulate
blood pressure and blood coagulation. But even more important, the
prostaglandins affect cell growth, metabolism, nerve-impulse
transmission, inflammation, and reproduction. There is evidence that
they can initiate labor during pregnancy by causing the uterus to start
contracting. Investigators now believe that the cramps may be due in
part to uterine contractions during menstruation for women who
have naturally high levels of these chemicals. Hot-water bottles,
heating pads, barbiturates, tranquilizers, and pain relievers like
DARVON or FIORINAL have little if any impact on prostaglandins so
it's no wonder the traditional remedies haven't worked very well. And
the old-timey non-prescription potions like LYDIA E. PINKHAM'S
VEGETABLE COMPOUND, HUMPHREY'S NO. 11, or CARDUI TONIC
didn't serve any better.

So far all this may seem pretty depressing. But don't give up.
Sometimes there really is a Santa Claus and this time he brought
some mighty powerful presents for women who have suffered from
killer cramps. Over the last few years a whole group of new drugs
have been developed which are very effective at shutting off the
body's manufacture of prostaglandins. The drugs are called non-

steroidal anti-inflammatory agents and they have become extraordinarily popular as first-line treatments for arthritis. Prescription products that possess the ability to reduce prostaglandin levels are MOTRIN (ibuprofen), NAPROSYN (naproxen), PONSTEL (mefenamic acid), and INDOCIN (indomethacin). The results of research on their effectiveness for relieving menstrual distress have been so promising you could call this a breakthrough. Experiments were carried out in such a way as to eliminate psychological influence. Double-blind tests were used so that neither the doctors nor the women receiving the medications knew if they were getting a real drug or a placebo.

The researchers discovered that placebos didn't provide much benefit, which confirms what we always knew, menstrual cramps *are* for real. Secondly, the investigators were unanimous in concluding that the drugs work.[8-10] By preventing the action of prostaglandins, these medications appear to provide significant relief for a large number of women. Not only was there calming of the cramps and reduction of the pain, an added bonus was less weakness, dizziness, nausea, leg cramps, and even decreased menstrual flow. And one of their big advantages is that you don't have to take the drugs continuously as you would birth-control pills (some of which also reduce prostaglandin levels). The medicine can be started at the same time the menstrual cramps occur and they can be stopped after only one or two days. But what about safety? Dr. Penny Budoff, one of the early researchers in this field recently discussed her research with PONSTEL:

> **I began the drug treatment at the onset rather than before menses for two reasons: (1) to prevent the inadvertent taking of the drug by an unknowingly pregnant patient, and (2) to medicate with the smallest possible effective dose. Drug safety has always been utmost in my mind. I have taken the drug myself during the past 3½ years, as have some 300 of my patients.[11]**

It was a reasonable alternative to narcotics, barbiturates, and birth-control pills. PONSTEL appears to be one of the safest of the anti-inflammatory agents available for the treatment of cramps. Our next choice would be MOTRIN followed by NAPROSYN. While no one has yet had a chance to look into the safety of long-term periodic use of these drugs it seems like a good bet that they are more effective and much less dangerous for severe cramps than most of the previous therapies. That does not mean that they are totally innocuous, however, and women whose cramps are mild or very sporadic may be better off trying aspirin or other less "powerful" means of alleviating their discomfort. Like most arthritis medications PONSTEL, MOTRIN and NAPROSYN may irritate the stomach, so anyone with a history of a peptic ulcer or gastritis should probably avoid the new treatment. And INDOCIN (which has not yet received FDA approval for treating menstrual cramps) can cause headaches, dizziness, and fatigue.

It is hoped the days of the incapacitation, hot-water bottles, and "It's all in your head" remarks are gone for good. It may be premature to say a revolution has occurred in the treatment of painful menstrual cramps but enough progress has been made so that no woman need feel guilty or humiliated ever again. And with a little luck the pain may disappear as well. As Dr. Budoff concluded, "there are now a large number of nonaddicting, nonsedating drugs that effectively alleviate the global problem of dysmenorrhea. That is good news for women."[12] Amen!

PREMENSTRUAL MADNESS

Now that we have scored one against cramps, how about that old bugaboo "premenstrual tension"? Some women really suffer before their periods. They may experience weight gain, fluid retention, irritability, impatience, anxiety, depression, breast pain, and severe headaches. And these symptoms can come on suddenly. One day everything is fine and the next day the whole world falls apart for no apparent reason. And nothing makes the discomfort worse than a condescending man who nods and with a knowing smile chalks the behavior up to pre-period bitchiness and warns the kids not to upset Mother since this is her "bad" week.

What can be done? Well, for an opener, stop feeling guilty! As usual, medical science has not devoted much attention to this subject. Our knowledge of the disorder has barely advanced out of the Dark Ages. There is a distinct possibility that women who suffer from premenstrual tension may be biologically different from their sisters who barely even notice a menstrual cycle. Just as we have only recently learned that women who experience dysmenorrhea have high levels of prostaglandins in their bodies, we may soon discover that pre-period problems are due to a hormonal imbalance. In fact, there is already some evidence that reduced progesterone levels might account for some of the symptoms, including fluid retention.[13] Another possibility is that the hormone prolactin is elevated and this may contribute to the problem. Unfortunately, these are just tantalizing leads. We will have to wait for some hot-shot investigators to get their act together and undertake some decent research before we find out exactly what is going on.

Even though medical science has lagged far behind in both interest and research the drug companies have not hesitated to fill the vacuum. Walk into almost any pharmacy in the country and you will find a section devoted to "feminine" products. Inevitably there will be "water pills" prominently displayed that promise great relief. One product called TRENDAR portrays an attractive woman trying to squeeze herself into her pants. In a tempting ad the reader is asked, "Can't get it together because of periodic puffiness? Take TRENDAR premenstrual tablets and wear your sleekest pants...your skinniest bikini and be your own sweet self." Another offering is AQUA BAN. It promises to help you "Lose excess body water, bloat and puffiness, relieve pressure-caused cramps, aches and tension due to premenstrual water build up...You'll look better, feel better...be brighter, more active and alert."

Fantastic! What more could you ask for? What is in this magic pill anyway? AQUA BAN contains 325 milligrams of ammonium chloride and 100 milligrams of caffeine. Dr. Laurel Ashworth, a consultant for the American Pharmaceutical Association, offered the following understatement: "The effectiveness of the 325- to 500-mg ammonium chloride doses present in various OTC (over-the-counter) preparations is questionable."[14] Another authority on non-prescription drugs, Dr. Neil Widger, also commented on the amount of ammonium chloride in AQUA BAN: "In order for this ingredient to be a diuretic, over four times this dose is required for most adults."[15] As for the caffeine, 100 milligrams is about as much as you get in a cup of brewed coffee. While it may provide a slight diuretic effect for some people it should be obvious that a cup of coffee is not particularly powerful and the effect wears off quickly. What's more, you might as well drink the real thing and at least enjoy the flavor. We're not any more impressed with the other ingredients you will find in most non-prescription "water pills." Extract of Buchu, Uva Ursi powdered extract, Hydrangea, and Pamabron are of doubtful value. If effective at all, they are merely a drop in the ocean.

Does all this bad news mean women will have to wait forever before they can diminish the discomfort? Not at all. If fluid retention and edema are a problem it would be prudent to start cutting back on salt a few days before you expect to start feeling bloated. If dietary discretion is too difficult or just not adequate you might want to go to the heavier artillery. Some women really do seem to benefit from "water pills." While there haven't been any decent studies on the value of *real* diuretics to reduce the edema formation and unpleasantness of premenstrual tension, there are enough testimonial reports by doctors and patients alike to warrant a short course with a prescription drug like hydrochlorothiazide (HYDRODIURIL) in a morning dose of 25 to 50 mg. If you use this drug be careful to eat foods high in potassium since the medication depletes the body of this crucial electrolyte. Potassium depletion may in turn make subsequent menstrual cramps more painful. Foods high in potassium and low in sodium include brazil nuts, dates, pecans, lima beans, bananas, apricots, whole ground cornmeal, blackstrap molasses, oranges and orange juice, winter squash, green peas, peaches, plums, wheat germ, walnuts, oatmeal, asparagus, almonds, avocados, potatoes, and peanuts.

Another drug worth considering is ALDACTONE (spironolactone). Some doctors have reported significant success with this diuretic in a dose of 25 mg three times a day for no more than five days. British researchers have claimed (in the *British Journal of Obstetrics and Gynaecology)* that ALDACTONE not only decreased the weight gain that commonly occurs with fluid build-up but reduced the mood symptoms as well.[16]

If you do go the diuretic route for premenstrual tension be very careful not to become "addicted." Regular use of these drugs by a healthy person can lead to a vicious cycle that may actually cause weight gain and water retention when the drugs are finally stopped. A condition called "idiopathic edema" (edema of unknown cause) may result that can stump doctors and lead to continued use of diuretics. In a marvelous article titled "Is 'Idiopathic' Edema Idiopathic?" (*The Lancet* February 24, 1979) some British researchers suggested that "intermittent edema of unknown cause in most, if not all, otherwise healthy women is due to their use of diuretics ... in other words, their edema is not idiopathic."[17] If you do become dependent on a diuretic it may take your body a week to ten days after you eliminate the drug before the weight gain and fluid build-up disappear and your body returns to normal. A mild diuretic like hydrochlorothiazide that is used for only a few days prior to menstruation should not cause any of these unpleasant problems.

If you would prefer to take the non-drug path there are a few options available. According to Dr. Robert Kinch, Professor of Obstetrics and Gynecology at McGill University, "Investigators have also reported achieving good results with the use of pyridoxine (vitamin B6). The patient is started on 40 mg, given daily throughout the month; this is increased by 20 mg each cycle until the patient is on a daily dosage of 100 mg."[18] Barbara and Gideon Seaman, M.D. in their book *Women and the Crisis in Sex Hormones* highly recommend calcium and magnesium supplements (dolomite) throughout the premenstrual week and during menstruation.

> **Each person will have to determine her own best dolomite supplement, but around six tablets a day, premenstrually and during menstruation, seems to help most people. Some need to go up to ten or twelve tablets, which somewhat exceeds the recommended allowance of 1 gram of calcium ... Calcium cannot be used properly without vitamin D, so on days when calcium is taken, 400 to 1,200 units of D should be added also."[19]**

It should come as no surprise that the medical establishment does not support this nutritional therapy, either for premenstrual tension or for menstrual cramps. Garold L. Faber, M.D., wrote in a question to the experts at the *Journal of the American Medical Association:* "A 26-year-old woman claims that calcium-magnesium tablets she has been taking for the past three months have brought her the first relief in ten years from menstrual cramps. Is there any validity to her claim?" The answer from the expert, Dr. Arpad I. Csapo, was unequivocal: "Calcium-magnesium tablets do not relieve dysmenor-rheic symptoms."[20] Even though there have been, to the best of our knowledge, no well-controlled studies on the use of calcium, Dr. Csapo is unbending and unquestioning in his total rejection of calcium supplements. Before we would be willing to make any such dogmatic statements one way or the other we would want some scientific research to back us up. The women's underground and overground health network has reported testimonial success with calcium-magnesium supplements. And the benefits of calcium for preventing weakening of bones (osteoporosis) in postmenopausal women is well documented. In our opinion dolomite tablets are certainly worth a try. If they work, great! If they don't, too bad. It is certainly one of the more innocuous treatments available, provided you don't overdo on the vitamin D.

There is one other possibility. While still experimental, it looks quite promising. Remember we mentioned that premenstrual tension may be partly caused by a hormonal imbalance. Some researchers believe that elevated prolactin levels may be responsible.

The pituitary gland sometimes goes haywire and secretes excessive amounts of this hormone. One bizarre result is called the amenorrhea-galactorrhea syndrome in which menstruation completely stops and there is continuous production of breast milk. Although this problem may be caused by a pituitary tumor (and this possibility must first be ruled out through medical tests) it can also occur spontaneously or when a woman stops using birth-control pills. According to a report in *Hospital Tribune,* Dr. John R. Tyson, Professor of Obstetrics and Gynecology at Johns Hopkins University School of Medicine, said that "A tremendous number of women who've been taking the contraceptive pills for a long time are affected. The disease (amenorrhea-galactorrhea) has taken on epidemic proportions."[21] Besides the continuous production of breast milk and the absence of a period, this condition is also often characterized by infertility.

So far this problem sounds awful, and it is. But hallelujah!—there is a remedy in sight. A new drug called PARLODEL (bromocriptine) can cut off the excessive secretion of prolactin and put an end to the symptoms. Numerous researchers have reported a success rate of 80 to 90 percent.[22, 23] They have also discovered that PARLODEL helps infertile women conceive.[24] Although it has been used extensively in Europe for this purpose it has not yet been approved for infertility treatment in the United States. (If pregnancy occurs the drug should be stopped immediately, just to be safe.)

The point of this hormone discussion is that some investigators believe excessive prolactin production may cause some of the symptoms of premenstrual tension. There is some hope that a drug like PARLODEL may be useful in putting an end to the problem.[25] Check with your doctor for the latest update on this intriguing research.

So to sum up, here are our recommendations. Try the nutritional options first. They are the least likely to cause complications. Dolomite, in a dose of around six tablets a day, seems like a sensible way to get a natural mixture of calcium and magnesium (people with kidney problems should check with a doctor first). And vitamin D (400 units) seems like a reasonable way to facilitate the calcium absorption. Pyridoxine (vitamin B_6) in a dose of 100 mg may also provide relief for premenstrual tension. If a sodium-restricted diet doesn't help prevent the bloating and puffiness it might be worth talking to a doctor about a diuretic. Our first choice would be Hydrochlorothiazide (25 mg) in the morning. And make sure you eat lots of potassium-rich foods—dates, pecans, limas, bananas, apricots, molasses, oranges, and so on. If that diuretic isn't particularly helpful our next bet would be ALDACTONE, 25 mg three times a day for no more than five days. If nothing works and life is still miserable, it may be worth discussing PARLODEL with your doctor. By the time you read this the FDA may have approved its use for menstrual problems as well as infertility. And if killer cramps put you out of commission for a day or two each month, a short course of either PONSTEL or MOTRIN should make life bearable again. Before taking any drug, make sure your doctor fully discusses potential side effects with you and then weigh the benefits against the risks. Good luck!

FEMININE HYGIENE HYPOCRISY

What, for goodness sake, is "feminine hygiene"? The dictionary defines hygiene as "a condition or practice conducive to the preservation of health, as cleanliness." So "feminine hygiene" must mean feminine cleanliness. What ever happened to "masculine hygiene"? Of course, we all know that "feminine hygiene" is nothing more than a euphemism for "intimate" or "personal" and these words in turn are euphemisms for genital products. The implication of all this is that women aren't clean, especially when it comes to their reproductive organs. That is patently ludicrous, but drug and cosmetic companies have a huge investment in keeping women uptight and insecure about their bodies. Each year approximately $100 million is spent on douches, "intimate" deodorants and other feminine "hygiene" products. Much of that money is wasted. Some of it may even mean higher bills later on.

Take feminine deodorant sprays for example. One lovely lavender container we found in the drugstore promised the following:

> MY OWN is the gentle spray deodorant formulated specifically for the outer vaginal area. MY OWN sprays on warm . . . Use it every day to feel fresh and confident . . . totally feminine all day, every day.

Balderdash! Confidence and femininity are certainly unlikely to result from such a product, and as far as we're concerned, neither is freshness. And to say any of these "feminine hygiene" sprays promote hygiene or cleanliness would be a perversion of those words. In fact, there is plenty of evidence that some of the "deodorant sprays for women" may actually cause irritations and allergic reactions in some people. Dr. Alexander Fisher, a dermatologist from the New York University School of Medicine, reported the following interesting cases:

Case 3. A 19-year-old woman acquired a mild pruritic [itchy] vulvar and perivulvar dermatitis after using a certain feminine hygiene spray for six months. Patch testing with the ingredients obtained from the manufacturer revealed a strongly positive patch test to isopropyl myristate [an emollient].

Case 4. A 40-year-old woman with known sensitivity to perfume had vulvar itching and dermatitis after the first application of a feminine hygiene spray. This patient had a strong positive reaction to the perfume supplied by the manufacturer. Three controls showed no reaction.

Case 5. A 29-year-old man acquired a penile and scrotal dermatitis each time he had had sexual intercourse with a woman who used a spray containing benzethonium chloride [an anti-bacterial agent]. Patch-test reactions. . . were strongly positive.[26]

The adverse skin reactions reported by Dr. Fisher are not isolated events. According to a consultant for the American Pharmaceutical Association, "The FDA receives many reports of adverse local reactions, all locally severe and all attributed to the use of these products. In most of these cases, systemic steroid treatment (oral cortisone-type drugs) was required even when the sprays were discontinued."[27]

Most of these products contain three ingredients—a perfume, an emollient to carry the fragrance, and a propellant gas to get the rest of the goo out of the can. Besides being capable of causing skin irritation there is some doubt that they are ever very effective as deodorants. And if a woman truly did have an objectionable vaginal odor, all such a product could do is mask the problem. Since a bad smell could be a warning of an infection, trying to cover it up might delay proper treatment.

Another bizarre craze recently created by the drug and cosmetic industry involves deodorized tampons. The rationale for such products is hard to imagine. There have been some gruesome reports in the medical literature of vaginal or cervical irritation associated with this kind of tampon use. A case history detailed in the *American Journal of Obstetrics and Gynecology* points up what can happen:

> A 16-year-old white virgin complained of urin-
> ary stress incontinence. She had used de-
> odorized tampons intermittently and chron-
> ically for 7 months ... During pelvic ex-
> amination a 2 by 3 cm. [3/4 in. by 1-1/5 in.]
> ulceration with a firm, raised border was
> observed on the right lateral vaginal
> wall ... The pathology report of biopsies was
> vaginal ulceration with acute and chronic
> inflammation. The patient was instructed to
> discontinue tampon usage. The ulcer healed in 5
> weeks without further treatment.[28]

While it's not entirely clear what causes tampon irritation, one
explanation is that the women are reacting to the chemicals in the
deodorized brands. Since the reactions tend to clear up after these
tampons are discontinued and reappear once they are introduced
again, we feel that this explanation is pretty sound. Good old-
fashioned soap and water will do more to promote hygiene than all
the deodorants in the world. Sensitive outer vaginal tissues deserve
gentle treatment and we can't think of a milder soap than DOVE. A
clean healthy body rarely produces an offensive smell. It's time we
stopped allowing ourselves to be snookered by companies that play
upon our insecurities in order to increase their profit margins.

DON'T OVERDOSE ON DOUCHES

Not very long ago we came across an extraordinary product—
LYSETTE LIQUID DOUCHE "with VAGINAL CLIMATE CONTROL."
That sounds a little as if it comes equipped with a thermostat.
LYSETTE promises to "cleanse, refresh and deodorize for complete
confidence" ... a little like the Tidy Bowl man. The list of ingredients
found in this product reads like a program at a chemist's convention:

> **Contains: Water, SD Alcohol 40, Teadodecyl-
> benzenesulfonate, Citric Acid, Sodium Citrate,
> Hydroxypropyl Methylcellulose, Thymol,
> Tetrasodium Edta, Menthol, Eucalyptus Oil,
> Propylene Glycol, Isopropyl Alcohol,
> Simethicone, Methylparaben, FD&C Blue No. 1
> And D&C Red No. 33.**

The vaginal tract is not impermeable to chemicals. In fact, just the
opposite is the case. The sensitive mucosal lining is highly capable of
absorbing almost anything which comes into contact with it. Drugs
and dyes can get into the bloodstream and circulate throughout the

body. And yet pharmaceutical and cosmetic companies have casually included such toxic chemicals as boric acid, methyl salicylate, and phenol in their products for vaginal use. Here is what one of the most authoritive reference books on toxicology (*Clinical Toxicology of Commercial Products*) says about one common chemical found in many douches:

> BORIC ACID—**Borates are still encountered as antiseptic agents despite their limited effectiveness. Powders, ointments, and solutions containing boric acid have long been prescribed for dermatologic disorders, eyewashes, gargles, urinary antiseptics, and diaper rinses ... The reputation of borates is so firmly entrenched that they are still readily available despite toxic potentialities reported as early as 1883. Acute poisonings have followed ingestion, ... enemas, lavage of serrous cavities [douching], and applications of powders and ointments to burned and abraded skin ... borates are rapidly absorbed from mucous membranes and abraded skin but toxic symptoms may be delayed for several hours ... Clinical findings commonly consist of gastrointestinal disturbances, ... skin eruptions, and signs of central nervous stimulation followed by depression.**[29]

In 1978 a panel of experts for the FDA concluded that "boron compounds (boric acid, etc.) are not effective in carrying out any of the OTC claims for active ingredients in vaginal douches or other non-contraceptive vaginal drug products, and that a serious question of safety exists with these ingredients at concentrations higher than preservative levels (preservative levels being less than 1 percent)."[30] And yet the American Pharmaceutical Association's 1979 edition of the *Handbook of Nonprescription Drugs* lists the following douches as containing boric acid: BO-CAR-AL, MASSENGILL DOUCHE POWDER, NYLMERATE II, PMC DOUCHE POWDER (boric acid, 82%) and V.A.[31]

Even if the safety of the chemicals included in douches weren't an issue there is still some question as to whether the practice of douching is itself harmful. Consider, for a moment, what douching is all about. You put some crazy conglomeration of chemicals into a rubber bag and let the liquid gush into your vagina. This creates pressure. There is considerable concern that the effect of this pressure may push bacteria and other beasties up into the uterus or change the flora and fauna of the reproductive tract in such a way as to make it more susceptible to infection. A report in the *New England Journal of Medicine* from the Yale New Haven Hospital raised a strong warning flag. The doctors noted that 90 percent of the women in their clinics who developed infections of the fallopian tubes or pelvic inflammatory disease (see pages 283-285) were "vigorous douchers." They concluded that "From our own data on gonorrhea and pelvic inflammatory disease, we look with strong suspicion at the douche as contributing to ascending infections by the gonococcus or whatever pathogens happen to be in the vagina."[32]

Many family doctors and gynecologists believe that a healthy vagina will take care of itself. Just as a mouthwash will not improve oral hygiene or eliminate the cause of bad breath, neither will a douche solve an odor problem. Itching, burning, or excessive discharge could well signal the onset of vaginitis. And in this instance the "remedy" could aggravate the condition by delaying diagnosis or causing inflammation.

VAGINITIS IS A VILLAIN

Almost every woman will, at some point in her life, probably suffer inflammation of the vagina. The symptoms include an irritating vaginal discharge, itching, burning, and painful swelling of the vagina and surrounding areas; sexual intercourse may become uncomfortable. Now, don't panic—not every discharge is cause for alarm. A healthy vaginal tract must maintain a moist environment and mucus is quite natural, especially before ovulation or menstruation. Birth control pills, pregnancy, and irritating chemicals (as in douches or deodorant tampons) may also cause a discharge. But chances are good that if you experience pain and itching along with the secretions, you've got problems.

There are three kinds of beasties that are primarily responsible for vaginitis. First come the **fungi.** You're probably more familiar with the term "yeast infection" to describe this problem. It is also sometimes called vaginal thrush or moniliasis but the real name for the varmint is *Candida albicans.* Second in line comes the wiggly **protozoan.** This nasty fellow is *Trichomonas vaginalis* or *"Trich,"* a difficult infection to eradicate. Last but not least comes the bully on the block, a **bacterium** called *Hemophilus vaginalis.* Until recently this infection was called "nonspecific vaginitis" because doctors weren't entirely sure which "blue meanie" was the responsible party. It didn't respond very well to traditional treatments either. But some new discoveries have pretty much knocked old "hemophilus" on his assophilus.

Well, how do you find out what you've got? We rather like the little acronym **COITAL** that doctor Marvin C. Rulin coined:

> **C** for *Color*
> **O** for *Odor*
> **I** for *Itching*
> **T** for *Thickness* or *Thinness* of discharge
> **A** for *Amount* of discharge
> **L** for *Look* of the mucosa[33]

There is overlap on some symptoms but a careful accounting of these signs can give the doctor some pretty good clues which when coupled with a microscopic slide examination should produce a diagnosis pretty quickly. Here are some rough guidelines that may help you tell the doctor what she needs to know.

Candida albicans (Yeast Infection)

> **C** The color is white.
> **O** The odor is minimal—logically enough may smell yeast-like.
> **I** The itching can be intense and unbearable!
> **T** The texture is THICK and lumpy and looks like cottage cheese.
> **A** The amount of discharge is scanty.
> **L** The look of the vagina and vulva is beefy red, often with swelling.

A smear test examined under the microscope should easily confirm the diagnosis of *Candida*. If yeast shows up without symptoms there is no cause for alarm though, since about 50 percent of healthy women have these fungi floating around in their vaginas and gastrointestinal tracts without any problems. This is why broad spectrum antibiotics like Tetracycline often bring on a yeast infection in that they disturb the delicate natural balance. By killing off the "goodies" along with the "baddies" the fungus is given an open sesame to take over. Women on birth control pills and diabetics are also more susceptible to infection and anyone who has recurrent bouts with *Candida* should have a urine sample checked to see if that is a reservoir for infection.

Let's say you are experiencing intense itching and a white, cottage-cheese type of discharge. The doctor checks the slide and sees the fresh fungi. Let's zap the buggers. There are three basic treatment options for handling yeast infections and they all involve "local" application of a cream or vaginal tablet. In other words, you don't swallow any pills. The first line of attack is usually with a drug called Nystatin. It is available in various brand-name preparations including MYCOSTATIN, NILSTAT, CANDEX and KOROSTATIN. The usual course of treatment with Nystatin is one or two vaginal tablets inserted daily for seven to fourteen days. If there is a recurrence some doctors recommend using the drug for the next two menstrual periods and a few days beyond. Side effects are minimal. Occasionally someone may be super-sensitive and develop a vaginal irritation, but that is unusual.

The two other drugs that are commonly employed in the treatment of *Candida* include MONISTAT 7 (miconazole) and GYNE-LATRIMIN (clotrimazole). The regular dose of MONISTAT 7 is one applicatorful of cream once a day at bedtime for seven days. Side effects are uncommon but burning, itching, or irritation of the vulva or vagina are a little more frequent than with Nystatin. The dose of GYNE-LATRIMIN is one vaginal tablet once a day at bedtime for seven days. Mild burning has been reported after insertion of the vaginal tablet but appears to be no more common than with Miconazole. Occasionally there may be a skin rash, mild cramps, and frequent urination as additional complications. One of these three drugs should do the job but if everything fails you could always fall back on an old standby, Gentian Violet. That lovely purple color will stain like crazy, but it may be worth the inconvenience to eliminate a stubborn case. Gentian Violet tampons (GENAPAX) may be less of a hassle for you than the same medication in vaginal tablet form.

Preventing recurrent yeast infections may require stopping birth control pills (if they are involved) or discontinuing broad spectrum antibiotics like tetracycline. If the sexual partner is responsible for reinfection, use of a condom should eliminate that problem. Cotton panties to cut down on heat and humidity may also be helpful and some people report benefit from an acidic douche (two tablespoons of vinegar to one quart of water). There is another possible treatment, but we hesitate to endorse it since there have been no well-designed experiments to test the benefit. Dr. Thomas E. Will, from the School of Public Health at the University of Minnesota, recently suggested that *Lactobacillus acidophilus,* a friendly bacteria used to culture yogurt and other milk products, could be helpful.[34] Taken orally every day for a few weeks the *Lactobacillus* may make the internal environment a little less hospitable for *Candida*. If you suffer recurrent infections it's certainly worth trying since this useful bacteria is about as safe as you can get. Following up on the same principle, some women's health groups recommend a yogurt douche—two to three tablespoons to a quart of water. Another possibility is the direct application of 3 milliliters of yogurt into the vagina with a plastic syringe. We will not vouch for any of these techniques until some significant research resolves the effectiveness issue more conclusively. But if it works for you, that's all that matters. One other paradoxical problem may contribute to a yeast infection. The drug of choice for wiping out *Trichomonas* and *Hemophilus* is FLAGYL. It can create conditions within the vaginal tract that lead to a yeast infection. So you might end up trading in your *Trich* infection for a yeast infection. This is pretty unlikely, but forewarned is forearmed.

Trichomonas vaginalis (Protozoan Vaginitis)

C The color is yellowish-gray-brown.

O The odor is quite unpleasant (stale or musty).

I Itching can occur, but is usually less severe than with a yeast infection. More vaginal than vulval itching.

T The texture is frothy.

A The amount of the discharge can be significant.

L The cervix has a strawberry appearance and the vulva may be fiery red.

You may experience all or none of these symptoms with *Trich*. There may be considerable burning and irritation and intercourse can be quite unpleasant. A microscopic slide exam should certify the diagnosis.

Proper treatment of this kind of vaginitis requires that the male partner also undergo therapy (or use a condom during intercourse) since he can act as a continual source of reinfection. Men don't usually suffer symptoms of trichomoniasis but they do carry it, so they can unwittingly keep giving it back to the woman.

Treating *Trich* is a giant problem. There is one drug and one drug only that is on every doctor's hit parade. It's FLAGYL (metronidazole) and it does work, no question about that. The dose is one 250 mg tablet three times a day for seven days in women and one 250 mg tablet twice a day for seven days in men. An alternative dosage regimen is what we call the "Big Bertha." Some reports suggest that a large dose (2 grams—eight tablets) taken just once will be almost as effective as the week-long program.[35] The problem with FLAGYL is not the dose or the temporary side effects, which may include stomach upset, nausea, loss of appetite, diarrhea, an unpleasant metallic taste, hives, dizziness, numbness, or tingling of the extremities, and occasionally joint pain. The real worry with this drug is its cancer-causing potential. This is a hot potato that no one wants to catch since the drug is the only effective agent available to clear up both trichomoniasis and non-specific vaginitis.

How dangerous is FLAGYL? Many different scientists have shown that FLAGYL is a "mutagen." This means that the drug has the ability to change the genes of certain types of bacterial cells when it is mixed with them in a test tube. That doesn't seem very bad, but when you consider that about 90 percent of the chemicals that are mutagens in these types of tests are able to induce cancer in animals, the evidence mounts. This is the type of test that got hair dyes and saccharin into trouble before they were tested in animals. Unlike saccharin, FLAGYL has been shown to be a mutagen at levels almost identical to those in the bloodstream of a woman taking the drug for severe vaginitis. Worse yet, in a very well done study by independent scientists FLAGYL was shown to cause cancer in mice when given to them in their food. This is serious indeed for it means that not only can the drug cause changes in test cells but it can cause cancer in live animals when given to them in reasonable doses.

Dr. Sidney Wolfe, health activist par excellence and head of Nader's Health Research Group, has petitioned the FDA on numerous occasions to ban FLAGYL (metronidazole) on the grounds that it is too dangerous. In a letter dated October 22, 1974 Dr. Wolfe made a strong plea:

> **We cannot imagine a larger or more solid body of cancer information on any environmental chemical than is now available for FLAGYL. This alarming additional evidence makes it clear that FLAGYL—long regarded in ignorance as a drug of little toxicity—is a lethal weapon against patients. It is prescribed over 2 million times annually, largely for the treatment of trichomonal vaginitis. If FDA has not the strength to act against *this* drug, it cannot be relied upon to act against *any* drug involving chronic hazards to patients.**[36]

Ouch! That's a powerful indictment. It should come as no surprise that The Food and Drug Administration denied the Nader group's petition to ban FLAGYL. In his answering letter to the Health Research Group dated October 21, 1975, FDA Commissioner Schmidt offered the following explanation:

> The FDA shares your concern over the car-cinogenicity of metronidazole in rodents. Nevertheless, the available evidence indicates that the total dose of metronidazole given to patients is of such a low order of magnitude, when compared to the life-span doses given to rodents, that the element of carcinogenic risk in treating trichomoniasis is very low. Further, it is our conclusion, which is shared by many experts and by our ob-gyn advisory committee, that trichomonal vaginitis is an important disease causing much suffering among its victims, and that metronidazole is the only drug currently marketed in this country which is effective for its cure.[37]

Where does all this leave you, the consumer? Probably confused and more than a little concerned. Nader's group says DANGER, BAN IT! Our favorite women's health book, *Our Bodies Ourselves,* says "WOMEN SHOULD AVOID THIS DRUG." The FDA says it's all we got and the benefit outweighs the risk. And we feel a little as if we're caught in the middle on this one. Neither the Health Research Group nor the folks from *Our Bodies Ourselves* offer much in the way of alternatives. A vaginal suppository that they recommend called FLORAQUIN is no longer available and even if it were there is toxicity associated with that drug too. No other treatment suggestions are offered except to prevent recurrences and these have been untested. Such ideas as "tub bathing throughout the menstrual cycle, loose clothing, and avoidance of tampons, ordinary douches, and vaginal sprays"[38] are reasonable. But we're afraid none of these techniques will do much for an acute attack, and if you're really suffering with an unpleasant vaginal odor, a yucky discharge, and severe itching, you want relief. Our feeling is that one "Big Bertha" dose of FLAGYL (eight tablets) may well be worth the risk. A recent study published in the *New England Journal of Medicine* titled "Lack of Evidence for Cancer Due to Use of Metronidazole" offers a small ray of hope that the controversy may have been blown up out of proportion.[39] The authors of the article found "no appreciable increase in cases of cancer" in women who took FLAGYL. But we do not feel this one report should allow us to let down our guard. Rather, we side with the medical experts from the highly respected and independent publication *Medical Letter* when they discussed the latest findings:

> *Conclusion*—**Metronidazole is a useful drug for treatment of trichomoniasis, amebiasis and**

> serious anaerobic infections. However, a recent negative follow-up study does not establish that the drug will not be carcinogenic in man. It would be prudent to use metronidazole as seldom as possible, and then in the lowest effective dosage for the shortest possible time.[40]

A final word of caution. Although FLAGYL has not been shown to cause birth defects, nevertheless we feel that it shouldn't be used during pregnancy. And NEVER drink alcoholic beverages (including beer and wine) while you are taking this drug. The result of this interaction can be most unpleasant indeed—nausea, vomiting, flushing, headache, and a general unwell feeling. Since this controversy is still unresolved keep reading your newspaper for latest developments and make sure your doctor is up to date on the latest developments.

NONSPECIFIC VAGINITIS

We are going to let you in on a little secret. We have been attributing "nonspecific vaginitis" to *Hemophilus vaginalis* because that is what the big boys (read honcho gynecologists) say about it, but in reality they don't truly know what causes this kind of infection. In the past doctors tended to throw all their unsuccessfully treated cases into the "wastebasket" of nonspecific vaginitis. It was a convenient catch-all. In that context the name "nonspecific" was quite appropriate. But lately they have been trying to pin all the blame on the bully boy *Hemophilus*. There is little doubt that Hemophilus lurks around these irritations but whether it is an innocent bystander or the guilty party is still up for grabs. For our purposes, however, let's go along with the "experts" and run a number on this nasty fellow.

Hemophilus vaginalis (Bacterial infection)

C Color me gray.

O The odor is musty and sour, kind of fishy—rather unpleasant.

I Neither itching nor burning is common.

T The texture is creamy, slightly foamy—a rather medium consistency.

A The amount of the discharge may be "profuse" or "copious"—in other words, lots and lots.

L The vaginal tract looks pretty good—no great changes.

You should be able to tell from the above description of *Hemophilus* that it doesn't deserve the bad name we gave it. It really isn't nearly as nasty as are *Trich* and *Candida*. Many patients have symptoms so mild that they don't even complain very much. Diagnosis is difficult since a microscopic slide exam doesn't always turn up something. And the cause of the infection? Once again, women are getting shafted. The disease is more often than not transmitted through sexual intercourse. Approximately 80 percent of the male sex partners of infected women will harbor *Hemophilus* in their urethras, and wouldn't you know it, they rarely experience any symptoms. So, just as with *Trich*, the man can keep reinfecting the woman unless he too is treated or uses a condom during intercourse.

In the bad old days *Hemophilus* was treated with an assortment of rather ineffective creams and antibiotics. Oral AMPICILLIN or DOXYCYCLINE (a type of tetracycline) was often tried but results were mixed. Tetracycline had a batting average of around 10 percent. AMPICILLIN tended to range from about 25 percent to 40 percent in effectiveness. Sulfa creams and BETADINE douches were virtually ineffective. But that is enough bad news and suspense. What will do the trick? Right, you guessed it (or you have a good memory), FLAGYL really knocks old *Hemophilus* out of the ball park—almost a 100 percent cure rate. [41] The dose that is used for both men and women is 500 mg twice a day for seven days. That's good news and bad news. It's nice to have something that will really cure the infection, but on the other hand it's difficult to justify such sledgehammer treatment for what is basically a mild disorder. So our recommendation? Well, you can always try the vinegar douche again (2 tablespoons to one quart of water) or you may want to give a good yogurt culture a chance. You can either insert the yogurt with a plastic syringe or use a douche. If these treatments don't work, and they may not, you could give AMPICILLIN a road test. It's a relatively safe drug (beware an itchy skin or a rash and be prepared for some stomach upset) and it certainly won't make you feel like Damocles with a cancer threat hanging over your head. The dose is 500 mg four times a day for seven days. If nothing works and the infection gets really bothersome, then FLAGYL might be worth considering, but only if both partners participate so there won't be any reinfection.

So there you be, the latest update on vaginitis. There are drugs to combat it but they involve problems. It would be helpful if the FDA resolved this cancer issue once and for all on FLAGYL so that we could use the drug in confidence, or else they should ban it and encourage research on something that might work as well without the risks. Any decision that you make about how to treat any of these infections should be made with full understanding of benefits and risks and your doctor should take some time to fill you in on the latest developments. This is a story that will continue to evolve.

HORRIBLE HERPES

No venereal disease causes women greater fear and trauma than herpes simplex virus type 2 (HSV-2). There's a cure for *Trich*. There's a cure for *Hemophilus*. There's a cure for gonorrhea. And there's a cure for syphilis. But genital herpes is a nightmare. A decade or so ago this disease was virtually unheard of. It was rarely found in the female genital tract and no one paid it much attention. But today HSV-2 is challenging gonorrhea for the dubious distinction of Big Number One in the venereal-disease sweepstakes and it is five times more common than syphilis. It has been estimated that at least 500,000 people become infected with herpes virus each year and twenty percent of the sexually active adult population has already had it. In all, there may be as many as five to ten million carriers who have come into contact with genital herpes at one time or another. [42]

Although HSV-2 is transmitted through sexual intercourse, men rarely suffer serious symptoms or complications. But as usual, women do. They suffer plenty. And what is insidious is that a woman can catch herpes from a man who shows no visible signs of the disease. The painful infection appears four to seven days after intercourse. At first there may just be a little itching and soreness. But soon there is redness and a small group of blisters or "vesicles" will develop over the top of the red area around the vulva. It can also occur inside the vagina and on the cervix where the lesions look very inflamed. After two or three days the blisters break down and form painful ulcers. Within a few days the ulcers crust over and slowly disappear in about ten days to two weeks unless they become infected with some other organism. If they do, the woman will often feel wiped out, almost as if she has the flu. She may develop a fever, a headache, joint pains, and if the sores become large enough she may have trouble urinating or walking. Antibiotics will knock out the secondary infection, but they won't do a thing for HSV-2. The shame, guilt, and ignorance that surround the "virus of love" only make matters worse.

So far, genital herpes sounds pretty unpleasant enough. But sadder still after you completely recover, the disease can keep coming back like malaria, even if you never again have intercourse with an infected male partner. The herpes virus is in your system and it may reappear unpredictably. No one knows exactly how this happens. One theory has it that the virus remains latent until something triggers an attack. Emotional upset, fever, menstruation, exposure to pesticides, depression, stress, or any other traumatic event may bring on an attack, though as time passes the recurrences tend to become less severe and with any luck may disappear entirely.

"Horrible herpes" is bad. The name fits. But we have saved the worst for last. Researchers have reported that there is an association between cervical cancer and HSV-2. No one knows whether the virus makes women more susceptible to cancer or whether the virus is just an innocent bystander that lurks around in dark corners. What we do know is that women who develop cervical cancer "are far more likely to have type 2 herpes virus antibodies than the general population or patients with other venereal diseases."[43] No matter what, anyone who has had a bout with herpes should have a pap smear every six months to a year, just to be on the safe side.

Up to now we have only discussed the problems a woman herself has to face with herpes. There is another legacy of this disease that could be the worst of all. When a woman with herpes becomes pregnant she must be extraordinarily careful. If there are any active sores within her reproductive tract during the delivery the baby could be exposed to the infection as it passes through the birth canal. Forty percent of the babies who acquire their mother's infections will develop serious brain damage or blood poisoning and many will die.[44] So if a woman or her doctor suspects a genital herpes infection the baby should be delivered by cesarean section within four hours after the water breaks or labor starts.

Disturbing, shocking, dreadful—herpes is all of these and more. And it happens to millions of nice folks like your neighbor across the street or cousin Jenny or your friend Bob. What about treatment? If we can cure syphilis and gonorrhea surely we should be able to do something about this horrible stuff. Unfortunately, there is more bad news. Most of the time doctors have been flying blind. They have attempted to pin the tail on the donkey and instead have ended up missing the target completely. Medical science has lagged far behind in its search for an effective treatment or cure, which is not to say doctors haven't tried. In fact they have thrown everything but the kitchen sink into the fray. In reviewing our files on herpes we came up with some extraordinary "remedies" recently reported in the medical literature, often with unwarranted enthusiasm. Here are just a few examples: NONOXYNOL 9 (a spermicide found in contraceptive foams), CHLOROFORM (local application), BCG (a tuberculosis inoculation), ETHER (local application), BETADINE (povidone iodine, an antiseptic found in douches), HERPIGON (an ointment of zinc, urea, and tannic acid), ZINC SULFATE (applied topically to the skin or on a soaked tampon), LEVAMISOLE (an oral medicine used to treat arthritis and intestinal worms), PHOTODYNAMIC INACTIVATION (red dye application coupled with exposure to light), and SALINE INJECTIONS (placebo treatment). [45-52]

Despite the doctors' initial enthusiasm there hasn't been much actual success. The work with zinc looks very promising but there is still a long way to go before it gets a green light. Some of the medical suggestions may actually cause more harm than good. The "photodynamic inactivation" process which involves puncturing the blisters, painting the sores with a red dye, and then exposing the lesion to light doesn't shorten the length of the disease nor does it prevent recurrences. At the same time it may alter the viruses' structure and make them potentially more dangerous as cancer promoters. People also get themselves into trouble when they try medicating with creams and ointments. Even antibiotic preparations can cause trouble. None of these treatments is effective and they could spread or prolong the disease. Some doctors have recommended sitz baths to soothe the pain but a few case histories recently published in the *American Journal of Obstetrics and Gynecology* make that bright idea look pretty poor:

> **Two young women with primary genital herpes were admitted because of extensive pustular lesions covering the entire perineum. Both patients noted a few painful lesions on one side of the labia minor. Their gynecologists prescribed frequent warm sitz baths three to four times daily, each of about 20 minutes duration. Within the next two to three days, marked extension of these painful lesions was noted. On admission, there were numerous painful ulcers, with foul exudate and exquisite tenderness. The labia were greatly swollen . . .**
>
> **Prolonged or frequent soaking tends to cause maceration of the normal skin. In the presence of herpes virus, new lesions may develop on the macerated area and local dissemination of the disease may occur. For this reason, wet compresses or hot sitz baths should be avoided in patients with active herpetic infection.** [53]

By now you may be ready to give up on "horrible herpes," but before you do we want to leave you with some good news. Dr. Herbert

A. Blough, a virologist at the University of Pennsylvania School of Medicine, has come up with some amazing preliminary results. In fact his work is so impressive you might call it a breakthrough. He dusted off an old antiviral drug called 2-DEOXY-D-GLUCOSE. For over twenty years it has been known that this agent could interfere with the multiplication of viruses in a culture. Work with animal models has been slow and unpredictable and no one ever tried the drug out on humans. Dr. Blough and his associate, Dr. Giuntoli, tested 2-DEOXY-D-GLUCOSE on thirty-six women with genital herpes.[54] Ninety percent of the patients who received the active compound experienced rapid improvement (within twelve to seventy-two hours), whereas control patients (who had received a sham treatment) did not get better until the disease had run its course (the standard ten days). What is impressive is that women improved regardless of whether it was their first infection with herpes or an old attack acting up. And better still, for most, there were no recurrences after 2-DEOXY-D-GLUCOSE. After more than three years only two women had experienced repeat attacks and the drug cleared those up quickly. So if initial success can be duplicated, one might even be able to call this compound a cure. To top the whole matter off, there are still no observed adverse reactions from the drug. Since it is applied topically to the surface of the skin there is little opportunity for absorption into the body and little risk of internal side effects. The bad news is that the FDA is dragging its feet. It will probably be more than a year before this twenty-year-old "experimental" drug becomes available and even that may be optimistic. But at least there's hope, which is more than we have been able to say for years.

Even if 2-DEOXY-D-GLUCOSE doesn't turn out to be the solution to the problem there is another drug waiting in the wings that offers even greater promise. ACYCLOVIR is a new antiviral drug developed by the Burroughs Wellcome drug company. All the initial reports suggest that this drug is extraordinarily effective against all herpes virus infections including shingles, cold sores, and genital herpes. It too seems to be remarkably nontoxic. So with a little luck and cooperation from the FDA we may see a "cure" for this terrible disease within a relatively short period of time.

URINARY TRACT INFECTIONS . . .WHO'S VULNERABLE?

Urinary tract infections are nasty. They are also exceedingly common, and affect women ten times more often than men. Despite the fact that doctors see this problem with great regularity, it is surprising how little they know about what triggers the condition. In the absence of sound scientific knowledge, a certain amount of mystique has arisen around this ailment. And drug companies tend to exploit some of the myths in their promotional campaigns.

One of the unproved assumptions has been graphically illustrated. In a recent medical-journal drug advertisement, beneath a bold headline that states, **"She's been feeling more pain than pleasure...,"** a young woman in her underwear looks uncomfortable. The titillating statement is followed by the declaration that **"Sexually active women are especially vulnerable to urinary tract infections."** The recommended solution, of course is a brand-name antibiotic, MACRODANTIN, emblazoned across the bottom of the page. And in the last picture the young woman is seen wearing a sexy evening dress with a big smile on her face and a young man nuzzling her. Clearly the drug did its job. She's feeling better and ready for romance.

A lot of doctors have bought the line that "sexually active women are more vulnerable to urinary tract infections." But as far as we know there never has been any good research to support this hypothesis. In fact, the assumption that promiscuity is a major factor in cystitis is contradicted by a recent research report published in the *Journal of the American Medical Association*. The investigators found that sexual habits were unrelated to the number of urinary tract infections (UTIs) experienced by the young women they studied:

> **The sexual habits of the patients [women with UTI] and controls [women without UTI] were strikingly similar. All patients and controls were heterosexual and sexually active... Both groups contained approximately the same percentage of women having frequent coitus... In both groups, more than 75% engaged in oral sex, while only a small percent included anal intercourse as part of their regular sexual behavior... Another factor related to sexual behavior that is significant is the difference in postcoital voiding between the two groups. The majority of controls (68%) frequently void within ten minutes of coitus, compared with only a small percent of the patients... Our study disclosed no direct relation between coitus and UTI apart from postcoital voiding.** [55]

These investigators also discovered another striking piece of information. Women who delayed urination for more than an hour after the first urge to go to the bathroom were far more likely to suffer the unpleasant symptoms of an infection.

What are the symptoms of cystitis? Most commonly there is burning or a painful feeling upon urination. Often you feel the need to urinate but the effort is unproductive. There may be low back pain and in some cases blood may appear in the urine. If there are chills, fever, nausea, and vomiting along with the pain there is a good possibility the infection is in the kidneys. No matter where the bacteria strike within the urinary tract it is imperative that you have a urinalysis and culture. Once upon a time the only way you could manage that would have been to take a urine sample to the doctor's office or a hospital laboratory. But times have changed. Today you can do it yourself. There are many different kinds of testing and culturing kits available and there is a marvelous book which will tell you everything you need to know in order to perform and interpret these tests. The book is called *How to Perform Your Own Urinalysis Without a Doctor for Under 50¢*. It is well-written, easy to understand, and a valuable resource for anyone with recurrent infections, diabetes, kidney disease, liver disease, or obstructive jaundice. The book is by Richard Anthony and it can be purchased by sending a check or money order for $9.95 to P.I. Industries Publishing Company, P.O. Box 949, Loveland, Colorado 80537.

Self-testing of urine can be extremely helpful. For one thing, many women delay a trip to the doctor, hoping that the burning and itching may go away. If they had a simple, cheap, and fast test available at home they would know immediately that an appointment was necessary. Urinary tract infections are also very common in young girls (second only to colds) and often the symptoms are not very obvious. Once cystitis grabs a foothold in the bladder the infection can migrate up to the kidney and cause permanent kidney damage. For this reason it is important to occasionally screen young children, especially if they have vague symptoms "such as failure to thrive, vomiting, fever, abdominal stress, or irritability."[56] Any unexplained fever that persists in a child less than three years old requires a urine culture almost automatically.

Self-testing is also important because sometimes the drugs that are given don't work. The bacteria responsible may be resistant to a particular antibiotic, and if the test strip continues to show the presence of an infection after treatment is initiated, you will know that you should get in touch with the doctor immediately. Finally, and perhaps most important of all, infections tend to recur. "Eighty percent of schoolgirls or women who are successfully treated for UTI and followed up with frequent urine cultures will experience a reinfection within two years."[57] For this reason it is important to run a test every once in a while just to make sure there hasn't been a recurrence.

You might think that doctors would be absolutely opposed to the idea of patients testing their own urine. That is probably true for many, but some liberated souls think it's a good idea. Dr. Calvin M. Kunin, writing in the *Journal of the American Medical Association*, concluded that people can use these self-diagnostic tests effectively.

> **In our view, the demonstrated reliability of dipping the strip by untrained subjects and the logistic advantages of self-testing offer great promise for use as a screening test for urinary tract infections in the general population, and for use in office practice... The results using three first-morning specimens indicate that it will detect almost 90% of persistent significant bacteriuria [UTI] without false-positive results... It may be the single most useful method currently available for screening large populations for urinary tract infections at lowest cost.** [58]

Dr. Kunin is referring to the "nitrite test." A small strip of plastic is dipped into a sample of urine collected first thing in the morning. Since about 95 percent of common urinary bacteria produce nitrite, the little reagent strip will turn pink (a positive result) in about 30 seconds if an infection is present. A number of companies manufacture this kind of test strip. You can get a package of three strips for a dollar from Ames. It is called MICROSTIX-NITRITE and if your pharmacist can't supply it you might try writing directly to the company: Ames Division, Miles Laboratories, Inc., P.O. Box 70, Elkhart, Indiana 46515.

If you really want to stock up or if you want test strips that will give you results for pH, protein, glucose, ketones, bilirubin, blood, nitrite, and urobilinogen you could ask for Ames N-MULTISTIX. Another company that makes a similar product called CHEMSTRIP 8 is Bio-Dynamics/bmc, 9115 Hague Road, Indianapolis, Indiana 46250. The factory price for a bottle of 100 N-MULTISTIX test strips from Ames is $21 and the factory price for a bottle of 50 CHEMSTRIP 8 test strips from Bio-Dynamics is around $10.50. That makes the cost per strip almost identical—21¢. If you send a check in the appropriate amount to the company they should honor your order, though it may take up to six weeks for delivery. Ordering from a local "Physicians and Surgeons" supply house (check the yellow pages) is more expensive, but definitely faster. Another source is your local pharmacy. No prescription is necessary. If the pharmacist doesn't have MICROSTIX-NITRITE or N-MULTISTIX in stock she should be willing to order one or the other, depending on your needs. Before using these strips, however, we really do recommend that you send for a copy of *How to Perform Your Own Urinalysis Without a Doctor for Under 50¢* by Richard Anthony.

If you *really* want to become sophisticated in your diagnostic technique you could also do a urine culture. This will also improve your diagnostic accuracy. Our favorite culture kit is called BACTUR-CULT. It is made by Wampole Laboratories, Division of Carter-Wallace, Inc., Cranbury, New Jersey 08552. The factory price for ten kits is $12.55 (order no. 55D1). Unfortunately, the company does not sell directly to consumers so you will either have to buy it from your doctor or get your pharmacist to order it from a distributor. The Ames Company also makes a culture pad test (MICROSTIX 3) which can be dipped in a first morning urine specimen and then incubated. Any bacterial infection shows up as a pink area on the pad. It can also be mailed to your doctor for confirmation. Twenty-five test kits cost $18.75 (factory price).

In our opinion, home testing of urine is great. It provides rapid information about infection, it confirms successful treatment, it cuts down on cost, and most important of all it enables the family to become actively involved. Any doctor should be delighted with this kind of help.

If you find that you've got an infection, what can you do about it? There are a number of very useful drugs that can usually eliminate the problem in rapid order. Sulfas are still the favorite therapy for a first infection and GANTRISIN (sulfisoxazole) heads the list. For people who are allergic to sulfa or when an infection recurs within two years many doctors use ampicillin (OMNIPEN, POLYCILLIN) or tetracycline (ACHROMYCIN V, ROBITET, SUMYCIN, etc.). Amoxicillin (AMOXIL, LAROTID, or POLYMOX) is also a strong contender. Unfortunately, amoxicillin is a little more expensive than a sulfa drug or ampicillin. When infections keep coming back time after time the doctor will probably choose a drug called BACTRIM or SEPTRA. Both medications contain a combination of two ingredients—trimethoprim and sulfamethoxazole. A prophylactic course with these big guns should clear up almost any tough infection. Good-bye UTI!

How about preventing a urinary infection in the first place? The researchers who discovered that women's sexual habits had little if anything to do with this problem also discovered that delaying urination was really the culprit. They suggest that women drink at least two quarts of fluid each day and make regular trips to the bathroom to urinate (about every two hours). Cranberry juice has the reputation of being very good and we certainly agree that it tastes terrific. Unfortunately, it does not have any special anti-bacterial properties. But if you can afford half a gallon a day, great! And after voiding always wipe front to back. It may be too soon to hope that these infections will be a thing of the past, but the proposed preventive program and the many effective medications available should help in turning the pain into nothing more than a memory for most women.

ESTROGEN THERAPY . . .AND THE FIGHT GOES ON

No single subject in medical science seems to have generated more controversy and more hostility than estrogen therapy. Researchers are confused, doctors are confused, and women are more confused than anyone else. There have been so many different stories circulated about it that it is hardly any wonder that many women are tempted to ignore the whole business. One set of investigators claim that their study proves estrogen is safe and that the other researchers are all wet. Another group comes up with exactly the opposite results and announces through the world press that the incidence of uterine cancer is much greater among hormone users. Whom are you going to believe? Well, we don't have any crystal ball or special insight so we can't predict what future research will reveal, but for now we have very little doubt. The weight of the medical literature definitely points toward danger.

Over the years millions of women have received estrogen prescriptions (like PREMARIN) from their doctors. The drugs were given to eliminate the symptoms of menopause, but many women also believed that the use of estrogen would help them stay feminine forever. In retrospect, it may seem ridiculous that a pill was offered as a fountain of youth, but it was an idea that had wide popularity. Although the early-warning flags were flying as long ago as 1954 it has only been within the last four years that the medical community started to sit up and pay attention. But even after the initial reports had surfaced many doctors chose to ignore or resist the cautions. The number of prescriptions written was incredible. Today it is almost impossible to ignore the handwriting on the wall. Additional reports have appeared in the journals leading to the overwhelming conclusion that estrogens are associated with a definite cancer risk.

Two of the latest investigations demonstrate more clearly than ever the magnitude of the problem. A study conducted by a group at Johns Hopkins University concluded that women who take these hormones longest have the greatest chance of cancer. [59] Women who used the drugs for more than five years were fifteen times more likely to develop cancer of the uterine lining than nonusers; women who used them for less than one year were only twice as susceptible as those who never used them at all. A group of doctors who studied women in western Washington State found that long-term users had at least a twenty-fold greater risk of developing cancer than nonusers. Here are their conclusions:

> **The long-term use of estrogens that appears to be needed to forestall the development of osteoporosis [weakening of bones] is unequivocally related to large increases in the incidence of endometrial [uterine] cancer. Lower dosages of estrogen are less hazardous than large ones among long-term users, but they produce a sizable excess risk nonetheless. [60]**

Amid all this gloom and doom there is still some room for optimism, even rejoicing. One of the world's foremost epidemiologists, Dr. Hershel Jick, and his associates from the Boston Collaborative Drug Surveillance Program analyzed data from a Seattle cancer study. Although they too found that "long-term replacement estrogen treatment is strongly associated with endometrial cancer," they also discovered that "discontinuation of estrogen intake is associated with a striking decrease in risk for endometrial cancer within six months."[61] In other words, when women stopped the hormone-replacement therapy there was a dramatic and almost immediate reduction in their risk of developing cancer.

So where does all this leave a woman who is suffering the severe symptoms of menopause? The decision to use any drug should be made with full knowledge of the benefits and the risks. Doctors have often avoided their responsibility to provide adequate information. The excuse is usually, "I didn't want to frighten her." Nonsense! That old chestnut went out with "Keep em' barefoot and pregnant." Women are intelligent and more than capable of making informed decisions, and many times it will be to use estrogen. Here are some letters we received from newspaper-column readers:

> **Menopause in some females is extraordinarily uncomfortable both physically and mentally. I**

> start feeling warm inside, like a fever, for a
> minute or two. Then my face starts to sweat.
> The hair on the back of my neck drips wet and
> my blouse sticks to my body. It's difficult to
> breathe, my complexion pales and the expres-
> sion on my face is total despair. I can endure a
> lot but this is ridiculous.
>
> I have had to give up playing bridge because of
> the need to leave my table and move about until
> the attack passes. I cannot go out to dinner, to a
> movie or sleep with anyone. I have a right to be
> comfortable.

Indeed she does! If she chooses to take estrogen that is her right and she should not be made to feel guilty or ashamed. The short-term use of estrogen for severe menopausal symptoms has a relatively low risk. But doctors and patients need to think more than twice before they decide to continue hormone therapy longer than one or two years.

OSTEOPOROSIS—WATCH OUT FOR THOSE BONES

One of the reasons that doctors give to justify prolonged administration of estrogen is that it will prevent osteoporosis, a weakening of bones that often comes with aging. What they often don't mention is that once a woman starts down the estrogen road she will probably have to keep taking it for the rest of her life if she wants to maintain the improvement. If she stops the drug she will forfeit any benefit she gained by rapidly losing bone. Within a few years she could well be in exactly the same place a woman who took no estrogens at all would have been.[62] The American physicians have lagged behind their British colleagues in this research. Here is what a group at the Mineral Metabolism Unit in Leeds, England had to say about their work:

> Lindsay et al. found that, in postmenopausal
> women, withdrawal of estrogen therapy is
> followed by a phase of rapid bone loss which
> largely negates the benefits, to bone, of estrogen
> therapy. Our observations on twelve post-
> menopausal women in whom we have se-
> quential measurements ... both during and
> after withdrawal of estrogen treatment confirm
> their findings.[63]

What is a woman to do? Osteoporosis is a crippler that leads to broken bones and much suffering. Approximately 500,000 fractures occur each year in postmenopausal women who suffer from this disease. But the significant risk of uterine cancer from estrogen is also a very real problem. This sounds very much like the old rock-and-a-hard-place type of decision. But it may not be as bleak as it appears. There is strong evidence that a lack of calcium could be an important factor in bringing on osteoporosis. Researchers at the Burke Rehabilitation Center in White Plains, New York, recently made some exciting observations:

> **The USDA survey of 5,500 "normal" females showed that in the age group of 45 years and over the estimated average calcium consumption approximated 450 mg. per day—about 50 percent *below* the 1974 RDA [recommended dietary allowance] of 800 mg. per day...There was a significant relationship of inadequate calcium intake to the incidence of osteoporosis, resulting in disabling fractures of vertebrae, long bones and hips of postmenopausal women. Investigations were initiated to determine the effects of dietary calcium intake on bone density... in postmenopausal women. Bone density increased with intake of calcium. Dairy products constituted the major source of calcium. The findings indicated that a daily intake of 800 to 1,000 mg. of calcium [a quart of whole or skim milk] is necessary to maintain normal or optimal bone health.[64]**

This research and that of many other investigators would lend credence to the idea that a regular calcium intake of 1 to 2 grams per day could slow or prevent osteoporosis from advancing. That is an awful lot of milk, especially if you have a hard time digesting dairy products. Many older folks lose their ability to digest milk sugar and will develop gas, indigestion, and diarrhea. Fortunately, there is now a product on the market called LACT-AID which predigests the milk sugar to eliminate this problem. But even with LACT-AID that is still mucho milk. If you can't pack away that much white stuff or eat lots of cheese regularly, we recommend dolamite tablets which supply calcium and magnesium. And since vitamin D is essential for adequate calcium absorption a dose of between 400 and 1,200 units has been suggested by the Chairman of the Department of Medicine at Albany Medical College of Union University, Dr. Stanley Wallach. He also recommends that exercise can help prevent osteoporosis from getting a foothold. He advises walking three miles a day if possible, riding a stationary bicycle, and swimming. The key to strong bones, then, is careful attention to diet and mineral supplementation coupled with vitamin D. This, together with lots of gentle exercise, could make estrogen treatment unnecessary.

WE'VE COME A LONG WAY

Sexist attitudes toward women's ailments can no longer be tolerated. Doctors must treat women's illnesses as seriously as they do men's. The days of the quick VALIUM fix for women are long gone. When psychological support is important women must build their own self-help networks. They can do the same thing to maintain good health. Drug commercials that play upon women's fears of insecurity and social unacceptability not only should be ignored, they should be eliminated. The FDA should get "feminine hygiene" sprays off the market along with other products that are counterproductive.

Although we have presented some "bad news" in this chapter there is also reason to be optimistic. New treatment for painful menstrual cramps should herald the dawn of a new day for millions of women. And suggestions for "premenstrual tension" may make the unpleasant condition easier to handle as well. Vaginitis can be cured, though there may be some risk associated with FLAGYL, the most effective medication available. "Horrible herpes" may become much less of a nightmare if the new/old drug 2-DEOXY-D-GLUCOSE lives up to its initial promise or the experimental medication ACYCLOVIR wins FDA approval. And for those women who have suffered from urinary tract infections, new home diagnostic techniques and a number of effective antibiotics should make the pain a thing of the past. There have been too many mistakes made for far too many years when it comes to treating women, but the times are changing. There is much reason to feel encouraged.

REFERENCES

1. Armitage, R. S.; Schneiderman, L. J.; and Buss, R. A. "Response of Physicians to Medical Complaints in Men and Women" *JAMA* 241:2186–2187, 1979.

2. Wolcott, Ilene. "Women and Psychoactive Drug Use." *Women and Health.* 4(2) Summer: 199–202, 1979.

3. Werble, Cole Palmer (ed). "Goyan Labels Minor Tranquilizer Advertising 'Sexist.' " *FDC Reports Drugs and Cosmetics* 41(48):8, 1979.

4. Lamy, Peter, P. "Influence of Gender on Drug Therapy." *Professional Pharmacy* 4(4):3–4, 1977.

5. Ibid.

6. Marx, Jean, L. "Dysmenorrhea: Basic Research Leads to a Rational Therapy." *Science* 205:175—176, 1979.

7. Ylikorkala, O., Dawood, M.Y. "New Concepts in Dysmenorrhea." *Am. J. Obstet. Gynecol.* 130:833—847, 1978.

8. Budoff, Penny Wise. "Use of Mefenamic Acid in the Treatment of Primary Dysmenorrhea." *JAMA* 241:2713—2716, 1979.

9. Hanson, Frederick W., Izu, Allen, and Henzl, Milan R. "Naproxen Sodium in Dysmenorrhea." *Obs. and Gynecol* 52:583—587, 1978.

10. "Drugs for Dysmenorrhea." *Med. Letter* 21:81—83, 1979.

11. Budoff, Penny Wise. "Mefenamic Acid for Dysmenorrhea." *JAMA* 242:2393—2394, 1979.

12. Ibid.

13. Kinch, Robert A. H. "Help for Patients with Premenstrual Tension." *Consultant* April: 187—191, 1979.

14. Ashworth, Laurel E. "Menstrual Products." in *Handbook of Non-prescription Drugs,* 6th ed. Corrigan, L. Luan, ed. Washington, D. C.: APhA., 1979, pp. 239—245.

15. Widger, Neil H. *Widger's Guide to Over-The-Counter Drugs.* Los Angeles: J. P. Tarcher, Inc., 1979, p. 131.

16. O'Brien, P. M., et al. "Treatment of Premenstrual Syndrome by Spironolactone." *British J. Obstet. Gynaecol.* 86:142—147, 1979.

17. MacGregor, G. A., et al. "Is 'Idiopathic' Oedema Idiopathic?" *The Lancet* 1:397—400, 1979.

18. Kinch, Robert A. H. "Help for Patients With Premenstrual Tension." *Consultant* April: 187—191, 1979.

19. Seaman, Barbara, and Seaman, Gideon. *Women and the Crisis in Sex Hormones.* New York: Rawson, 1977, pp. 142—144.

20. Questions and Answers. "Relief of Dysmenorrhea." *JAMA* 242:285, 1979.

21. White, Kristin. "Bromocryptine is Ok'd in U.S. for Amenorrhea Rx." *Hospital Tribune* Oct., 1078, p. 4.

22. Ibid.

23. Pharmacy. "Parlodel Signals Breakthrough for Treating Amenorrhea/Galactorrhea." *Chain Store Age/Drug Edition* 54(9):126—127, 1978.

24. Henahan, John. "Bromocriptine Helps Infertile Women Conceive." *Medical Tribune* 19(32):3, 1978.

25. Kinch, op. cit.

26. Fisher, Alexander A. "Allergic Reaction to Feminine Hygiene Sprays." *Arch. Dermatol.* 108:801—802, 1973.

27. Hoag, Stephen G. "Feminine Cleansing and Deodorant Products." in *Handbook of Nonprescription Drugs* 6th ed. Corrigan, L. Luan, ed. Washington, D. C.: APhA, 1979, pp. 259—267.

28. Barrett, Kathryn F., et al. "Tampon-Induced Vaginal or Cervical Ulceration." *Am. J. Obstet. Gynecol.* 127:332—333, 1977.

29. Gosselin, Robert E., et al. *Clinical toxicology of Commercial Products.* 4th ed. Baltimore: Williams and Wilkins, 1978, pp. 63—64.

30. Tentative Findings of the Advisory Review Panel on Contraceptives and Other Vaginal Products. Information Copy. "OTC Contraceptives and Other Vaginal Drug Products." November 1978, Document 0712A.

31. Hoag, op. cit., p. 267.

32. Neuman, Hans H., and DeCherney, Alan. "Douching and Pelvic Inflammatory Disease." *N. Engl. J. Med.* 295:789, 1976.

33. Rulin, Marvin C. "Tips for Better Management of Vulvovaginitis." *Modern Medicine* 47(16):50—59, 1979.

34. Will, Thomas E. "Lactobacillus Overgrowth for Treatment of Moniliary Vulvovaginitis." *Lancet* 2:482, 1979.

35. Dykers, John R. "Single-Dose Metronidazole for Trichomonal Vaginitis." *N. Engl. J. Med.* 293:23, 1975.

36. Wolfe, Sidney, and Johnson, Anita. Health Research Group. Letter to Food and Drug Commissioner Alexander Schmidt, October 22, 1974.

37. Schmidt, Alexander M. Commissioner of Food and Drugs. Letter to Health Research Group, October 21, 1975.

38. The Boston Women's Health Book Collective. *Our Bodies, Ourselves.* New York: Simon and Schuster, 1976, p. 138.

39. Beard, C., Mary, et al. "Lack of Evidence for Cancer Due to Use of Metronidazole." *N. Engl. J. Med.* 301:519—522, 1979.

40. "Metronidazole (Flagyl)." *Medical Letter* 21(22): 89—90, 1979.

41. Carlson, E. J., and Yankee, D. E. "Promise Her Relief From H. Vaginalis." *Patient Care* Jan: 54—58, 1979.

42. "Herpes Patients Fight Medicine's Empty Cupboard." *Medical World News.* July 23, 1979, p. 27.

43. Rulin, op. cit., p. 59.

44. Ibid.

45. Donsky, Howard J. "Nonoxynol 9 Cream for Genital Herpes Simplex." *N. Engl. J. Med.* 300:371, 1979.

46. Kern, Arthur B., and Schiff, Bencel L. "Treatment of Herpes Simplex Infections." *Arch. Dermatol.* 113:1463, 1977.

47. Willis, William F. "A Cure for Recurrent Herpes Simplex." *Arch. Dermatol.* 114:1096, 1978.

48. Woodbridge, Peter. "The Use of Betadine Antiseptic Paint in the Treatment of Herpes Simplex and Herpes Zoster." *J. Int. Med. Res.* 5:378—381, 1977.

49. Fahim, Mostafa, et al. "New Treatment for Herpes Simplex Virus Type 2 (Ultrasound and Zinc, Urea, and Tannic Acid Ointment). *J. of Med.* 9:256—263, 1978.

50. "Early Clinical Results Show Topical Agent Effective vs. Genital Herpes." *Hospital Practice* 14(1): 44—53, 1979.

51. Chang, Te-Wen, and Fiumara, Nicholas. "Treatment with Levamisole of Recurrent Herpes Genitalis." *Antimicrobial Agents and Chemother.* 113:809—812, 1978.

52. Kaufman, Raymond H., et al. "Treatment of Genital Herpes Simplex Virus Infection with Photodynamic Inactivatin." *Am. J. Obstet. Gynecol.* 132:861—869, 1978.

53. Chang, Te-Wen. "Local Dissemination of Herpes Simplex Following Soaking or Sitz Bathing." *Am. J. Obstet. Gynecol.* 131:342—343, 1978.

54. Blough, Herbert A., and Giuntoli, R. L. "Successful Treatment of Human Genital Herpes Infections with 2-deoxy-D-glucose. *JAMA* 241:2798, 1979.

55. Adatto, Kiku, et al. "Behavior Factors and Urinary Tract Infection." *JAMA* 241:2525—2526, 1979.

56. Kallen, Ronald J. "UTI: Treating the First Infection and Avoiding the Second." *Mod. Med.* 47(19): 28—38, 1979.

57. Adatto, op. cit., p. 2526.

58. Kunin, Calvin M., and DeGroot, Jane E. "Self-Screening for Significant Bacteriuria." *JAMA* 231:1349—1353, 1975.

59. Antunes, Carlos M. F., Stolley, Paul, et al. "Endometrial Cancer and Estrogen Use." *N. Engl. J. Med.* 300:9—13, 1979.

60. Weiss, Noel S., et al. "Endometrial Cancer in Relation to Patterns of Menopausal Estrogen Use." *JAMA* 242:261—264, 1979.

61. Jick, Hershel, et al. "Replacement Estrogens and Endometrial Cancer." *N. Engl. J. Med.* 300:218—222, 1979.

62. Lindsay, R. "Bone Response to Termination of Estrogen Treatment." *Lancet* 1:1325—1328, 1978.

63. Horsman, A., et al. "Effect on Bone of Withdrawal of Estrogen Therapy." *Lancet* 2:33, 1979.

64. Albanese, Anthony A., et al. "Osteoporosis: Effects of Calcium." *American Fam. Physician* 18(4):160—167, 1978.

7

Contraceptive Update

The Pill: More bad news ● Infected by the IUD: Pelvic Inflammatory Disease and microwave ovens ● Spermicidal scandals: Radium, mercury, and boric acid poisoning ● Vaginal suppositories: over-promoted and unreliable. Comparing spermicidal foams. ● (Re) Introducing the cervical cap ● Success with condoms ● Vasectomy update: Some disturbing news ● Home pregnancy tests: Reliable or rip-offs?

Women are no dummies! Despite the fact that doctors and drug companies have been pushing birth control pills and IUDs for years, women have begun to say NO to the risks of these methods of contraception. Between 1975 and 1978 the number of prescriptions filled for the Pill dropped from 64 million to 49 million, a decrease of about 23 percent.[1] Why the sudden decline? Instead of casually accepting the doctor's recommendation for contraceptive methods people have had more opportunity to think for themselves. For one thing, the FDA required that a Patient Package Insert be provided with every prescription. This informational brochure described a long list of scary side effects that many physicians had been unwilling to discuss. Even the former Commissioner of the FDA, Dr. Donald Kennedy, got into the act. When asked what he would tell the female members of his own family if they asked him about birth control pills he responded that he would advise them to "find another method." Given an opportunity to evaluate the benefits and the risks for themselves, a lot of women have said thanks but No Thanks!

Perhaps many couples have been re-evaluating women's use of oral contraceptives because some large-scale investigations resulted in data that was hard to ignore. British researchers from the Royal College of General Practitioners studied 46,000 women over many years.[2] They discovered that the females using the Pill had a death rate five times higher than those who had never used this method of birth control. And women who had been using these drugs for more than five years had a mortality rate ten times that of the non pill-takers. What was particularly startling was that the excess deaths from oral contraceptives were significantly greater than "the mortality from complications of pregnancy in the controls, and was double the death rate from accidents."[3] Until this report was published family planning agencies could always fall back on the argument that getting pregnant was a lot more dangerous than taking the Pill. That doesn't hold water anymore.

What is the latest update on oral contraceptives? About all we can say is the bad news just keeps rolling in. In 1973 Dr. Janet Baum, a pathologist at the University of Michigan, discovered seven cases of liver tumors in young women on oral contraceptives. At first the medical profession was skeptical. No one wanted to accept the possibility that there might be a connection between the Pill and these extremely dangerous tumors. Dr. Baum tried to publish her findings in the *Journal of the American Medical Association,* but was flatly rejected. Five years were lost before the U.S. medical establishment woke up to reality. In a justifiably angry letter Dr. Baum socked it to the conservative fools.

> To the Editor.—I was both amused and annoyed at an article in the medical news section of *The JAMA* (231:451, 1975) concerning the possible association of hepatic [liver] cell adenomas tumors and oral contraceptives.
>
> In 1970 when I wrote the first paper on the subject, on the basis of three cases, I submitted it to *The Journal* for publication. It was rejected with a comment to the effect that the possible relationship was ridiculous and that possibly I should write up the case histories as interesting case reports and forget about the rest of the article. In 1973, after I had seen four more cases, I rewrote the article and submitted it to *Lancet,* a British publication; it was published in the Oct. 27, 1973 issue.
>
> I am glad to see that editors of *The Journal* have finally recognized the possible significance of this problem.
>
> As Dr. Mays and I have both pointed out, the tumors often rupture spontaneously, causing massive, if not fatal, intra-peritoneal hemorrhage.[4]

Although it took the medical establishment a long time to recognize the gravity of the situation, once the word was out other physicians began detailing their own experiences and articles appeared with increasing frequency in the medical literature.[5, 6] Both benign and malignant cases have been reported. A recent account published in *Medical World News* brings us up-to-date on current thinking with regard to the relative risk of developing these liver tumors:

> **Women 27 or older who have been on the Pill four years or more run at least 200 times the normal risk of liver tumors, according to an epidemiology study reported to the American College of Obstetrics and Gynecologists here. And women under 26 years old who have used oral contraceptives (OCs) four years or more are 19 times as likely to develop the tumors... All OC users should have liver palpation as part of physical exams and should be taught to report abdominal masses or pain... The association between OCs and hepatoma seems stronger than that between cigarettes and lung cancer.[7]**

Now well over 100 cases of liver tumors have been documented.[8] And the prediction is that we should expect approximately 280 cases each year as a result of the use of birth control pills.[9] This all came as a great surprise to the medical profession. It shouldn't have. As far back as 1966 a British pathologist reported the appearance of liver tumors in rats that had received estrogen. Dr. Carolyn Lingeman, from the National Cancer Institute has emphasized, "Results of these tests in animals should have received more attention before these drugs were pronounced to be 'safe.'"[10]

Liver tumors aren't the only "new" complication that has recently turned up. In 1978 researchers from the University of Iowa reported for the first time that oral contraceptives could stimulate growths within the pituitary gland in susceptible individuals.[11] This may lead to a loss of menstruation. A more subtle but conceivably more devastating consequence of the Pill was reported in the *American Journal of Obstetrics and Gynecology* by Dr. Francis J. Kane:

> **A review of available clinical studies indicates that 10 to 40 percent of oral contraceptive users may suffer mild to moderate depression syndromes. Clinical and animal data indicate that a variety of mechanisms may be involved, includ-**

ing alterations in folate, pyridoxine, and vitamin B$_{12}$ metabolism ... The evidence summarized would seem to point to the occurrence of mild to moderate depressive states characterized by tiredness, lethargy, sadness, and sometimes accompanied by loss of interest in sex.[12]

Sex—the big mystery. Surprising as it may seem, there has been relatively little research directed toward the effect of birth control pills on libido. One of the few studies that has been carried out was done at Wesleyan University. The investigators compared the sexual habits of women using different methods of contraception. Those who relied on non-pill techniques (such as foam, IUDs, diaphragms, or whose sexual partners used a condom) appeared to initiate sexual activity more often than women who used oral contraceptives. The peak in sexuality seemed to coincide with ovulation and the researchers hypothesized that since the Pill suppressed ovulation it might also have an inhibiting effect on sexual arousal. (News Front. "Sex Drive in Women Peaks at Ovulation." *Modern Medicine* 47(7):37, 1979).

As if all this weren't bad enough, other research has shown that young women using birth control pills have significantly higher levels of cholesterol and triglycerides in their blood.[13–15] Add this to the discovery that the Pill can raise blood pressure and one could make a very strong case that a lot of women may have a greater risk of developing arteriosclerosis, coronary heart disease, and heart attacks, especially as they get older.

Now if that ain't getting zapped, you tell us what is? Yet for many women oral contraceptives may be the only reasonable or acceptable means of contraception. If each woman makes that decision with a complete understanding of benefits and risks, then fine. Oral contraceptives shouldn't be foisted on women by patronizing doctors or planned-parenthood enthusiasts who think they can decide what is best for someone else. Unfortunately, too often that has been the case. An article in the *American Journal of Public Health* titled "Efficacy Information in Contraceptive Counseling: Those Little White Lies" let the cat out of the bag. The investigators found that family-planning personnel "do indeed appear to place the methods they actively dispense in an extremely favorable position." While "counseling" their clients about various methods of contraception the

Clinicians bias their effectiveness rates toward the IUD and Pill and against the condom and

> **foam. Stated more bluntly, clinicians seem to respond to questions about effectiveness in a manner that is biased toward the methods they provide and against traditional methods.**[16]

This policy is unforgivable! As you shall see, "traditional" methods of birth control may be a whole lot safer and more effective than the "professionals" have been letting on.

INFECTED BY THE IUD

The letters "PID" seem pretty innocuous. Even the words "pelvic inflammatory disease" are not overly disturbing. Who knows, it could be a doctor's delicate way to describe menstrual cramps. We only wish it were so. Actually, PID is dreadful—and much worse than inflammation. It's a serious infection—within the fallopian tubes, ovaries, or uterus. At first, symptoms may be barely noticeable. There may be some spotting or bleeding between periods and maybe even some cramping. As the infection takes hold abdominal pain gets worse and there may be a vaginal discharge. A low-grade fever may occur and if nothing is done an abscess could result that might be life-threatening. Even if the disease doesn't get out of hand and treatment is successful the possibility exists that a woman will be left sterile.

It used to be that doctors thought pelvic inflammatory disease was a result of VD. Gonorrhea was considered the culprit and obviously this wasn't the sort of thing "nice girls" ever had. They were wrong. While gonorrhea can lead to PID it is responsible for less than half the cases.[17] What doctors didn't realize was that IUDs were responsible for an extraordinary number of infections. A recent follow-up study by the Gynecology Advisory Committee of the FDA revealed that young women who wear IUDs and have not had children "have a rate of infection three to five times that of women of the same age who don't wear IUDs."[18] And more often than not the infections were *not* caused by gonorrhea.

Recently it has been estimated that there are over 500,000 cases of PID each year in the United States. A team of physicians from the University of Washington calculated that, of that number, 110,000 cases or 22 percent were attributable to the IUD.[19] Without even trying to determine the human suffering such a rate of infection might cause, the researchers attempted to assess the cost in dollars and cents of this number of cases. Based on obsolete data the figures are still staggering:

> Rendtorff and associates calculated that the direct medical costs of treating acute PID averaged $233 per case in 1973. Thus, 110,000 cases of IUD-associated PID cost over $26 million in that year. If time lost from work and other indirect medical costs are included, the cost of treating PID increased to $402 per case. The inclusive cost of 110,000 cases of IUD-associated PID would be $44 million in that year.[20]

That was a long time ago. The cost of health care has since gone through the stratosphere and the number of IUDs in use has increased as well. Today the figure could well have doubled.

What do all these facts and figures mean in more human terms? Here is a real case history from the records of Grady Memorial Hospital in Atlanta, Georgia. A 28-year-old woman with one child had a LIPPES LOOP in 1967. In 1969 the little thread attached to the IUD disappeared and the doctors inserted a SAF-T-COIL to help in locating the loop. Both devices were left in after both IUDs were located within the uterus. Over the intervening years the woman experienced "several episodes" of PID but apparently they were treated successfully. Her last "episode" proved fatal:

> By history obtained from the family, it was determined that the patient had had several days of abdominal pain and distention, fever, and nausea and vomiting before being brought to the surgical emergency clinic in a stuporous state on May 3, 1977. Shortly after arriving in the facility the patient had a cardiac arrest, was resuscitated, and was evaluated by the surgery service...The patient was taken to the operating room after stabilization, and laparotomy [abdominal surgery] revealed a massive pelvic abscess that had ruptured and spilled 1,500 c.c. [1.6 quarts] of free pus into the abdominal cavity...
> The patient died within 24 hours of admission after six cardiorespiratory arrests.[21]

No one knows why women wearing IUDs are more susceptible to PID. Some investigators have suggested that bacteria, fungi, and other beasties migrate up the tail of the device (the thread that is connected to the IUD to facilitate removal) from the vagina and enter a normally sterile uterus. Other researchers believe that the IUD itself leads to a low-grade inflammatory process within the uterus— some sort of chronic, non-specific infection not serious enough to cause clinical symptoms—and that this is in fact what produces the contraceptive effect. If the infection gets out of control pelvic inflammatory disease might result. Whatever the cause, PID requires prompt treatment with antibiotics. But therein lies a paradox. If the IUD is not removed the possibility exists that the antibiotics will reduce the contraceptive effectiveness.[22,23] One of our readers from Fresno, California, wrote to us in 1979 to document her own experience with antibiotics and an IUD:

> **I had my IUD inserted in April of 1977. In May 1978 I was put on several medications by my family physician for walking pneumonia. I had a period 6-12-78. On 6-19-78 my gynecologist put me on AZOGANTRISIN for a bladder infection. By July I felt pregnant, and sure enough, I had a baby in March, 1979.**
>
> **What perplexes me is that my gynecologist could give no explanation as to why I became pregnant. I asked him if it was due to the antibiotics and he said "Nah!" He'd never heard of it. I saw him again this week, and again he denied that the antibiotic could be at fault. His nurse** *laughed at me* **and said, "That's a new one—I've never heard of that."**
>
> **I have several friends on IUDs: One friend conceived while on antibiotics—her obstetrician said it was due to the antibiotics and to use another method of birth control if she ever uses antibiotics again.**

Unfortunately, there has been very little research devoted to the problem of IUD contraceptive failures. The medical literature contains several case histories of women who became pregnant with an IUD in place when they were given steroids like CORTISONE or PREDNISONE.[24] If pregnancy is prevented through an inflammatory or infectious process it is only logical to assume that drugs which interfere with that process (antibiotics or anti-inflammatory agents) may reduce contraceptive effectiveness. As you probably know, this drug/device interaction is further complicated by the fact that it is extremely dangerous for a woman to become pregnant with an IUD in place. Septic abortions, blood poisoning, and even deaths have been associated with IUD-related pregnancies. In 1979 a Denver jury awarded a woman $6.8 million because the DALKON SHIELD she was using led to a miscarriage that almost caused her death. The A. H. Robins Company, maker of the DALKON SHIELD, has paid out over $40 million to settle approximately 2,400 claims that have been brought against this banned IUD. But any similar device would be equally dangerous if a woman became pregnant. So it would make good sense for a woman to use a back-up method of contraception if she has to take a drug that might reduce the effectiveness of her IUD.

Now, are you ready for something really bizarre? A friend of ours, Dr. V. Georges Hufnagel, one of the finest Ob-Gyns you will ever find anywhere, told us a story that made our hair stand on end. In her practice of medicine, Georges came across some cases of women who had their uteruses singed while standing in front of a microwave oven. (We promised weirdness!) It seems that these ladies were wearing a CU-7 IUD. Since this device contains a copper wire wrapped around plastic it is susceptible to the microwave radiation that may leak from the oven. The result is that the IUD heats up, and whammo—a nasty burn. The moral of the story—make sure your microwave oven doesn't leak radiation or don't stand in front of it wearing an IUD.

"MANNING" THE BARRICADES

Let's hear it for the barrier methods of contraception! Ever since the introduction of the Pill and the IUD these traditional forms of contraception have had to take a back seat. Condoms, diaphragms, cervical caps, and spermicidal foams are among the most underrated and unappreciated techniques for preventing pregnancy. As we've already seen, family-planning personnel have tended to downplay their desirability and emphasize their ineffectiveness. But women can and do think for themselves. As Pill use has declined, the popularity of these "old-fashioned" methods has soared. In 1975 pharmacies filled prescriptions for only 503,000 diaphragms. By 1978 that figure had jumped to 1,205,000—an increase of almost 140 percent.[25] And now that condoms have come out of the closet (and from behind the counter) the hard fact is that sales have skyrocketed! While solid data is hard to come by there is significant evidence that women are major condom purchasers. The trade journal *American Druggist* reports that "one out of every eight condom purchasers in U.S. drug stores today is a woman; ... in stores where condoms are on open display, women account for an even larger proportion of purchasers—15%." A recent survey carried out by Consumers Union revealed that "the condom is no longer an exclusively male-controlled method. Seventy-five percent of our women respondents reported that they purchased condoms, at least occasionally."[26]

One reason that barrier methods of contraception are becoming increasingly popular is that people are waking up to the fact that they are more effective than previously thought. A recent review article in the *American Journal of Obstetrics and Gynecology* offered the following statistics:

> **Data for the diaphragm suggest that the failure rates even among teen-agers, may be much lower than originally thought (possibly as low as 5 percent[27] or 13 percent) and that women willing to use the methods should be so encouraged.[28]**

A consultant to the *Journal of the American Medical Association* offered even greater support: "A few minutes of instruction and more time for practice will equip a woman with a reliable (97%) contraceptive that has no systemic side effects."[29]

And let's not forget the condom. A doctor with the Bureau of Venereal Disease Control from the New York City Health Department recently chastised his colleagues for underestimating the value of this traditional technique:

> **Modern improvements in condom design, convenience, and sensitivity have to a large extent gone unnoticed by the public and many physicians, while its occasional failures both as a contraceptive and as a prophylactic against sexually transmitted disease are greatly exaggerated. Repeated studies showing it to be, if properly and consistently used, 97% effective as a contraceptive[30] and notably effective in preventing gonorrhea as well as most other sexually transmitted diseases are disregarded.[31]**

The ability of barrier contraceptives to assist in disease prevention should not be taken lightly. There is evidence that oral contraceptives may actually increase the likelihood that a woman will catch gonorrhea from an infected male partner.[32] And the IUD can turn a "simple" case of the clap into a disaster by spreading the infection into the uterus and tubes. We have already detailed the complications of pelvic inflammatory disease, not the least of which can be sterility. "Old-fashioned" methods, on the other hand, can dramatically cut down on VD. When couples rely on a diaphragm, foam, or a condom the woman is about ten times less likely to become infected with cervical gonorrhea than if she used the Pill or an IUD.[33]

SPERMICIDAL SCANDAL
(They glowed in the dark)

Now before you come away with the impression that our enthusiasm for barrier contraceptives clouds our objectivity, strap on your seat belt and prepare for a story that will shock your sensibility! For the last couple of hundred years it has been taken for granted that the lining of the vaginal tract is relatively impervious to chemicals. Without any evidence, researchers and physicians assumed that you could stick just about anything into the vagina and it would not be transmitted to the rest of the body. No one even bothered to consider the possibility that radium or other toxic material would be absorbed. Radium? Now hold on—would anyone in her right mind ever put radium into the vagina! No, but in an effort to create spermicides, researchers came up with some pretty toxic combinations. We came across a "special note" in a 1944 issue of *Human Fertility* that blew our minds:

> A tube of CHLORADIUM VAGINAL JELLY received from the manufacturer was analyzed at the radioactivity center of the Massachusetts Institute of Technology and found to contain 1.9 micrograms of radium element. Dr. Joseph C. Aub, of the Collis P. Huntington Memorial Laboratories, stated that if this quantity were stored in the body it might eventually cause radium poisoning. It is known that only a portion of the radium contained in the jelly would be absorbed from the vagina and only a small part of that absorbed would be retained. Since, however, the use of material for contraception customarily involves repeated use and quantities which would greatly exceed that in one tube, it would seem unwise to use radium-containing materials for such a purpose.[34]

Is that an understatement or what? Were those people insane? It is hard to believe that rational human beings would actually have used radium, a radioactive substance, as a spermicide, but the name of the product speaks for itself—CHLORADIUM VAGINAL JELLY. But that was in 1944, you say, they didn't know any better in those days. Like hell they didn't! An article published in 1943 titled "Protection of

Radium Dial Workers and Radiologists from Injury by Radium"
provided plenty of warning:

> **In 1924, Blum identified radium as the respon-
> sible agent in an occupational poisoning
> case...When taken into the body radium
> behaves like calcium. A portion of the ingested
> radium eventually is deposited in bones...In
> chronic radium poisoning, where the body
> contains 1 to 10 micrograms of radium fixed in
> the skeleton, there are usually no clinical
> symptoms until some five to fifteen years after
> the exposure....**
>
> **Based on these observations, a committee
> called together in 1941 by the National Bureau
> of Standards tentatively established 0.1 micro-
> grams of radium fixed in the body as the toler-
> ance value for humans.[35]**

One tube of CHLORADIUM VAGINAL JELLY contained almost 20
times the amount of radium allowed for occupationally exposed
workers back in 1941. Today, standards are much stricter. We now
know how dangerous even low-level radiation exposure can be.
Because radium has a half-life of 1600 years and will remain in bone
almost indefinitely, the maximum level permitted in *air* is
0.000000000003 micrograms. CHLORADIUM had over a million times
this permissible level. God knows what happened to the women who
used this brand of spermicidal jelly. Lung and bone cancer are only
two possible malignancies that can result from contact with this
highly toxic material. Radium wasn't the only dangerous chemical
that has been used in these kinds of products. In fact, as recently as
1978 it was possible to purchase vaginal suppositories and douches
that contained either mercury (as phenylmercuric acetate in
LOROPHYN) or boric acid. Both chemicals are extremely toxic and
both can easily be absorbed from the vaginal tract in substantial
concentrations. What is so extraordinary is that this information has
been available since 1918 if anyone had bothered to look.[36] It seems
that the old attitude that contraception was the woman's problem led
many male researchers and physicians to overlook the possibility of
toxicity.

It took the Food and Drug Administration almost sixty years to
wake up to the potential dangers of spermicidal suppositories that
contained these and other known toxic ingredients. In 1978 our
"guardians" issued a report that received virtually no publicity but

nevertheless had devastating implications. The experts concluded that mercury could be absorbed from vaginal contraceptive preparations and is "potentially hazardous to the fetus and the breast-fed infant ... the Panel does not consider them to be safe."[37] That isn't the half of it! If a woman accidentally became pregnant while using one of these spermicidal suppositories or jellies the possibility exists that the fetus would be born with a birth defect in the form of "delayed neurologic or intellectual damage" that might not show up for years. The "experts" didn't think the mercury exposure would be dangerous to the women themselves, but we think differently. All forms of mercury are poisonous if absorbed into the body. And because this chemical accumulates slowly over time a woman might not even be aware that she was slowly developing toxicity. Signs of mercury poisoning are insidious and often hard to detect. They include mental depression, irritability, fatigue, loss of appetite, anemia, and insomnia. It's easy to see how such symptoms might be classified as psychosomatic complaints by a physician and either ignored or treated with VALIUM. We may never know whether or not thousands of women experienced low-level mercury toxicity from their spermicidal jelly.

Boric acid is another baddie in spermicides. It has been used as an eye wash and as an antiseptic in ear, nose, and throat preparations. And it has been used in spermicidal suppositories (ANVITA). The medical literature is full of reports of boric-acid poisonings. Toxicity manifests itself as nervous system depression, skin rash, stomach upset, and diarrhea. As with mercury, boric acid can cause birth defects and since it could be absorbed from the vagina in early pregnancy when a woman may not realize she is pregnant, the hazards hardly seem worth the benefits, especially since the drug's effectiveness (as a spermicidal agent) has not even been established.

By now you may be getting pretty depressed. We have shot down birth control pills, the IUD, and after a big build-up we have even criticized spermicidal chemicals. But all is not as bleak as it appears. After years of indifference and inactivity the FDA has finally moved to eliminate most of the nasty chemicals from spermicidal creams and jellies. Be careful, though, there may still be a few holdovers on pharmacy shelves that contain mercury or boric acid (ANVITA containing both these chemicals was still available in 1979). **READ LABELS!** The good news, however, is that the current favorite ingredients, nonoxynol 9 and octoxynol, appear safe and effective. Basically, these chemicals are nothing more than fancy detergents. While the experts don't really know how they work to kill the sperm, one possibility is that they "dissolve" them to death. While the "oxynols" may occasionally cause a local irritation in sensitive persons there have been no reports of toxicity. That's not to say they are perfectly harmless—there have been reports of women who experienced burning and itching after inserting a spermicidal suppository and even some male partners have reported irritation after intercourse, but to date the incidence of these side effects appears low. And compared to the kinds of problems we have discussed earlier, one would have to say that these reactions are in a completely different class when compared to liver tumors and PID.

The drug companies have not missed an opportunity to capitalize on the apparent safety of spermicides. Recognizing that women are becoming more and more anxious about the Pill and the IUD, manufacturers of the ENCARE OVAL and SEMICID (spermicidal suppositories) have exploited this fear to push their products. Advertisements appeared in college newspapers and women's magazines emphasizing safety:

THE MOST TALKED ABOUT
CONTRACEPTIVE
SINCE THE PILL

Women using ENCARE OVAL say they find it an answer to their problems with the Pill, IUD's, diaphragms, and aerosol foams . . .

ENCARE OVAL is free of hormones, so it cannot create hormone-related health problems—like strokes and heart attacks—that have been linked to the pill. And, there is no hormonal disruption of your menstrual cycle . . . Safer for your system than the pill or IUD.

Now you can say goodbye to the Pill, the IUD, diaphragms, foams, creams and drippy jellies. SEMICID is here. SEMICID contains no hormones, so none can enter your system. Unlike the IUD, SEMICID can't penetrate the uterine wall. SEMICID is seldom irritating and can be purchased without a prescription.

What's wrong with that? Not a thing! In fact, we only wish the condom makers would be more active in following the lead of the spermicidal promoters. So far, so good, but the makers of the ENCARE OVAL really blew it when they moved away from the safety issue and started pumping the effectiveness of their product. In a slick three-page color ad that appeared in many medical journals they really got carried away. Three nude women (medical journal ads are often rampantly sexist) were featured with their testimonials: "I'm worried about taking the pill"—"I can't use an IUD"—"The diaphragm is just too much trouble." The ad claimed to introduce "A NEW CONCEPT IN CONTRACEPTION":

> ENCARE OVAL is a new and different vaginal contraceptive. The potent spermicide nonoxynol-9 is contained in a special base that melts at body temperature . . . In a recent West German survey of 287 physicians prescribing ENCARE OVAL, only 43 pregnancies were reported after 10,017 women completed 63,759 months of use. This represents a pregnancy rate of approximately 1 per 100 women years. (*Modern Medicine*, January, 1978)

Baloney! That ad was blatantly misleading. For one thing, they made it appear that the product was really unique ("new and different"), when in reality nonoxynol-9 has been the primary spermicide in such old favorites as DELFEN FOAM, CONCEPTROL, and EMKO for years. But even worse was the implication that ENCARE OVAL was 99 percent effective. While it's true that the "Oval" is different from foams, jellies, and creams in that the suppository can be inserted without an applicator and probably is less "messy," there is real doubt that it is any more effective than these older products. In fact, it may be *less* effective! The claims of effectiveness were based on a study done in Germany, which, according to the Food and Drug Administration "was poorly assembled and consists largely of testimonial evidence."[38] Physicians were paid to fill out questionnaires that had been distributed by representatives of the drug company. That just ain't kosher.

What is the success rate of spermicides used alone? According to the experts who have carried out the really extensive, well-designed investigations, spermicidal products are about 85 percent effective. That is to say, 15 out of 100 women could expect to become pregnant using this method of birth control over one year.[39,40] Yuck! That doesn't sound so hot. And it sure as heck doesn't come close to the 99-percent figure the ENCARE OVAL company was advertising in the beginning. But even if 85 percent doesn't look super-terrific, don't panic. Those statistics represent something called "use-failure" rates—the actual success rate depends on many factors—motivation, experience, convenience, partner acceptability, and so on. A particular method of birth control may *theoretically* be quite effective, but if used carelessly or only occasionally the actual failure rate may be significantly higher. There have been a zillion studies carried out in recent years in order to evaluate both the "use" as well as the "method" failure rate. Some studies have shown spermicidal failure to be as low as 1 percent while others have produced dismal "use-failure" rates of almost 30 percent.[41,42]

Not only can motivation and experience influence contraceptive effectiveness but so can the brand you select. Not all spermicides are created equal. Even if they contain the identical active ingredient there may be significant differences in relative potency. Some may disperse rapidly within the vagina while others fizz and foam slowly. With ENCARE OVAL one of the big selling points was the no muss, no fuss, no foam—just a simple vaginal suppository. But there's a catch. The couple has to wait after insertion before they initiate or resume lovemaking, or they could get into big trouble. Masters and Johnson (of *Human Sexuality* fame) recently evaluated the spermicidal effectiveness of the ENCARE OVAL in a sophisticated laboratory setting.

> **Following placement of the contraceptive, an unlubricated latex rubber dildo was introduced intravaginally by the female study subject who then manipulated this manually in a fashion simulating coitus. This method was employed to duplicate the mechanical thrusting with attendant dispersal of the contraceptive product that ordinarily occurs during sexual intercourse... Maximal spermicidal effectiveness was found between 5 minutes and 1 hour after insertion of the vaginal contraceptive... In contrast, tests at 30 seconds, 1 minute, and 3 minutes after contraceptive insertion showed poor spermicidal effectiveness... At test intervals more than 1 hour following contraceptive insertion, spermicidal effectiveness was diminished.[43]**

In order to get around this problem, the makers of the ENCARE OVAL offer the following recommendation: "IMPORTANT—WAIT TEN MINUTES after insertion to assure proper dispersion, which is necessary for contraceptive protection." Seems simple enough until you think about it. A lot of couples may find it too difficult to delay or interrupt their lovemaking to watch the clock. As Masters and Johnson pointed out in their article, "This disadvantage is not found with aerosol foam products that achieve maximal intravaginal dispersal within seconds after insertion."[44] And if a woman inserts the suppository in advance of intercourse she will also have to keep an eye on the clock to make sure she doesn't go over the one-hour limit at which point the effectiveness diminishes. Masters and Johnson also found that "preliminary testing done in the simulated female superior coital position points toward diminished spermicidal effectiveness in this situation."[45] In case that didn't make any sense (sex researchers love to use big words that no one can understand) what they were saying is that if the woman is on top during love-making the ENCARE OVAL may not work as well. Bummer!

Another important difference between various products is the concentration of chemical spermicide. The following table provides a quick summary of the concentration of nonoxynol-9 in various popular brands:

Concentration of Nonoxynol-9 in Spermicides[46]

Delfen Foam...................	12.5	percent
Koromex Foam	12.5	percent
S'Positive Suppository	10.0	percent
Because Foam.................	8.0	percent
Emko Foam...................	8.0	percent
Dalkon Foam	8.0	percent
Delfen Cream.................	5.0	percent
Conceptrol Cream	5.0	percent
Semicid Suppository	5.0	percent
Encare Oval Suppository	2.27	percent

Spermicidal concentration should not be the primary criterion for selecting a particular brand. There are other factors that can also influence overall effectiveness. Nevertheless, after evaluating various tests that compare the relative potency of different products, we have concluded that DELFEN FOAM is the most effective product available on the market today.[47]

DIAPHRAGMS AND CERVICAL CAPS

Diaphragms are messy, there's no denying that. You have to smear them with spermicidal cream or jelly which occasionally can lead to problems. Not too long ago a friend phoned us in the middle of the night in a panic. Seems that she had filled her diaphragm in the dark and as soon as she inserted it she knew something was very wrong.

There was a strange burning sensation that wouldn't go away. Upon investigation she discovered that she had made a dreadful mistake and used toothpaste instead of spermicidal jelly. We calmed her down, assured her that it was not an emergency, and recommended a douche in order to wash out the **Crest**. Such mistakes are probably rare, but some women do experience irritation from the jelly itself. About the only solution to this problem is to experiment with various brands that contain different ingredients. With some luck it may be possible to find one that doesn't produce any irritation. A cervical cap may offer another solution—more about that later.

How good are diaphragms? As usual the statistics vary greatly. Some researchers have found that anywhere between 10 and 30 women out of a hundred may become pregnant over the course of one year. But other researchers have found as few as 2.4 pregnancies per 100 woman-years of use.[48] This data is a little misleading, however, because it does not include women who were new users. Pregnancy risk is far greater during the first five months of use, when a woman is still new to the method. With practice it is conceivable such a success rate is achievable, especially if the diaphragm is fitted properly, is periodically rechecked for size, and the health provider has done a good job teaching how to insert and check its position.

As for the cervical cap, it is an unsung heroine in the barrier contraceptive arsenal. It has been ignored by the FDA and avoided by the major drug companies. The rubber cap fits snugly over the cervix and while significantly smaller than the diaphragm it too works by preventing sperm from wending their way up into the uterus. Unlike the diaphragm, it does not require spermicidal jelly (unless a woman wants double insurance) and it can be worn for days or even weeks at a time. But where are they—why is access to cervical caps so restricted in this country when they are widely used in Europe? According to Barbara Seaman, co-founder of the National Women's Health Network, drug companies "make more money from sperm-killing ointments used with diaphragms than from the diaphragms themselves, and fear cervical caps would cut into spermicide sales because less ointment is needed with them. Physicians don't like cervical caps because it takes them an hour to show patients how to use them. It's faster to write a prescription for pills."[49]

Because cervical caps have been unavailable in this country for so many years there has been little research done on their contraceptive effectiveness. The FDA recently recommended that the device should be banned, presumably because they lacked sufficient data to compare caps with other forms of contraception. This is a real shame if, as Seaman says, the cap is one of the safest, cheapest, and most convenient methods of birth control in existence. Fortunately, many research institutions are now testing cervical caps and a dentist from the University of Chicago recently developed a unique model that can be molded to exactly fit the woman's cervix. These inexpensive, custom-fitted "Chicago Caps" can be worn for months at a time because they have a one-way valve which permits menstrual flow. So the future looks very rosy for this old-fashioned contraceptive technique.

HOORAY FOR CONDOMS!

Condoms are great! They are surprisingly effective, they can dramatically reduce the incidence of venereal disease, they take the contraceptive responsibility off the woman, and best of all, they are SAFE for the health of both parties. And that is a Safe with a capital S! There are so many different condom products available that even a person who is allergic to latex rubber or a particular lubricant can find an option that is suitable. Another important advantage is availability. Unlike the Pill, the IUD, the diaphragm, or the cervical cap, condoms do not require a physician or a prescription. Today the corner drugstore almost inevitably has a large supply visible right up front. It wasn't always that way.

Once upon a time condoms were illegal—that's right, actually banned—in the United States. Anti-condom laws were passed by most states and in 1873 Congress itself acted to prevent their sale or use. Even local municipalities got into the act and over two hundred cities outlawed condoms. In fact, it was often illegal to even *tell* someone that there was such a thing as a condom that could prevent pregnancy. Until only a few years ago condoms were kept well hidden behind the counter in most pharmacies. (It wasn't until 1975 that a federal court struck down any law which barred open display of condoms as unconstitutional).

It's easy to understand why people were reluctant to use condoms as a method of birth control. There was the widespread belief that condoms weren't very effective. Although ranked higher than spermicides alone or even the diaphragm, most authorities list a 10 percent use-failure rate. But a recent article in *Consumer Reports* offers some exciting new statistics:

> **In three British studies covering 686 woman-years of experience, the use-failure rate for condoms was 4 percent; the method-failure rate (omitting pregnancies due to nonuse and**

misuse) was 1 percent. A 1 percent method-failure rate does not mean one pregnancy for each 100 occasions of use. It means only one pregnancy in every 100 women per year. Assuming two uses per week for each woman, that is one pregnancy in *10,000* occasions of proper use.[50]

The key to success with condoms is conscientious use. And that means every time you do it. During a marathon lovemaking session you better be prepared to use a *new* condom for each *act* of intercourse. And if you want even more protection, double up—both partners can take responsibility if the woman uses spermicidal foam while the man uses a condom. This is probably only necessary when a woman is most fertile—around the middle of her cycle. Excessive, but as the saying goes, "Buckle up for safety."

Now we can almost hear you saying, "Well, if condoms are such a good idea why don't more people use them?" They don't because condoms have a few disadvantages, mainly that they interrupt lovemaking and they can reduce physical sensation. A friend of ours once complained that using a prophylactic was comparable to going to bed with galoshes on. While a turn-off for many men, it could be a blessing for others. According to Masters and Johnson, premature ejaculation is a relatively common problem for men (and obviously for women as well). By reducing sensation, condoms may actually prolong intercourse and indirectly improve sexual pleasure for both partners. And new manufacturing techniques have reduced thickness without sacrificing quality.

Which brings up the matter of how a consumer goes about deciding what kind of condom to buy. There are so many products on the market with so many bizarre features that it is hardly surprising many middle-aged, middle-class folks get a little nervous when it comes to purchasing prophylactics. For example, there are textured, contoured, and ribbed models. Condoms come lubricated and unlubricated, with and without reservoir tips, in all the colors of the rainbow. And the names are wild enough to shock a scarecrow—BAREBACK, AROUSE, EXCITA, FIESTA, GALLANT, NON STOP, ROUGH RIDER, STIMULA, and CLIMAX. Condoms have come a long way from the days of the grungy little dispensing machines (found in gas-station men's rooms) that furtively advertised "for the prevention of disease."

If you really want to get the lowdown on condoms we recommend that you order a back issue of *Consumer Reports*. The October 1979 publication will tell you practically everything you ever wanted to know about this method of birth control. In addition, the experts from Consumers Union laboratory tested various brands and made excellent recommendations. Based on their research we feel comfortable endorsing NUFORM, TROJANS PLUS, FOUREX CAPSULATED, CONCEPTROL SHIELDS, HORIZON NUDA, EXCITA, FEATHERLITE WITH NATURSOL, HORIZON STIMULA, RAMSES, and SHEIK (Nos. 28 and 54). But please don't hold us responsible if a goof- up occurs. Nothing is perfect. Experiment and make the experience one of shared responsibility. If you select an unlubricated brand (and we think that is a good idea) don't use VASELINE or any similar product since it can weaken latex rubber. Stick with a safe, water- soluble lubricant like K-Y JELLY. For more detailed information on condoms send $1.25 to Subscription Director, Consumer Reports, P.O. Box 1000, Orangeburg, New York 10962, and request Volume 44, Number 10, October 1979.

VASECTOMY UPDATE: VILIFIED OR VINDICATED?

When we wrote *The People's Pharmacy* there were only a few early warning signs that disturbed us about vasectomies. Some doctors had voiced concern that men with vasectomies would be more prone to thrombophlebitis, arthritis, or multiple sclerosis, and would be more susceptible to infection. To date none of these fears have been substantiated and most appear unfounded. We were lulled into a possibly false sense of security and to be quite candid we had decided not to say another word about vasectomy in this new book. But before we gave up completely it seemed prudent to check with an expert. And Dr. Nancy J. Alexander, an investigator in reproductive physiology at the Oregon Regional Primate Research Center in Beaverton, Oregon fits that bill.

Dr. Alexander is in the very forefront of research into the immunological aftereffects of vasectomies. She and her associate, Dr. Thomas Clarkson, have come up with some fascinating discoveries. But before we get into their results, let's fill in some background so you can understand why this immune issue is so important. Just because the doctor cuts and ties a knot in the vas (the tube that carries sperm) doesn't mean the sperm factory goes on strike or cuts back production. The machinery continues turning out millions and millions of little sperm which keep piling up at the surgical barricades. What happens to them? Well, they don't just disappear. Usually they are ejaculated and never actually come into contact with the body's internal environment. But after a vasectomy, bits and pieces of sperm leak out of the tubes and are absorbed into the body. When these remnants encounter the immune system they are rejected just as if they were a foreign substance.

So, big deal. Unfortunately, it may be a big deal. Whenever you tinker with the immune system there is some cause for alarm and Dr. Alexander's research should make everyone sit up and take notice. She and her associates found that 50 percent of the monkeys developed atherosclerosis (hardening of the arteries) after vasectomies. They also found signs of potential kidney damage.[51–53] It is not entirely clear how all this happens but according to Dr. Alexander an "immune complex" may form between the antibodies and the sperm remnants. Apparently they glom together and then are deposited in the walls of arteries and in the kidneys. What are the implications of this monkey research for humans? To correctly report Dr. Alexander's statements here is an excerpt of our conversation:

People's Pharmacy: **If 50 percent of the men who have undergone vasectomy react in a similar manner as have your monkeys, is there the possibility that ten, fifteen, or twenty years later a man might have a higher incidence of atherosclerosis and kidney disease?**

Dr. Alexander: **Yes, if men do indeed respond in a similar fashion. However, there is no information yet available as to whether men and monkeys respond equally.**

People's Pharmacy: **And what is your recommendation to a man considering a vasectomy?**

Dr. Alexander: **Well, I am undoubtedly biased since I am so close to the studies. Based on what we know and the many things that we don't know at the present time my feeling is that he would be wise to wait several years until more information is available, especially since there are alternate methods of contraception available. I certainly feel that anyone who has a genetic predisposition—has parents who died of stroke or heart attack at an early age—should not get a vasectomy at the present time. Perhaps further studies will demonstrate that vasectomy has no ill effects, but certainly such studies are necessary before a green light can be given.**

People's Pharmacy: Wow! That's pretty heavy. What has been the result of your research and hasn't it scared some folks? What do you tell someone who has already had a vasectomy?

Dr. Alexander: Some urologists have stopped doing vasectomies or are counseling their patients or are not doing them on certain individuals. Unfortunately, our studies require an extended time frame so further information will not be immediately available. We can only describe the current state of the research.

People's Pharmacy: For a surgical procedure that has been performed on millions of men isn't it shocking that there are so many unanswered questions?

Dr. Alexander: There is no perfect contraceptive. Based on the current state of knowledge, one must weigh the pros and cons and decide what is most appropriate. Finding potential side effects associated with vasectomy is no different than the possibility of side effects associated with drugs.

People's Pharmacy: Might there be some reason for men who had a vasectomy and then began to develop atherosclerosis, coronary artery disease, kidney disease to consider having the vasectomy reversed [vasovasostomy]?

Dr. Alexander: Could be. Dr. Clarkson and I are doing a study and part of our study involves trying to determine whether that is the case in monkeys.

People's Pharmacy: Here's a question on another tangent. We've received a large volume of mail from women who are concerned about tubal ligation. What's your opinion on the safety of that procedure?

Dr. Alexander: There should be no problem. The reason for that is there is only one egg produced compared with millions and millions of sperm. Presently, except for the surgical risk it seems as if it may be the safest method of permanent contraception available.

And there you have it. We stopped the presses for that one because we felt it was so important. Since this surgery became popular millions of men around the world have had vasectomies. According to a recent editorial in the *Lancet* (a British medical journal), "there is a fast-growing trend towards male sterilization, and at present rates a good 10% of the husbands of women now aged 25–34 will be vasectomized by the time the wife is 35. In the United States about a million male sterilizations are now done each year. In India six million men were sterilized in 1976. Although the procedure is generally regarded as simple, effective, and safe, questions have been raised about possible long-term effects, resulting from antibody reactions to sperm and from hormonal imbalance or altered blood coagulation."[54]

It should be pretty obvious by now that we have more questions than answers. It may turn out that this is all a tempest in a teapot. We certainly hope so. But for a procedure that is being performed on so many men it is frightening that we do not know the long-term consequences of vasectomy. This isn't just a gap in our knowledge, it's a vast chasm. Most people are totally unaware that surgical procedures are poorly regulated. We agree with Dr. Alexander when she suggests that men wait a few years before going ahead with this operation. With any luck we will learn that our fears were unfounded. But if the early warning signs hold up—YIKES!—the dynamite could blow. Let's all keep our fingers crossed that this is one powder keg which just fizzles out.

PREGNANCY TESTS—RELIABLE OR RIP-OFF?

Whoops! Missed period. Could just be late, but with each passing day the anxiety level mounts. Am I or am I not pregnant? Once upon a time to answer that question a woman had to make an appointment with a doctor, submit to a pelvic examination, and provide a urine specimen. The whole schmeer might run as much as fifty dollars and take up a good chunk of the day and mistakes could still occur. If the answer came back NO it seemed like a tremendous waste of time and money. Today the corner drugstore carries do-it-yourself pregnancy tests with such reassuring names as PREDICTOR, ACU-TEST, ANSWER, DAISY 2 and E.P.T. (EARLY PREGNANCY TEST). They generally sell for between $8 and $11, and sales are booming. It's hardly any wonder— no waiting, no doctor, no pelvic examination, and no big bill. Seems wonderful, but are they really as good as the manufacturers claim?

The home pregnancy kits work on exactly the same principle as the most commonly used laboratory tests. As soon as a woman becomes pregnant, the placenta, which will be the fetus's "lifeline," begins to develop. As it grows, it secretes a hormone called HCG. If the urine contains this hormone the test will be positive and, in most cases, the woman is pregnant. (There are special situations where disease or drugs like major tranquilizers or methadone could foul up the test.) So far everything appears fine, but there is a clinker. Most laboratories recommend that a woman wait six weeks after her last period before coming in for a pregnancy test. An analysis done sooner than this is not very reliable. Despite this caution, the drugstore pregnancy kits encourage earlier testing and proudly tout 97 percent accuracy. And therein lies the rub. If the do-it-yourselfer comes up with a positive result (a brown doughnut-shaped ring at the bottom of the test tube) she can be 97 percent sure she is pregnant. So far this sounds accurate enough, but if the results are negative, there's still about one chance in four that you're pregnant when the test results say you are not.[55]

The sense of security a negative test produces can turn to ashes if a woman discovers a month later that the test was wrong. The earlier the kit is used, the more likely it is to produce this sort of "false negative" result which, for certainty's sake, requires retesting at a later date. So now, instead of only costing ten dollars you have to ante up to twenty in order to be absolutely sure the negative results were correct. There is another disadvantage to the home pregnancy tests. The directions are a little complicated and they must be followed meticulously for accurate results. A woman who is panicked about the possibility of an unwanted pregnancy (for example, a teenager unable to admit to the family doctor that she is sexually active) may find it difficult to concentrate on following the instructions exactly, and the test is not reusable.

So what's the bottom line on this thing? Are the do-it-yourself tests worth the time and money? We think they are, but with some qualifications. While we are in favor of any tools that give consumers greater involvement and power in their own self-care, we don't like to have people throw away money unnecessarily. A wise woman should first check in her community to compare costs of the home tests against laboratory fees. There are many agencies (Planned Parenthood, county health departments, women's clinics, the YWCA) that will provide a pregnancy test free of charge and with utmost confidentiality. Even the local hospital or a private doctor may charge less than the cost of a drugstore pregnancy kit and many doctors will run the test without requiring a physical exam. You can leave a urine sample and call back the same afternoon for the results.

But if you are one of those people who would just rather "do it myself," or if the home pregnancy test is cheaper or laboratories are not accessible, here are a few guidelines. Be patient. Wait a reasonable amount of time after your missed period before rushing out to buy a kit. (Two weeks should be the minimum.) Be sure to follow the instructions exactly. It is important that the urine specimen be the first of the morning (when HCG levels are highest) and the container you use should be clean. Even a hint of detergent can mess up the results, so rinse the jar with water at least six times and let it dry the night before.

If it is essential to know in less than two weeks you should have a new "radioreceptor assay" test done by a qualified laboratory. For all practical purposes it is 100 percent accurate and can give you an answer almost before your period is overdue. The test may cost a little more ($15 and up) and it does require donating a little blood instead of just providing a urine sample. But if you have to know immediately, the radioreceptor assay is for you. If time is not that crucial the home pregnancy test seems adequate.

WHO KILLED THE GRAY GOOSE?

What does the future promise in terms of birth control? Don't hold your breath waiting for a male Pill. There are still too many glitches in that gulch. What has been tried either reduces libido or makes the breasts grow. There are advocates of "natural" methods of contraception and they may promote astrology or some other wacko technique. The proponents of the mucus method may have something going because cervical mucus does change in consistency around the time of ovulation. A woman can be taught to feel this difference and when coupled with a careful temperature chart can certainly improve upon the old rhythm method. One of these days there will be some kind of litmus-paper test that will enable a woman to test vaginal secretions and precisely determine time of ovulation. As promising as these ideas are, "rhythm" still makes us a little nervous when it is all that is used. Combine it with some other contraceptive, however, and you can feel fairly secure.

What *is* the **right** method of birth control? Well, if you haven't learned from reading this chapter that there is no one "right" method for everyone, then you wasted a lot of time. Making a decision about contraception is very difficult. Inevitably, you end up with the dilemma of benefit versus risk and this is a very individual matter. Some people want effectiveness above all else and using the Pill is the only way they can have peace of mind. Others are so concerned about safety that even a small risk of serious side effects is enough to frighten them away from oral contraceptives or an IUD. We will not make any recommendations, but we will tell you where our heads are at. We're scaredy cats, and give us those good old-fashioned barrier contraceptives any day. You, dear reader, are on your own. Good luck on any method you may select!

REFERENCES

1. The Los Angeles Times-Washington Post News Service. "Pill Use Declining." *The Durham Sun* Nov. 3, 1979, p. 14-A.

2. Royal College of General Practitioners, Oral Contraceptive Study. "Mortality Among Oral Contraceptive Users." *Lancet* 2:727–731, 1977.

3. Selected Abstracts. "Mortality Among Oral Contraceptive Users." *JAMA* 239:790, 1978.

4. Baum, Janet, K. "Liver Tumors and Oral Contraceptives." *JAMA* 232:1329, 1975.

5. Mays, E. Truman, et al. "Hepatic Changes in Young Women Ingesting Contraceptive Steroids." *JAMA* 235:730–732, 1976.

6. Nissen, Edward D.; Kent, Deryck R.; and Nissen, Steven E. "Etiologic Factors in the Pathogenesis of Liver Tumors Associated with Oral Contraceptives." *Am. J. Obstet. Gynecol.* 127:61–66, 1977.

7. "High Hepatoma Risk for Women on Pill Four Years or More." *Medical World News* 19(15):13–14, 1978.

8. Ibid.

9. Rooks, Judith Bourne, et al. "Epidemiology of Hepatocellular Adenoma." *JAMA* 242:644–648, 1979.

10. Lingeman, Carolyn Harvey. "Evaluating Carcinogenicity of Oral Contraceptives." *JAMA* 236:1690, 1976.

11. Sherman, Barry M., et al. "Pathogenesis of Prolactin-Secreting Pituitary Adenomas." *Lancet* 11:1019–1021, 1978.

12. Kane, Francis J. "Evaluation of Emotional Reactions to Oral Contraceptive Use." *Am. J. Obstet. Gynecol.* 126:968–972, 1976.

13. Wallace, R. B., et al. "Altered Plasma-Lipids Associated with Oral Contraceptive or Estrogen Consumption." *Lancet* 2:11–14, 1977.

14. Roth, M. S., et al. "Effects of Steroids on Serum Lipids and Serum Cholesterol Binding Reserve." *Am. J. Obstet. Gynecol.* 132:151–156, 1978.

15. Bradey, Douglas D. "Serum High-Density-Lipoprotein Cholesterol in Women Using Oral Contraceptives, Estrogens and Progestins." *N. Engl. J. Med.* 299:17–20, 1978.

16. Trussell, R. James; Faden, Ruth; and Hatcher, Robert A. "Efficacy Information in Contraceptive Counseling: Those Little White Lies." *Amer. J. Pub. Health* 66:761–767, 1976.

17. Cunningham, F. Gary, et al. "Evaluation of Tetracycline or Penicillin and Ampicillin for the Treatment of Acute Pelvic Inflammatory Disease." *N. Engl. J. Med.* 296:1380–1383, 1977.

18. News. "HEW, FDA Issue Follow-Up Report on IUDs." *Am. Fam. Physician* 20(3):197–200, 1979.

19. Eschenbach, David A; Harnisch, James P.; and Holmes, King K. "Pathogens of Acute Pelvic Inflammatory Disease: Role of Contraception and Other Risk Factors." *Am. J. Obstet. Gynecol.* 128:838–849, 1977.

20. Ibid.

21. Hager, David W., and Majmudar, B. "Pelvic Actinomycosis in Women Using Intrauterine Contraceptive Devices." *Am. J. Obstet. Gynecol.* 133:60–63, 1979.

22. Dikshit, Suhasini, and Ledger, William J. "A Role of Antibiotics in the Contraceptive Effectiveness of an Intrauterine Foreign Body in the Rabbit." Unpublished Report.

23. Wrenn, T. R.; Weyant, J. R.; and Bitman, J. Abstracts, *Society for the Study of Reproduction* 3:23, 1970.

24. Zerner, John; Miller, Buell A.; and Gestino, Michael J. "Failure of an Intrauterine Device Concurrent with Administration of Corticosteroids." *Fertility and Sterility* 27:1467–1468, 1976.

25. Los Angeles Times-Washington Post News Service. "Pill Use Declining." *Durham Sun* Nov. 3, 1979, p. 14-A.

26. "Condoms." *Consumer Reports* 44(10):583–589, 1979.

27. Lane, M. E., et al. "Successful Use of the Diaphragm and Jelly by a Young Population: Report of a Clinical Study." *Family Planning Perspective* 8:81, 1976.

28. Rosenfield, Allan. "Oral and Intrauterine Contraception: A 1978 Risk Assessment." *Am. J. Obstet. Gynecol.* 132:92–106, 1978.

29. Lieberman, E. James. "Teenage Sex and Birth Control." *JAMA* 240:275–276, 1978.

30. Hatcher, R. A.; Stewart, G. K.; et al. *The Condoms* Contraceptive Technology, 1978–1979, New York, Irvington, 1978, pp. 85–88.

31. Felman, Yehudi M. "A Plea for the Condom, Especially for Teenagers." *JAMA* 241:2517–2518, 1979.

32. Johnson, J. W. C. "Gonorrhea in the Female," in Rovinsky, J. J. (ed): *Davis Gynecology and Obstetrics.* New York, Harper and Row, 1974, vol. 2, chap. 59.

33. Keith, Louis, et al. "Cervical Gonorrhea in Women Using Different Methods of Contraception." *J. of American Venereal Disease Association* 3(1):17–19, 1976.

34. Spermicidal Times. "Special Note." *Human Fertility* 9(1):11, March, 1944.

35. Evans, Robley, D. "Protection of Radium Dial Workers and Radiologists from Injury by Radiation." *The Journal of Indust. Hygiene and Toxicology* 25(7):253–267, 1943.

36. Macht, D. I. "On the Absorption of Drugs and Poisons Through the Vagina." *J. of Pharmacol. and Exp. Ther.* 10:509–522, 1918.

37. Tentative Findings of the Advisory Review Panel on Contraceptives and Other Vaginal Drug Products—Information Copy, November, 1978.

38. "Encare Oval Overpromoted." *FDA Drug Bulletin* 8(3):20–22, 1978.

39. Vaughan, B.; Trussell, J.; Menken, J.; and Jones, E. F. "Contraceptive Failure Among Married Women in the United States, 1970–1973." *Family Planning Perspectives* 9(6):251–258, 1977.

40. Vessey, M., et al. "A Long-Term Follow-Up of Women Using Different Methods of Contraception—An Interim Report." *J. of Biosocial Science* 8(4):372–427, 1976.

41. Population Information Program, The Johns Hopkins University. "Spermicides—Simplicity and Safety are Major Assets." *Population Reports* 7(5):H94–H95, 1979.

42. Paniague, M. E.; Varllant, H. W.; Gamble, C. J. "Field Trials of a Contraceptive Foam in Puerto Rico." *JAMA* 177:125, 1961.

43. Masters, William H.; Johnson, Virginia, E.; et al. "In Vivo Evaluation of an Effervescent Intravaginal Contraceptive Insert by Simulated Coital Activity." *Fertility and Sterility* 32(2):161–165, 1979.

44. Ibid.

45. Ibid.

46. Huff, James, and Hernandez, Luis. "Contraceptive Methods and Products." In *Handbook of Nonprescription Drugs* (6th ed), ed. Corrigan, L. Luan, Washington, D. C.: APHA, 1979, p. 256.

47. Homm, R. E., et al. "A Comparison of the In Vivo Contraceptive Potencies of a Variety of Marketed Vaginal Contraceptive Dosage Forms." *Curr. Ther. Res.* 22(4):588–595, 1977.

48. Vessey, M., et al. "A Long-Term Follow-Up of Women Using Different Methods of Contraception—An Interim Report." *J. of Biosocial Science* 8(4):373–427, 1976.

49. New York Daily News. "Greed Blocking Birth Control Device?" in *The Charlotte Observer* Aug. 2, 1979, p. 3-A.

50. Consumers Union. "Condoms." *Consumer Reports* 44(10):583–588, 1979.

51. Alexander, Nancy J. "Immunological Aspects of Vasectomy." In *Immunological Influence on Human Fertility,* B. Boettcher, ed. New York: Academic Press, 1977, pp. 25 — 46.

52. Alexander, Nancy J., and Anderson, Deborah J. "Vasectomy: Consequences of Autoimmunity to Sperm Antigens." *Fertility and Sterility* 32:253 —260, 1979.

53. Editorial. "Safety of Vasectomy." *Lancet* 2:1057—1058, 1979.

54. Ibid.

55. "The e.p.t. Do-It-Yourself Early Pregnancy Test." *Medical Letter on Drugs and Therapeutics* 20(8):39 — 40, 1978.

Drugs and Children

... **Into my memory shall run**
The thought of the child I love best,
Undressed and ready for bed,
Or hiding behind the door,
And cautiously peeping out;
Or stubbing his toe and falling,
And crying a little and climbing up on my lap,
To hear the story of the three bears over again.

—Sarah N. Cleghorn

Nothing in the world brings greater anguish to a parent than a sick child. Whether it be the pain and itch of poison ivy or the high fever of a nasty cold, you feel helpless and inadequate, and the urge to do something is overpowering. Giving a child medicine is almost always the quickest, surest way to feel that you're taking remedial action. But although the act of administering a drug makes a parent feel better, the remedy might not be particularly helpful and might actually do more harm than good.

Shopping for children's drugs is a little like skipping through a minefield. Pharmacy shelves are filled with ineffective, inappropriate, and downright dangerous medications. Now it doesn't bother us a whole heck of a lot if an adult is stupid enough to be snookered by slick advertising and take some worthless cold remedy. That's an independent decision. But it really raises our ire when a well-meaning parent encourages a trusting toddler to swallow a potentially hazardous concoction. Not all the criticism should be leveled at mothers and fathers, however. Part of the blame lies with the drug companies that seem to care more about the health of their profits than the well-being of their customers. Part of the blame lies with pharmacists for selling worthless or dangerous remedies when they should know better. And part of the blame lies with doctors who through ignorance or stupidity prescribe damaging drugs for children.

ANTIBIOTICS AND YOUR CHILD

The classic example of physician incompetence is the continued prescribing of tetracycline for young children, especially for relatively minor illnesses such as bronchitis or sore throat. (Rocky Mountain spotted fever is the only case for which tetracycline is undeniably the best choice.) Doctors have known for approximately twenty years that this broad-spectrum antibiotic has serious and long-lasting side effects when given to pregnant women, nursing mothers, or children under the age of eight. Tetracycline can produce an ugly stain and deformity in developing teeth that will last a lifetime. This is just the most obvious and most permanent adverse reaction. It can also interfere with normal bone growth, cause stomach upset, produce "bulging fontanel [skull] syndrome," precipitate a rash, and lead to fungal superinfections which may manifest themselves as vaginitis, proctitis, or thrush. Since 1972 the following warning has appeared in bold letters in the package inserts that accompany every preparation of tetracycline sold in the United States:

> **The use of drugs of the tetracycline class during tooth development (last half of pregnancy, infancy, and childhood to the age of 8 years) may cause permanent discoloration of the teeth (yellow-gray-brown). This adverse reaction is more common during long-term use of the drugs but has been observed following repeated short-term courses. Enamel hypoplasia has also been reported. Tetracyclines, therefore, should not be used in this age group unless other drugs are not likely to be effective or are contraindicated."**

The warning is reasonably clear. Most high-school graduates should be able to comprehend the drift of this message, so you would assume that someone who made it through college and medical school would have it knocked. Just to reinforce the point a little further, the Committee On Drugs of the American Academy of Pediatrics concluded in 1975 that besides the unpleasant side effects tetracycline produced, it had virtually no role in modern treatment. Their verbatim conclusion titled "Requiem for Tetracyclines" went like this:

> There are few if any reasons for using tetracycline drugs in children less than 8 years old. This class of antibiotics is capable of producing many adverse effects, two of which are specific for younger children and one of which is irreversible. Accordingly, it is difficult to justify the continued availability of drop or syrup formulations of tetracyclines. As long as they continue to be marketed, physicians who care for children should make every effort to discourage their use and curtail prescribing tetracycline for pediatric patients. [1]

In case you missed it, the pediatricians were making a plea for the removal of liquid tetracycline, since this kind of formulation appears to encourage inappropriate prescribing for small children. It wasn't until 1978 that the FDA got around to proposing the removal of "pediatric drops" from the market. Tetracycline syrups are *still* available despite the pediatricians' recommendation to the contrary.

The sting in this story is that doctors continued to prescribe tetracycline in huge quantities even after the dangers were widely known. In 1977 researchers from Vanderbilt University Medical School in Tennessee wrote in the *Journal of the American Medical Association* that "tetracycline continues to be prescribed widely for young children."[2] They studied the prescribing patterns of doctors participating in the Tennessee Medicaid Program. To their consternation they discovered that "more than one fourth (27%) of all physicians who cared for young children prescribed tetracycline during the two study years."[3] Even though they were dealing with a small sampling of children (less than 10 percent of all children under eight) they found that over 4,000 had received over 7,000 prescriptions for this antibiotic. They concluded their article with this devastating comment:

> While the magnitude of actual toxicity due to the misuse of tetracycline in this age group

cannot be ascertained from our data, exposure of
young children to these risks is inappropriate.
The prescribing of tetracycline to children under
8 years of age remains widespread; the requiem
for tetracyclines was sadly premature.[4]

If you aren't outraged about what you have just read then you
should have your head rebored. The continued prescribing of
tetracycline for young children isn't just shocking, it's criminal. Quite
honestly, we don't understand why the FDA continues to allow drug
companies to market these syrups given the fact that "eliminating
liquid formulations would decrease the strikingly large number of
inappropriate prescriptions for young children."[5] The excuse given is
that older people require their medications in liquid form. But that
just does not wash. Between July 1978 and June 1979 the National
Disease and Therapeutic Index recorded use of tetracycline liquid
preparations. It was found that 60 percent of the prescriptions for
these drugs were written for children between the ages of zero and
nine while people over sixty-five received only a paltry 6 percent.
Even more astonishing is the fact that 80 percent of the liquid drugs
in the tetracycline family (like AUREOMYCIN, DECLOMYCIN, TER-
RAMYCIN, and VIBRAMYCIN) were given out to children. How so
many doctors have somehow managed to miss or ignore a message
that has been bannered so widely for so many years is a mystery to us.
Perhaps if the suggestion that appeared in the *Yearbook of Drug
Therapy* were taken seriously, things would change:

> **Antibiotics continue to be a group of drugs for
> which questionable prescribing persists. Sig-
> nificant numbers of physicians apparently are
> still not aware that tetracycline stains teeth,
> inhibits bone growth and promotes enamel
> hypoplasia, fungal superinfection, gastroen-
> teritis, phototoxicity, rash and bulging fontanel
> syndrome in young children. If irrational pre-
> scribing by physicians continues to be docu-
> mented, some unpalatable form of control will
> be instituted or the privilege will be transferred
> to clinical pharmacists.[6]**

Because tetracycline is available in so many different brand-name
preparations it is virtually impossible for parents to know whether
they are giving their child this type of antibiotic unless a physician
tells them. Here is a table that lists most of the major sources of this

drug. By referring to this table you can double check to make sure your doctor hasn't slipped up and inadvertently prescribed tetracycline to your youngster:

BRAND-NAME ANTIBIOTICS
CONTAINING TETRACYCLINE

Achromycin	Oxy-Tetrachel
Achrostatin V	Paltet
Amer-Tet	Panmycin
Amtet	Partrex
Anacel	Piracaps
Aureomycin	Retet
Bicycline	Robitet
Bristacycline	Rondomycin
Centet	Sarocycline
Cycline-250/500	Scotrex
Cyclopar	SK-Tetracycline
Comycin	Steclin
Declomycin	Sumycin
Declostatin	T-Caps
Desamycin	T-125/250
Doxycycline	Terramycin
Doxy-II	Terrastatin
Doxychel	Tet-Cy
Duratet	Tetra-C
Fed-Mycin	Tetrachel
G-Mycin	Tetrachor
Kesso-Tetra	Tetra-Co
Lemtrex	Tetracyn
Maso-Cycline	Tetralan
Maytrex	Tetram
Mericycline	Tetramax
Minocin	Tetrex
Mysteclin-F	Trexin
Nor-Tet	Urobiotic
Oxlopar	Uri-Tet
Oxy-Kesso-Tetra	Vectrin

It may seem that we are making a mountain out of a molehill on this tetracycline issue. We think not. The effects can be far more devastating and long-lasting than is generally appreciated. According to a report from the National Institute of Health, "The tooth discolorations, ranging from yellow through brown and gray, usually result in acute embarrassment to young children. They sometimes lead to considerable psychological damage."[7] A distraught mother who wrote to our newspaper column, "The People's Pharmacy," feels the pain almost as much as her daughter:

> **My teenage daughter has lived with ugly yellow stains on her teeth for many years. She would like to start dating but her embarrassment about smiling or showing her teeth is making her terribly self-conscious. The stain was caused by an antibiotic called tetracycline that the doctor prescribed for an infection when she was two. Is there any kind of toothpaste she can use which will make the stain go away so she won't feel so insecure?**

Unfortunately, there is no toothpaste available which can undo the doctor's blunder. But that doesn't mean something can't be done. According to Dr. Edgar W. Mitchell, Assistant Secretary of the Council on Dental Therapeutics for the American Dental Association, there is a way to cover up tetracycline-stained teeth. The discoloration can be masked either of two ways.

> **In the bleaching technique, a concentrated solution of hydrogen peroxide is carefully applied with heat to the tooth surface. Several applications may be required before favorable results are seen. Also it is usually necessary to treat the teeth again in a few years to maintain the lighter color.**[8]

Please keep in mind that this technique requires the skill of an experienced dentist. The other procedure involves the "careful placement of acrylic—or porcelain jacket crowns—on the front teeth. A disadvantage is that these crowns must be remade every 3 to 5 years until the patient is about 20 years of age."[9] They may also need replacement periodically after that. Some dentists coat the teeth with resins that are bonded to the etched surface. No matter which approach is tried, you can count on the fact that it will cost you a bundle and take lots of time in the dentist's chair. If you would like to receive information about these procedures, you can request a free brochure titled *Bleaching of Vital Teeth* by sending a self-addressed, stamped envelope to:

American Association of Endodontists
P.O. Box 11728
Atlanta, Ga. 30355

DRUGS DURING PREGNANCY AND CHILDBIRTH

The inappropriate prescribing of tetracycline for children is unforgivable. Fortunately, the long-term result is primarily cosmetic. Although stained teeth may be a source of embarrassment, they do not usually affect dental health. Other prescribing patterns, however, may do considerably more damage. Ever since the Thalidomide tragedy the dangers of indiscriminate administration of drugs to pregnant women has been obvious. The March of Dimes has made every effort to advise women and health professionals about the potential problems drugs can cause during gestation. Nevertheless, women still run to the drugstore and self-medicate and doctors continue to hand out too many medications. Writing in the *American Journal of Diseases of Children,* Dr. Gail Udkov, an M.D. from the Department of Pharmacology and Toxicology at the University of Rochester School of Medicine, had this to say about her colleagues:

> **Despite the knowledge that drugs ingested by pregnant women may have untoward [undesirable] effects on the developing fetus or be handled differently by the newborn, worrisome prescribing patterns continue. A recent prospective study of a middle-to-upper class population of gravid [pregnant] women found a mean intake of 9.6 (range, 1 to 37) drug preparations during pregnancy, with a mean of 6.4 prescribed by the physician.[10,11]**

Until recently what we were mainly concerned about with drugs was the possibility that they would cause gross malformations—a child born with a cleft palate or a deformed limb. The hazards of alcohol abuse during pregnancy have been highly publicized following widespread recognition that a cluster of physical abnormalities in conjunction with mental retardation may result. But new research has raised a completely different and, in some respects, even more sinister specter. There is growing concern that many drugs may affect behavior and intellectual ability. This kind of drug-induced damage leaves no visible mark. An apparently healthy baby is born and parents breathe a sigh of relief that all is well. The child appears to grow normally and it is easy to miss or ignore subtle signs that indicate all is *not* as well as it should be. There have been reports that anesthetics such as nitrous oxide, ether, or trichloroethylene used during labor may cause behavioral deficiencies in some children. We don't have a firm grasp on all the kinds of behavior affected, but these children may show a lag in their ability to sit or stand, have a shorter attention span, have difficulty coping with complex tasks, and manifest signs of hyperactivity.[12] As they grow they may be slow to develop language and learning skills and have problems with memory and judgment.

What has made research into this question so incredibly difficult is that the true extent of the problem may not rear its nasty head or be noticed until the child reaches school and by then it is virtually impossible to trace the factors that could be responsible for poor performance. One large-scale investigation has attempted to get at this thorny issue by evaluating the impact of pain relievers and anesthetics used during labor and delivery. The results have sparked a fire storm of controversy within the medical community, especially among obstetricians and anesthesiologists. Dr. Yvonne Brackbill of the University of Florida and Dr. Sarah Broman of the National Institute of Neurological and Communicative Disorders and Stroke (NINCDS) teamed up to analyze the data from a study of 53,000 babies born between 1959 and 1966. This immense study (called the NINCDS Collaborative Perinatal Project) collected data from twelve teaching hospitals across the United States.[13] Besides keeping careful track of all medications and anesthetics used during delivery, researchers monitored the children's behavior and neurological development through age eight. The study was completed in 1974 and the results were first reported in *Science* magazine in 1978:

> **When the babies in these studies were tested at 4 months, 8 months, and 12 months of age, those whose mothers were heavily medicated lagged in this development of the ability to sit, stand, and move about. They were also deficient in developing inhibitor abilities, such as the ability to stop responding to redundant signals, to stop crying when comforted, and to stop responding to distracting stimuli. As they grew older, their development of language and cognitive skill lagged or was impaired.[14]**

These results have been roundly criticized by anesthesiologists, obstetricians, statisticians and perinatologists.[15] One professor of obstetrics and gynecology at Harvard Medical School, Dr. Emanuel

Friedman, described the report this way: "In tone, it is shrill and strident, leaving no doubt about the authors' preconceptions." There have been charges, counter-charges, and rebuttals and at times the language used by these respected researchers has been hot and heavy. It's easy to see why. Most women receive pain relievers or some kind of anesthetic during labor and delivery. One report has it that "now 95 percent receive these drugs."[16] Have these medications been causing harm? One can only wonder. Serious objections have been raised about the statistical techniques Brackbill and Broman used. So far there is more controversy than facts, and we will just have to wait to see what evolves, but there is reason to be concerned about the lack of information at this stage. Dr. Brackbill summarized the problem succinctly:

> **Although FDA procedures require proof of safety and efficacy before a new drug is cleared for clinical use, most drugs used for childbirth have not been approved for that purpose on any grounds; nor has any drug approval been based on tests that measure early neuro-behavioral effects on infants or predict later central nervous system dysfunction.**[17]

Women are rarely informed about what kinds of pain medicine they will receive during their labor and delivery. If an anesthetic has to be used, no one has mentioned the name ahead of time or described how it will work. All that must change! Recent research on animals demonstrates that DARVON (propoxyphene), synthetic sex hormones, PONDIMIN (fenfluramine), or VALIUM given during pregnancy can have significant effects on the offspring's behavior.[18] Does this mean that a woman should never take a drug during her pregnancy or during a difficult delivery? Of course not! There are times when a drug is absolutely necessary. But a careful balance must be struck and women (and men) must be informed about risks as well as benefits. As usual, the Committee on Drugs of the American Academy of Pediatrics says it best:

> **The committees recommend that until further studies are available, it would be advisable to avoid the use of drugs or drug dosages that are known to produce significant changes in neurobehavior of the infant. This statement does not mean that the patient in labor should be denied reasonable relief of pain by analgesic**

or anesthetic agents, but rather that the
minimum effective dose of these agents should
be administered when indicated. Moreover the
committees recommend that the physician discuss with the patient, whenever possible before
the onset of labor, the potential benefits and
side effects of maternal analgesia and anesthesia on both the mother and the infant.[19]

So before a woman gets close to experiencing labor pains she should
be absolutely sure she learns what all the contingencies may be. If a
pain reliever has to be used or an anesthetic given she should know
what she will receive and find out what is known about adverse
effects. With some planning and forethought childbirth can be made
safe for both mother and baby.

CASHING OUT ON COLD REMEDIES

So far we have been dumping on docs for prescribing inappropriate
drugs to children and pregnant women. But moms and pops can be
equally at fault. They really get bummed out when they see a snuffly
sneeze or hear a horrible hack and so they badger doctors for
unnecessary antibiotics like penicillin when little Jason or Jennifer
has a cold. If they are turned down by a conscientious doctor who
knows that antibiotics do absolutely nothing for viral infections the
parents may head for the local pharmacy where they can stock up on
all sorts of useless or harmful concoctions without a prescription. The
drug companies are more than delighted to supply anxious adults
with armloads of glop that will merely help alleviate useful
symptoms. Useful? You heard right! Most of the symptoms that
accompany a cold serve a constructive purpose (if nothing more than
to keep you off the streets where you will spread it around to others).
But more on that later.

Many of the popular products on pharmacy shelves are pitched
directly at the "kiddie" market. For example, there is CONTAC JR.
(with a 20-proof alcohol content, cherry flavor, and three active
ingredients, not counting the booze). Capitalizing on their "famous"
name, McNeil Labs bring your children CO TYLENOL FORMULA FOR
CHILDREN (also with three ingredients and 14-proof alcohol). You
can find a host of products with such names as BABY COUGH SYRUP,
CHILDREN'S HOLD 4 HOUR COUGH SUPPRESSANT, and KIDDIES
PEDIATRIC. Many of the cough and cold remedies for youngsters
have questionable ingredients. For example, CREOMULSION FOR
CHILDREN has creosote and ipecac (expectorants of unproved

efficacy), cascara (a laxative), menthol, white pine, wild cherry, and alcohol. There is little valid evidence that any of these ingredients will even suppress a bad cough. Antihistamines are another common constituent in cold remedies. They provide little if any benefit, and they can cause problems. Antihistamines typically produce drowsiness in adults but quite the opposite side effect may occur in some children. Experts for the American Pharmaceutical Association described what could happen:

> **A paradoxical effect frequently seen in children is CNS [central nervous system] stimulation rather than depression, causing insomnia, nervousness and irritability (e.g. phenindamine). For this reason antihistamines must be used cautiously in children with convulsive disorders.**[20]

As discouraging as it is to find so many unnecessary ingredients in children's cold remedies, it is downright disheartening to discover that there is one ingredient that could be fatal. CAMPHOR is the baddie and it should have been eliminated years ago. It is found in chest rubs, nose drops, and some cough remedies. Familiar products that contain camphor include VICKS VAPORUB, VAPOSTEAM, DRISTAN LONG LASTING VAPOR NASAL MIST, SINE-OFF ONCE-A-DAY, SINEX, VA-TRO-NOL, and VICKS INHALER.[21] It is also found in the antiseptic CAMPO-PHENIQUE which is used for fever blisters and cold sores. The Committee on Drugs for the American Academy of Pediatrics has taken a strong stand against camphor. Here are some of their observations:

> **Reports of camphor poisonings have appeared in the literature for more than 100 years. The National Clearinghouse of Poison Control Centers reported over 494 cases in 1973, of which 415 were in children less than 5 years old.**
>
> **Camphor is readily absorbed from all sites of administration, and several reports cite camphor intoxication secondary to vapor inhalation or skin absorption. A near-fatal case in a 6-month-old infant occurred after rubbing of the chest and nose with an ointment containing camphor, menthol, and thymol.**
>
> **Conclusions:**
> **1. Camphor has no established, therapeutic role in scientific medicine.**

2. **Camphor has potent, serious toxicologic actions; the ingestion of relatively small amounts has proven fatal.**

3. **Although accidental oral ingestion is the most common route of intoxication, significant quantities can be absorbed percutaneously [through the skin] and via inhalation.**[22]

In 1976 an FDA panel of experts recommended that if camphor is included as an ingredient in cold remedies, the label should contain this warning: "For external use only. Do not take by mouth or place in nostrils."[23] One cold remedy that contains camphor, SAVE-THE-BABY, not only doesn't include such a warning; it actually recommends internal use and placement in nostrils. According to the manufacturer, Vetree Products, Ltd., SAVE-THE-BABY is useful for:

> **Relief of certain symptoms of spasmodic croup, coughs, nasal irritation and congestion, throat irritation, bronchial irritation and muscular soreness of the chest, all when due to colds. For best results use SAVE-THE-BABY 'good and warm.'**
>
> **For relief of nasal irritations and nasal congestion associated with colds—rub nose with SAVE-THE-BABY and apply to nostrils.**
>
> **In severe cases where relief does not follow in half an hour, give SAVE-THE-BABY internally, following dosage direction given above [children over one year old—15 drops or one-half teaspoonful], and repeating every half hour until relieved (not more than six doses), or until the doctor arrives.**
>
> **Internal dosing may cause vomiting, but this should occasion no alarm as it helps to clear the phlegm and helps return to normal breathing.**
>
> *Beware Of Imitations.*
> *Accept No substitutes.*[24]

The instructions to take internally and repeat every half hour until relieved (up to six doses) are absolutely mind-boggling given the FDA admonition warning specifically against such dosing. Even more incredible is this drug company's casual dismissal of vomiting, since vomiting may be the first sign of camphor poisoning. According to the most knowledgeable pediatricians, "With mild poisoning, gastrointestinal tract symptoms are more common than neurologic, and include irritation of the mouth, throat, and stomach. *Vomiting may be the only symptom, or it may precede or follow other symptoms.*"[25] (Italics ours.) We find it paradoxically fitting that the label on the SAVE-THE-BABY box contains this not so amusing cop-out:

> **The name "Save-The-Baby" is not intended to imply that the product will "save babies," but rather that it is efficacious in those conditions for which it is recommended.**

We have serious doubts that the product is effective and are much more concerned that it might damage babies rather than save them. Camphor should be eliminated from all over-the-counter products and parents should be reluctant to use any medication that contains this ingredient, including chest rubs. In the first three months of 1979 there were 290 reports of camphor emergencies, an increase of 17 percent over 1978.[26] "The FDA advisory panel recently decided that camphor has no known therapeutic uses and that it is unsafe in concentrations higher than 2.5%."[27] The following products continue to be sold in levels that exceed that amount: CAMPHORATED OIL, CAMPHO-PHENIQUE, CAMPHOR SPIRITS, SOLTICE-HI-THERM ANALGESIC BALM, BEN-GAY CHILDREN'S RUB, SOLTICE QUICK-RUB, SAYMAN SALVE, VICKS VAPORUB, PANALGESIC, HEET, SOLTICE QUICK RUB (CHILDREN'S), and SLOAN'S LINIMENT. Until the FDA gets off its duff and assumes its responsibility to protect our children, parents will have to be vigilant and take on the job themselves.

What should you do when your child has a cough? If you want to be safe, do absolutely nothing. Coughing is useful. As bad as it sounds to an adult, a cough helps keep air passages open by clearing away excess gunk in the lungs. What's more, the combination of ingredients in many of the cough remedies on the market is totally irrational. More often than not they contain expectorants which are theoretically supposed to help loosen mucus and aid in expelling phlegm. (But how many youngsters can master the gruesome technique of coughing up the stuff?) Simultaneously, the same products usually contain a cough suppressant which is supposed to prevent expectoration and keep mucus stuck in the lungs anyway. Just for good measure they throw in an antihistamine to thicken mucus and make it even harder to get up. To say these ingredients are working at cross purposes would be a superb understatement. What's more, many of the most popular products contain four or five active ingredients. These "multi-symptom" cold remedies are an ad man's dream come true and a concerned consumer's nightmare.

For this reason many medical authorities blast the use of these products. A panel of experts for the FDA recommended over three years ago that drug companies should limit the number of active drugs they put in any given product to three. You might think a conscientious firm would heed the recommendation. Not bloody likely when you consider the stakes of this business. Americans spend approximately **one billion dollars** each year on cough/cold items.[28] Perhaps one of the most cynical products introduced *after* the FDA panel recommendation was COMTREX. Not only did the manufacturer (Bristol-Myers) ignore the suggestion to limit the number of ingredients, the company actually flaunted their inclusion. The product contains five active ingredients, including a pain reliever, decongestant, cough suppressant, and an antihistamine, not to mention a whopping 40-proof alcohol liquid preparation. In a pitch to pharmacists the company placed the following ad in the trade publication *Drug Topics:*

> COMTREX really caught on with people who caught colds. In fact, COMTREX is the most successful new product introduction in the history of the general cold remedy category.
> Part of that success is because all over America people have discovered COMTREX is a different kind of cold reliever. It's a multisymptom cold reliever that all by itself helps relieve more symptoms than most other products.
> And part of that success is due to the heavy advertising we've put behind COMTREX. Highly effective print and television campaigns that gave 8 million people a reason to buy COMTREX in just one year. And we'll be duplicating our first year effort in the upcoming cold season. . .
> And isn't that the kind of success you want to put on your shelves?[29]

Pharmacists may choose to put COMTREX on their shelves but we would not choose to put it in our bodies or the bodies of our children. We would prefer to follow the recommendations put out recently by the Committee on Drugs of the American Academy of Pediatrics:

> A cough is usually a mild symptom of the common cold, but even in this instance clearing of secretions is probably beneficial.
> A productive cough [one that brings up

> phlegm] in acute illness and a nonproductive
> cough (as in influenza, the convalescent phase
> of pertussis [whooping cough], and so forth)
> should be suppressed only when repeated bouts
> of coughing result in emesis [vomiting], exhaus-
> tion, or insomnia. (A truly "nonproductive"
> cough is unusual in infants and young children.)
>
> In general, regardless of the etiology or
> duration a productive cough should not be
> suppressed, and treatment should be directed
> toward mobilizing secretions. Nonmedical
> approaches (e.g. physiotherapy, hydration, and
> so forth) are the most likely to be beneficial.[30]

If your young person truly does have a non-productive cough that
won't respond to a piece of hard candy or a humidifier and is
seriously disturbing his sleep or keeping him home from school, then
here are some simple guidelines to follow. For children more than one
year old the American Academy of Pediatrics recommends single-
ingredient preparations that contain either codeine or dex-
tromethorphan. Unfortunately, you really have to hunt to find
products that contain just one single ingredient. In all our research we
have been able to locate only two brands that satisfy us (except for
generic codeine): SILENCE IS GOLDEN (paradoxically made by the
same Bristol-Myers of "Multi-Symptom" fame) and TRICODENE
DM. Products that come close enough to satisfying our high standards
to warrant a recommendation include ST. JOSEPH COUGH SYRUP FOR
CHILDREN, SYMPTOM 1, ROMILAR CHILDREN'S COUGH SYRUP, HOLD
4 HOUR COUGH SUPPRESSANT (LOZENGES), and SUCRETS COUGH
CONTROL FORMULA.

TEASPOONS ARE FOR TEA—NOT FOR MEDICINE

Just because you have finally found an acceptable cough medicine
doesn't mean your worries are over. One of the big problems with
liquid medicine (of any variety) is that you have to measure out the
correct dose. Since most prescription and over-the-counter medicine
for children comes in liquid form correct dosing is extremely
important. But don't count on the instructions you find on the label.
For example, the COMTREX bottle suggests that for "children 6—12
years: ½ the adult dose in medicine cup provided (1 TBLS.)" In our
opinion, that is a pretty broad recommendation. A scrawny six-year-
old can differ significantly in drug sensitivity from a stocky twelve-
year-old, just as a 95-pound grandmother can differ from a 248-

pound football player. The "one for all" type dose strikes us as patently preposterous.

Even if detailed dosage instructions were provided, you would still have to get the stuff from the bottle to the mouth correctly. This may seem like a simple act but believe us, it is fraught with obstacles. For one thing, your little gremlin may not be in a mood to cooperate. And for another, it takes a mighty steady hand to fill a spoon to the brim and then transfer it intact to a waiting mouth. Think about it for a minute—even when you take stuff yourself, how many times have you spilled the medicine before you could slurp it? If so, that was an incorrect dose! But even assuming you have nerves of steel and a steady hand and are able to get the medicine from bottle to mouth in one perfect swoop, chances are excellent that you will still be administering a totally inaccurate dose. The reason is that while ordinary teaspoons are fine for tea they're terrible for medicine. A medical teaspoon should be *exactly* 5 ml. but the spoons you've got lying around in the kitchen drawer may not come close to that. According to the Committee on Drugs for the American academy of Pediatrics:

> **Teaspoons are particularly poor measuring and administering devices. The measured capacity of the teaspoon has been shown to be within the range of 2.5 to 7.8 ml. In addition, teaspoons are a poor delivery device because they tip easily. Furthermore, the same spoon, when used by different persons, may deliver from 3 to 7ml.**[31]

If anything, the pedes may be underestimating the problem. Several studies of spoons used by families to administer medications have found that a teaspoon might hold as little as 2 ml or up to about 10 ml. If your physician's prescription for a tablet were so vague that you might take anywhere from one to four pills, you would be justifiably alarmed. But that is about what happens when you pick a kitchen spoon at random.

These discrepancies can muck up an entire treatment program. For one thing, not enough medication may be given to cure an ailment. Investigators have found that some children's ear infections did not go away because they were not given an adequate dose of antibiotic. Other families have complained that the ten-day supply of liquid medicine runs out by the eighth day and have criticized the pharmacist when they have to purchase another entire bottle. This is not only expensive, but the person receiving such heavy-handed spoonfuls runs the risk of adverse effects from an overdose.

So what is the answer to the dilemma of the kitchen spoon? If the blasted thing is inaccurate what's better? Glad you asked that question. The measuring spoon found in most kitchens is—it delivers an accurate teaspoon dose, if you can get it down without spilling any. There also are some products on the market that will eliminate the muss and fuss *and* insure proper dosing. For example, there is a medical spoon available with a hollow calibrated handle (much like a test tube) that tells you the precise dose from one-quarter to two teaspoons. We have had ample opportunity to try the spoon on our three-year-old and can testify that it eliminates a lot of uncertainty, struggle, and spills. Even more accurate are the oral syringes that measure up to two teaspoons. (You can't put a needle on the end, so there is no possibility of abuse.) If your pharmacist is on the ball he or she will have these products available. If you wish to order directly there are two major companies that will supply them for a minimal cost. You can write to:

Robbins Associates, Inc.
1151 Rupp Drive
Burnsville, Minnesota 55337

OR

Apex Medical Supply, Inc.
9701 Penn Avenue South
Minneapolis, Minnesota 55431

The cost of the "EZY-DOSE SPOON," calibrated eye dropper, or oral syringe each costs about $1.00—$2.00. In our opinion this small investment is certainly worth the expense whether you have to give a liquid antibiotic or a cough medicine.

SORE THROATS

Mommy, it hurts! That's a familiar refrain when a child has a scratchy throat. Since we've all been there ourselves at one time or another we know how painful a bad sore throat can be. As usual, the temptation to *do something* is overwhelming. And as usual, the drug companies stock pharmacy shelves with all kinds of tempting and inappropriate products. There are lozenges and gargles galore and selecting a particular brand is a little like playing Pin the Tail on the Donkey. Used to be we believed that the awfuller it tasted the better it must be. For years, LISTERINE had the inside track for both flavor and sales. But the claim that LISTERINE would relieve sore throat symptoms was only a smart-sounding slogan. As we mentioned in Chapter 1, the Federal Trade Commission took the Warner-Lambert Company to court for false and misleading advertising. The case was as long, drawn-out, and bitter as they come. But when the FTC finally won, the company hypesters had to stop advertising LISTERINE for the treatment of sore throats—better still, they actually had to use prime-time television to tell folks that gargling with LISTERINE wouldn't do a blasted thing for their sore throats.

Unfortunately, LISTERINE isn't the only product deserving that kind of attention. You could practically eliminate the use of all sore-throat products and you would be none the worse for wear. In fact you would probably be better off. None of the products available can cure or shorten the duration of an infection and some may actually cause more harm than good. Throat lozenges almost inevitably contain a local anesthetic called benzocaine. Theoretically this ingredient should be able to reduce symptoms if provided in a strong enough concentration. But take heed of what the American Pharmaceutical Association has to say:

> **Benzocaine is beneficial in diminishing sore throat symptoms in concentrations of 5—20%. Concentrations of less than 5% are not considered beneficial. There are currently no OTC [over-the-counter] preparations containing an effective benzocaine concentration.[32]**

Even if benzocaine was added in a concentration that was strong enough to do something there would be reason to avoid it. For one thing, the drug could cause an allergic reaction and just add to your child's sore-throat misery. For another, covering up serious sore-throat symptoms is dangerous. These symptoms are sending out an important message. It is difficult if not impossible to tell the difference between a garden-variety virus infection and a nasty strep throat without a culture. And an untreated strep infection (group A beta-hemolytic streptococci) can, if ignored, occasionally lead to rheumatic fever or kidney disease. That is why doctors justifiably emphasize the importance of taking cultures and initiating antibiotic treatment. What's more, penicillin will do absolute wonders for this kind of bacterial sore throat. The antibiotic will wipe out symptoms quickly and prevent serious complications from developing, if you follow through on a full ten-day regimen.

But there is no reason to truck your sick child to the doctor's office in order to get that culture. Why expose the youngster to an office full of other sick kids, and if she or he really has a strep infection why expose others to a contagious disease? What you can do is obtain the throat culture yourself. That's right, you can learn to swab your own child's throat. All you need is some training and cooperation from your physician. Now if all this sounds a little hard to believe, just note the results of some studies presented to the American Academy of Pediatrics:

> Over a ten-month period, 142 parents volunteered to take part in the study. A medical student or child health associate showed parents how to take a throat culture and supervised a trial swabbing in the office. The parents took home a kit containing a sterile dacron swab and a sealed filter-paper strip. Seventy-nine parents got a culture from their child at home when they suspected strep infection. The student or health associate took a duplicate culture the same day either at the home or in the office. All cultures were mailed to a state lab for analysis . . .Of the 79 duplicate cultures obtained from the first group, the results agreed in 77 instances or 97.5% of the time . . .
>
> Johns Hopkins Associate Pediatrics Professor Harvey P. Katz found that mothers' positive strep cultures agreed with those taken by professionals in 136 of 137 paired home-vs.-clinic cases.[33, 34]

Those results are extremely impressive. It is unlikely you would get any better agreement if you had two health professionals collect the samples. What this means is that you can find out quickly and easily if your child requires antibiotic treatment and once the therapy is initiated you can check with another swab to make sure it has been successful. You can cut down on office visits, keep your child comfortable at home, and save money to boot. Why not talk it over with your doctor next time you visit? If you get a green light you can take home a tongue depressor and a sterile swab and be ready next time a bad sore throat strikes. Of course, you'll have to run the culture into your pediatrician's office for analysis but that's easier than bundling up a sick child. And if, as is likely, the throat turns out to be a viral infection, just stick to the salt-water gargle (one-half teaspoon in a warm eight-ounce glass of water). Don't throw away money on expensive and useless medications.

FIGHTING A FEVER MAY BE FOOLISH

Parents freak when children develop a fever. At the first sign of an elevated temperature most people reach for the aspirin bottle because once the mercury in the thermometer creeps above the magical 98.6 mark we assume the kid is sick. But what is a fever in the first place? And does it deserve the bad rep it's developed over the years? Body temperature is a very personal thing. Although the average is 98.6 there is no reason to get worried if your level hangs in at 97 or even 99. Your temperature is set by an incredibly sensitive internal thermostat and (talk about climate control!) the body does a fantastic job of regulating the internal environment under all sorts of extremes in external temperature fluctuation.

When you develop an infection your body's defensive armies go into action. White blood cells are mobilized from all over and rush to the battlefront. As they start knocking off the bad guys (viruses and bacteria) they begin manufacturing a special chemical called "endogenous pyrogen" which is a fever producer. This substance heads for the brain, which is where your body's thermostat is located. Once it arrives at your climate-control center endogenous pyrogen resets the thermostat at a higher level. Immediately the message is spread throughout the system—*conserve heat.* Blood vessels in the skin start to constrict. The effect is a little like running your car with the radiator disconnected. That may seem a ridiculous analogy, but it is much more realistic than you would ever imagine. The skin is a remarkably sensitive temperature regulator. In the summer when the weather gets really warm you sweat a great deal and your blood vessels dilate like crazy so the circulating blood can be cooled by the passing air. Your car keeps its engine cool by circulating water through the radiator where it too is cooled by the air. If you were to reset the car's thermostat higher, or by chance disconnect the radiator entirely, the temperature inside the engine would climb rapidly. Well, when blood vessels start to constrict that is basically what happens: less blood is exposed to the cooling effect of air, and core temperature in your internal engine starts climbing. And if endogenous pyrogen sets the thermostat really high (say 102 to 104), you will have chills and need to pile on the blankets. Your muscles will start contracting, which will probably make you shiver, raising temperature even more. Your skin will feel hot and dry and again the heat conservation system is working smoothly because the less you sweat the more heat will be retained.

So, what difference does it make if your body does go to extreme measures to raise temperatures? Just this. A fever makes you feel yucky. Muscles and joints ache, eyes get glassy and you want to stay in bed. Right! Now you're beginning to see the light. For one thing, a fever keeps you off the streets and is a nice evolutionary adaptation to keep you from spreading whatever crud you picked up to everyone else on the block. But a fever does something else that may be much more important than inducing rest. Dr. Matthew Kluger, a professor of physiology at the University of Michigan, reported that when reptiles and fish develop a fever after a bacterial infection, their survival rate is improved. Attempts to lower body temperature by using aspirin actually increased mortality. It is his belief that a moderate fever may be beneficial and adaptive rather than harmful.[35] One of the proposed explanations to account for the positive effect of a fever is that it causes iron levels in blood to fall. Bacteria have problems surviving if iron falls low enough. Drs. Charles Dinarello and Sheldon Wolff from Tufts University School of Medicine made the fascinating discovery that a similar mechanism may take place in humans:

> **In our laboratory we have found a similar drop in blood iron levels in people with natural fevers and in volunteers given experimental fevers, and we have further explored the connection between fever and iron levels in animals. The substances that induce experimental fever in people have two effects in mice: they lower blood iron levels and bolster the animals' resistance to infection. This increased resistance to infection may be related, as it is in the lizard, to levels of iron so low that microorganisms cannot grow.[36]**

Of course there is little doubt that a very high temperature can be dangerous and deserves treatment. Further research on birds, mammals, and eventually humans will be required before we know for sure whether or not a fever is a useful adaptive response.

The moral of this tale is, relax, pop. A fever is only a symptom. You don't have to make heroic efforts to bring down a mild elevation in temperature. What IS important is what's causing the fever. Giving aspirin may make the child feel better temporarily, but it won't shorten the duration of the infection. Only Mother Nature and a strong immune system can do that.

ASPIRIN AND YOUR CHILD

Now please don't get us wrong. There is certainly a place for aspirin. When a child really feels miserable because of pain or a fever you ought to provide some relief. But what about the dose? How much baby aspirin is right for your youngster? You would think that there would be a ready answer for such a simple question. We hate to disillusion you one more time, but you guessed it, there is a surprising lack of unanimity among the "experts" when it comes to figuring out proper dose. In fact, that is putting it mildly! A recent article published in *The Journal of Pediatrics* titled "Aspirin for Infants and Children" revealed some amazing information.[37] The authors mailed a questionnaire to 5,724 pediatricians. Of the 2,296 doctors who responded it was surprising to see how widely they differed in their prescribing practices. Some doctors recommended aspirin every three hours while others preferred every four or six hours. Some recommended 65 milligrams (mg) for each year of age while others thought 81 mg was right. Many doctors recommended one baby aspirin tablet for each ten to fifteen pounds of body weight but a significant minority believed a higher dose was necessary. And the physicians relied on many different methods for calculating dose.

It is hardly surprising that there is such variability among physicians. The standard reference books that doctors rely on to determine dose also disagree. The pediatricians were almost unanimous, however, in agreeing that the current labeling dose for children's aspirin is inadequate. After analyzing the survey, the investigators observed:

> **The labeled dosage schedule that has long been on pediatric aspirin preparations is at variance with the recommendations in authoritative medical references, studies demonstrating antipyretic [fever lowering] effectiveness in children, and the prescribing habits of pediatricians . . .**
>
> **Aspirin is the most widely used antipyretic-analgesic in pediatric practice in the United States and, when properly used, is safe and effective. For some years, however, widely divergent dosage schedules for children have been recommended by various authors and apparently used by practicing pediatricians. Such a multiplicity of dosage instructions would be expected to cause confusion among parents, perhaps contributing to the administration of improper dosages which could result in salicylate intoxication.[38]**

One of the problems with dosage instructions that are inadequate is that parents may unintentionally "double up" the amount they give or repeat a dose too often. As a fever starts to climb or the pain returns, the temptation is strong to give another couple of tablets after only three hours. This can lead to aspirin toxicity which is very dangerous in children.

How do you find the solution to this Chinese puzzle? If you want to take the quick and easy way out you could follow the FDA's shotgun recommendations. Here are the broad guidelines they suggest:

RECOMMENDED DOSE OF BABY ASPIRIN TABLETS

AGE OF CHILD	NUMBER OF 81-MG TABLETS/4 HOURS	DOSAGE IN MG EVERY 4 HOURS	MAXIMUM DOSE PER 24 HOURS
Under 2 Years	Physician Only	—	—
2 to under 4	2 tablets	160	800
4 to under 6	3 tablets	240	1200
6 to under 9	4 tablets	320	1600
9 to under 11	5 tablets	400	2000
11 to under 12	6 tablets	480	2400

Children over twelve can take 8 baby aspirin tablets (81 mg or 1 1/4 grains each). It is recommended that not more than five dosages in 24 hours be used unless the doctor specifies otherwise.

Using this chart makes us a little nervous. As you can see, the age categories are fairly general. A six-, seven-, and eight-year-old would all receive the same dose, four tablets. That does not take into account the tremendous variation in size and body weight that can occur. A short, underweight six-year-old can really differ from a chunky child of eight-and-a-half in his ability to absorb medication, but with this formula they would be treated the same. So if you would like to be more precise in your calculations, pay attention. We are going to provide you with a formula that will allow you to determine a dose that corresponds to your child's weight.

The doctors who ran the pediatricians' aspirin survey concluded that an appropriate dose of aspirin in children should be kept "between 10 and 20 (preferably 15) mg/kg."[39] That seems complicated even if you translate it into the word equivalent "milligram per kilogram," especially since "baby" or "children's" aspirin is often labeled in an archaic measurement called grains (1 1/4 grains to be

exact; versus 5 grains for adult aspirin). As far as we are concerned
grains belong on the farm so let's convert 1 1/4 grains to metric
units—81 milligrams. So far so good, but who knows how much their
child weighs in kilograms? Okay, enough is enough. Calculating a
dose of *15 mg/kg* is not too hard (divide the child's weight in pounds
by 2.2, then multiply that times 15 for the total dose). But if your
child is sick you are in no mood to start converting and figuring, so we
have done that for you. To make matters simple this dose comes out
to **1 baby aspirin for each 12 pounds of body weight.** So if Junior
weighs 24 pounds, he should get two tablets (81 mg each); 36
pounds, 3 tablets, and so on. Of course it is guaranteed that your
young person won't weigh a convenient increment of 12 pounds so
you will probably have to get out the old calculator and divide by 12.
If Junior is 30 pounds, divide by 12 and you arrive at 2 1/2 tablets. If
he is 39 pounds, divide by 12 and you get 3 1/4 tablets. It isn't easy to
cut a child's aspirin into neat fractions, but with a little diligence you
should be able to come up with something pretty close.

Before you start giving the medication, recall some words of
warning. "Every four hours" means just that. Do not start cutting
corners by giving aspirin every three or three and a half hours. And
remember, aspirin can be irritating to the stomach. Even if you give it
in chewable, yummy orange flavor, make sure your child washes it
down with a good-sized glass of liquid. Not only will this reduce the
likelihood of irritation, it should speed absorption into the
bloodstream. And if you are ever in doubt about the severity of the
situation always call your doctor!

EARACHES: OH, THOSE OTITIS BLUES

If your young person hasn't had at least one ear infection by the
time she or he reaches the age of two you must be living a charmed
life. Otitis media, as the doctors call it, is extremely common. In fact,
this may be a gross understatement. Dr. Jerome Klein, Director of the
Division of Pediatric Infectious Diseases at Boston City Hospital,
calls "the incidence of middle ear disease 'staggering.'" Of approximately 3.3 million infants born in the United States last year, he
predicts that nearly one third will have three or more separate
episodes of otitis media by the age of 2 years."[40] If misery loves
company you can take assurance from the fact that many other
parents have gone through exactly what you've experienced.

Although there are lots of theories as to why young children are
more susceptible to ear infections than older children or adults, we're
still in a twilight zone when it comes to hard facts. Whatever the

cause, ear infections are a mess. For one thing, they can hurt like the devil and for another they could lead to serious complications if left untreated. If the infection gets "loose" and hits the nervous system, meningitis can occur and that's pretty scary. A far more common problem is loss of hearing. Even a small impairment during the learning years can interfere with language development and social adjustment. So don't take a child's earache lightly.

Although only a doctor can determine the severity of ear disease, with some motivation, a little practice, and a doctor who is a good teacher parents can become skilled in the use of an otoscope—the little funneled flashlight a doctor uses to check out the eardrum. If your child is one of the susceptible ones who seems to develop an infection every time you turn around, it might be worth investing in an inexpensive instrument. "Inexpensive" is a relative term in this instance—no medical equipment is really cheap. Your rock-bottom, no-frills otoscope will run about $40. If your doctor will show you how to look at the ear when your child is healthy, you can check for telltale differences in the appearance of the eardrum when he has a cold or complains of an earache.

Since ear infections are serious business they deserve prompt treatment. And antibiotics are the answer. There was a time when **Penicillin** was the drug of choice. But that was in simpler days when the bacterium responsible for most infections in the ear was pneumococcus. Times have changed and today, a lot of doctors are worried about something called *H. influenzae*. Now this rather benign-sounding bug bears no relation to influenza or a viral infection. *H. influenzae* is a bacterium and a nasty one at that. And what is so bothersome is that it is becoming resistant to antibiotic treatment. **Ampicillin** and **Amoxicillin** (AMOXIL, LAROTID, POLYMOX, ROBAMOX, TRIMOX, and WYMOX) used to be guaranteed winners for nearly all ear infections. **Amoxicillin** has a slight edge because, with a lower dose, the levels of medication in the child's bloodstream are higher. But if you want **Amoxicillin** to really do a good job it should be taken on an empty stomach with a large glass of water (and that includes the liquid medicine as well). Side effects to be alert for with **Amoxicillin** include stomach upset, nausea, vomiting, and diarrhea. A skin rash is also a possibility. If your child is allergic to **Penicillin** avoid **Amoxicillin** since it is chemically similar and could produce a life-threatening reaction. And always follow the doctor's instructions to give the full course of medicine even if improvement is quick and dramatic following initial doses. Otherwise the beasties could come back stronger than ever.

Now, unfortunately, the little buggers of *H. flu* are getting "stronger" and so might survive a usual regimen. Fortunately, the resistance hasn't become so widespread that these "cillin" drugs are no longer useful, but the warning signs are there. There is, however, a new back-up antibiotic and it is rapidly becoming a first-line approach—Cefaclor (CECLOR). Not only will it knock nasty pneumococcus on its butt, but it produces a strong cure rate against *H. influenzae.* Other alternatives include BACTRIM or SEPTRA, or either **Penicillin** or **Erythromycin** and sulfa (for example, GANTRISIN). If your doctor has her ear to the ground she will know what is happening in the community and what combination is most effective.

URINARY-TRACT INFECTIONS IN CHILDREN

Parents rarely think about children when cystitis or infections of the kidney, bladder, or ureter are mentioned. It's a "woman's problem," isn't it? Wrong! Infants and young children are also susceptible to urinary-tract infections and more than most parents realize. Symptoms to be alert for include frequent urination, burning or pain when urinating, wetting pants or the bed long after potty training finally succeeds, and urine that is cloudy or red. What is more insidious, however, is that there may not be any symptoms at all. And infections that are not treated may develop into kidney disease in later years.

The first thing an alert parent can do to prevent a urinary-tract infection from getting out of hand is to be alert for symptoms. But since that is a catch-as-catch-can sort of thing the real solution is to periodically test for infection at home. This sort of screening doesn't require expensive equipment (like the otoscope) nor does it require special training. Anyone could get the hang of it in about three minutes. There are two tests you can do. The first is simple as all get out and costs less than thirty cents. A little dip strip is immersed in a urine sample taken early in the morning. If the color changes to pink in a minute or less, it is a sign of nitrite in the urine which in turn is a sign of a bacterial infection. For more information on how to obtain and use these dip-strip tests turn to page 269. Another alternative is the culture kit. With this handy-dandy device you can actually culture your child's urine at home. You collect the first urine sample of the morning in a clean container and pour it into a special tube which has a "yummy" substance only bacteria could love to feed on. Then you pop the tube into a small home incubator and if the little buggers are there they will grow and multiply. Twenty-four hours later you can actually count the bacteria colonies and interpret the test. Even without an incubator you can do this analysis by letting the tube stand at room temperature (68° to 77° F.) for 32 to 48 hours. Coupled with the nitrite dip-stick test you will be armed with valuable information for your doctor. This home culture kit is called BACTURCULT (see page 268 for advice on how to find it). Now we grant you, this all sounds pretty dicey. But read the results of a study published in the journal *Clinical Pediatrics:*

> **The false-negative rate in home culturing was 3.9%, and the false-positive rate was 13.5%. These rates were not much different from those obtained in the clinic when tests were done under conditions similar to those in the home. In fact, parents, on evaluation, were found to be essentially as accurate as medical investigators in interpreting test results.**
>
> **The combination of tests thus appears to improve the accuracy of home culturing.[41,42]**

If you still doubt your ability to do it all yourself, there is another kit that allows you merely to collect a urine sample, "inoculate" a culture medium, and then take it to the doctor's office the next morning for analysis. The value of the home tests is that they produce accurate results that can establish if an infection exists and if it is responding to antibiotic treatment.[43,44] Since the tests are simple, inexpensive, reliable, and easy to use, a parent could check a child's urine if there has been a susceptibility to infection. Because urinary-tract infections are quite common in children (second only to colds and infections in the upper respiratory tract) and because they may not always produce obvious symptoms, these tests may be very helpful in preventing chronic infections from getting out of hand. Obviously, this sort of testing requires cooperation from the family doctor.

There are a few tricks that may help prevent infections from occurring in the first place. Bubble bath is *OUT.* You should also teach little girls to wipe from front to back when going to the bathroom. Perhaps most important of all, never encourage a child to "hold it in." When the cry "I have to pee" is heard, make every effort to comply. Delayed urination may set up conditions that promote infection in later years. And the more liquids you can pump into the children the better off they will be, as long as you avoid sweet stuff like soda pop.

DREADFUL DIARRHEA

Before we even get into this subject, let us state our prejudice clearly. We don't believe an occasional bout of the "crud" is worth getting very excited about. In general, childhood diarrhea is a self-limiting problem that will disappear in twenty-four to forty-eight hours. This does not mean it should be ignored. Diarrhea *can* be a symptom of something more serious — appendicitis, parasites poisoning, or whatever. More often than not, however, a garden variety case of diarrhea can be controlled by feeding the child only clear liquids for twenty-four hours. Ginger ale, flavored gelatin mixtures, or cola should help replace fluid and provide minerals. If you really want to get sophisticated we recommend PEDIALYTE or LYTREN (available in your local pharmacy). These are liquids that come in cans, carefully formulated to balance salts and minerals which have been depleted.

You may be wondering, is there any remedy that will *really* stop the runs fast? Sorry! Once again our therapeutic nihilism rears its head. We do not believe that vigorous drug treatment is beneficial in most cases of children's diarrhea. What about that good old standby KAOPECTATE, you ask. Surely something as basic as kaolin and pectin can't hurt. Well, there is some question about how effective that combination really is in controlling diarrhea. What's more, one of our favorite pediatricians, Dr. Catherine DeAngelis, writing in an excellent book called *Pediatric Primary Care* had this to say on the subject: "The use of kaolin or pectin preparations like KAOPECTATE should be discouraged. They taste bad, may cause vomiting, and are generally not effective."[45]

LOMOTIL (diphenoxylate and atropine) has long been the doctor's favorite drug when the trots turn into the runs. It is a special favorite of folks who travel to countries where "turista" is a way of life. While we're not all that wild about giving LOMOTIL to adults (since suppressing diarrhea may be counterproductive in many instances), we are positively paranoid about giving this drug to children. It has been responsible for not only poisoning in children but also some deaths.[46] Here is what the *Medical Letter* had to say:

> LOMOTIL can relieve the symptoms of acute gastroenteritis in children, but it can also mask the signs of dehydration and cause fatal toxic reactions. Since children become dehydrated more rapidly than adults, and may be particularly susceptible to the toxic effects of atropine and diphenoxylate, use of this combi-

nation for treatment of diarrhea in children is
hazardous.[47]

If you are absolutely obsessed with treating an acute attack of
diarrhea in your child you may want to discuss the drug called
CALCIUM POLYCARBOPHIL with your doctor. One study reported that
this drug "is a safe and highly effective agent for use in treatment of
acute nonspecific diarrhea in children and was superior to the kaolin-
pectin control."[48]

COPING WITH CONSTIPATION

We are now treading on sacred territory. An extraordinary number
of people believe that a bowel movement a day is essential to health
and they make heroic efforts to keep their children "regular." Here is
a letter from a reader of our newspaper column that should help
illustrate what the long-term effects of such a policy can be:

> I am dependent on a laxative for a bowel
> movement. I take two tablespoonfuls of
> PHILLIPS MILK OF MAGNESIA every couple of
> days depending on how I feel. So I have about
> two movements each week. Have been doing this
> for many, many years.
> I am now 71 and have had open heart surgery
> and am a diabetic. *No* thanks to my mother,
> have constipated all my life. She insisted I use a
> laxative everyday. Would like to hop off this
> merry-go-round but I'm beginning to think I am
> too old to worry about this habit any more.
>
> H. R. in Baltimore

We're inclined to agree with H. R. that at this stage in his life he
might as well throw in the towel and accept his "addiction." There is
little doubt that overreliance on laxatives has caused his constipation.
After seventy years of chemical stimulation, his gut has given up.
This case may be extreme but why start your child down this road?
There is nothing that says a BM which takes place only once every
two or three days is harmful and there are cases where a young person
does just fine once a week. As long as there is no blood in the stool
and passage is not painful or difficult there is no reason to become
preoccupied with bowel function.

If you are concerned and the nagging suspicion that all is not right
won't go away, then by all means check it with your pediatrician. She
will usually recommend increasing fluid intake with lots of juices. A

diet high in bulk and roughage is also a good idea. You can't go wrong with prunes, lots of leafy vegetables, and bran flakes. Of course getting these foods into the tyke is a whole other matter and we will leave that chore up to you. If all else fails, let your doctor recommend a laxative or stool softener rather than making this complicated choice on your own.

If you insist on pushing us to the wall we would probably give in eventually and comply by trying to steer you away from danger rather than offering great enthusiasm for any product. For an infant during the first year who has suddenly become constipated, MALTSUPEX is about as innocuous as a laxative can be. It is an extract from barley malt and is much more gentle than most other highly promoted "gentle" products. For babies over one month old the dose is one to two teaspoonfuls in the day's feeding. Children can take one or two teaspoonsfuls in milk or in cereal once or twice a day, although as they get older they may not like the look of this malt and may object when they see the milk turn color. Can't say we blame them. A child who is holding his stool in for such a long time that he has an accident periodically may also warrant a short course with a laxative. MINERAL OIL (not given at meal time), SENOKOT, or even MILK OF MAGNESIA may help temporarily, but DO NOT get into the habit of relying on chemical stimulation. Your child could end up like our 71-year-old friend from Baltimore.

BAFFLING BELLYACHES

Tummy troubles are as common in children as tulips in the springtime. From the time they hit four until they reach ten the chances are very good that you can count on a stomachache to "liven" up your day periodically—and at the worst possible moment. Why do children get bellyaches? If we could answer that we would make a lot of pediatricians green with envy. Even stomach pains that come back time after time and make life miserable for everyone are hard as the dickens to diagnose.

Your average kid-type stomachache usually hurts in the general area of the belly button. Pediatricians don't usually get terribly nervous about this sort of thing if the child keeps playing and continues to eat and sleep normally. What does worry the docs is when the pain becomes constant and with a specific location rather than in an amorphous area. If the pain can be pinpointed away from the bellybutton area proper it deserves prompt attention. Other warning signals you should take very seriously include a pain that wakes a child up at night or is associated with a fever, significant loss of appetite, or a marked weight loss. Any of these symptoms require extensive evaluation in order to locate the cause of the trouble.

What about the regular old, undramatic bellyache that comes and goes? What should be done? The less the better! Do not resort to high-powered drugs like belladonna, barbiturates, or antispasmodics. Pediatricians at Boston's Children's Hospital offer this sound advice:

> **In general, avoid giving medicines like aspirin or paregoric to relieve pain. These medicines are not all that effective in relieving pain and may conceal a problem deserving medical attention. It is perfectly safe and often helpful for you to apply a hot-water bottle to the child's belly and have him lie down until you see exactly which way things are going. These simple measures are about as far as we suggest that you go in attempting to relieve the discomfort.**[49]

If the stomachache seems to be related to some heavy head stuff or anxiety your young person is going through, it might be helpful to talk things out and find out what the problem is. One of your basic trouble spots could well be mealtime itself. If you find yourself shouting "Eat, eat, EAT" every time your kids sit down at the dinner table and your pleas are met with stubborn resistance, maybe it is time to analyze your tactics. If the little gremlin is growing normally chances of starvation are slim. Backing off from the battle cry may turn the table on the tummyaches and improve eating in the long run. Having lived through it all ourselves we know how difficult such restraint can be, but somehow everyone seems to survive.

There is another possibility to explain those baffling bellyaches. Your child may be having problems with milk and dairy products. A surprising number of children lack an enzyme called lactase which is necessary for digesting milk sugar (lactose). Many adults suffer from this problem ("lactose intolerance") as well, and something as simple as a bowl of ice cream or a glass of milk, for example, can cause tremendous discomfort—diarrhea, gas, bloating, and cramps. Even someone who was able to drink milk as a young child may not be able to do so as a teenager or an adult. For reasons that are totally unclear it appears that the lactase enzyme that is necessary to handle milk sugar can begin to peter out at different ages. Because symptoms may vary in severity and because it may take longer than an hour for the pain to start, many children and adults don't associate their digestive-tract problems with dairy products.

So what's the solution to this predicament? Well, if you want to find out whether those recurrent stomachaches are caused by lack of lactase, all you have to do is eliminate milk and dairy products from your child's diet for a couple of weeks. If the symptoms begin to disappear you have just shamed Sherlock Holmes with your detective skills. If you go back to adding milk products to the diet and symptoms reoccur, you know you have struck paydirt.

Does this mean the child will have to go through life without drinking any more milk? Absolutely not! There is a marvelous product available called LACT-AID that contains the enzyme lactase. When the powder or liquid is added to milk it pre-digests a large proportion of the milk sugar and will eliminate problems for most people. LACT-AID can be purchased in many pharmacies or health-food stores, but if it is unavailable in your area you can order it directly from the manufacturer. Write to the Sugar Lo Company, P.O. Box 1017, Atlantic City, New Jersey 08404 for price information. If your child has been missing school because of chronic stomach pains caused by lactase intolerance, your problems should be just about over.

THE "OTHER" SCHOOL DRUG PROBLEM

**No more pencils, no more books,
No more teachers' dirty looks.**

That wonderful old refrain we used to sing on the last day of school may have to be revised. The school's personnel themselves may deserve some dirty looks on the issue of drugs in school. We're not referring to illicit drugs like marijuana or alcohol, but common and accepted ones like antibiotics, allergy remedies, pain relievers, and asthma medicine. A big part of the problem is just in getting people — parents, teachers, and children — to recognize that medications dispensed in school can spell trouble. Many schools do not have nurses; they must rely on teachers, secretaries, or administrators to give medications. Often these well-meaning people are not aware of the proper use of the drugs they are dispensing. More often than not the school lacks a medication policy and no one knows who should be responsible for administering a drug or recording it.

An associate of ours, Susan Spalt, a registered nurse with a degree in public health, has pointed out that schools have to deal with two distinct situations: first, they must keep medication on hand to treat children for emergencies which may occur during school hours; and second, they are expected to carry out medication regimens begun at home. Susan's survey in her local district turned up a variety of "routine supplies" kept on hand and administered under a variety of disorganized "plans" in schools. These ranged from antibiotic ointments and steroid creams to pain relievers and menstrual products. In addition, parents often send their kids to school with a wide assortment of prescription drugs and over-the-counter remedies. Susan found students taking asthma medication or antibiotics as well as nose drops and cold remedies. She even found one student storing a bottle of incorrectly labeled seizure medicine in the school secretary's desk. None of the schools Susan studied had any information about the reasons for administering these medical supplies, possible side effects, correct dosage, or proper administration of the medications that were stored in school facilities.

This casual approach can be incredibly dangerous. Some children are allergic even to something as "innocent" as plain aspirin. They may develop asthma or hives in response to a "safe" dose. If the wrong dose of a drug were given, unwanted side effects could easily result. Drug interactions also pose potential hazards. A child taking medication for bed-wetting or hyperactivity can run into real trouble if given an apparently innocuous cold remedy.

Another problem with routinely handing out drugs is it reinforces children's ideas that there is a pill for every ill. It's bad enough that television commercials constantly blare forth this message. While children need to learn which symptoms require medical treatment, they also ought to learn that there are other ways to deal with aches and pains besides popping a pill.

You can help to change this situation in your community. First, if your child is in elementary school find out about the first-aid and medication policy at his school. If no formal plan exists a health committee made up of health professionals, school staff, and parents should be formed. Here are some guidelines established by the Committee on School Health of the American Academy of Pediatrics:

> **Ideally, all medication should be given at home ... Any student who is required to take prescribed medication during regular school hours should comply with school regulations. These regulations should include the following:**
>
> **1. Written orders from a physician should detail the name of the drug, dosage, time interval that the medication is to be taken, and diagnosis or reason for the medication to be given.**

2. Written permission should be provided by the parent or guardian requesting that the school district comply with the physician's orders.

3. Medication should be brought to school in a container appropriately labeled by the pharmacy or physician.

4. One member (or a team) of the staff should be designated to handle this task, ideally the health personnel if available.

5. A locked cabinet should be provided for the storage of medication.

6. Opportunities should be provided for communication between the parent, school personnel, and physician regarding the efficacy of the medication administered during school hours.

Nonprescription medication, e.g., aspirin, ointments, cold tablets, should not be given without prior written permission of parent or guardian.[50]

Many of these problems could be eliminated entirely if sound information on correct methods of self-care and proper use of medications were introduced in school health classes. Unfortunately, these programs are often pretty dull and few teachers are themselves adequately informed about drug products.

TAKING IT ON HOME

So much for lectures and dirty looks. There are many topics that haven't been covered in this chapter. Pediatric pharmacology is a subject that requires a whole book. For example, we did not get into the quicksand of hyperactivity or bed-wetting. If you want to learn about our thinking on those subjects we recommend you take a look at *The People's Pharmacy.*

Although we haven't touched more than the surface in this chapter, we have managed to discuss some pretty important topics. You now know how to protect your children from tetracycline-stained teeth. You learned about birth defects—not those you can see, but the intellectual or behavioral defects that may not show up for years after a child is born. You know that shopping in the pharmacy for non-prescription drugs is a little like playing Blind Man's Bluff, but a lot more dangerous. Cold remedies, like so many over-the-counter drugs, may be counterproductive and in some cases even lethal when given incorrectly to a child.

By now you know that we are not just careful when it comes to recommending drugs for young people, we are super-cautious. There have been too many mistakes made by well-meaning adults and too many adverse reactions. Children can't defend themselves against adult ignorance. They must trust us when we insist the medicine is good for them but such faith may be unwarranted. Everyone wants children to get well as quickly as possible, but we have got to learn to question the doctor just as rigorously when he gives us a prescription for our children as when he gives us a prescription for ourselves. Doctors do make mistakes and when they are busy they may not take the time to calculate a child's dose carefully and precisely. One study carried out by physicians at the University of Southern California Medical Center discovered that an alarming number of prescriptions contained omissions or outright errors.[51] In fact, of the 2,213 prescriptions they examined (from an emergency room in a local hospital) only 5 percent were acceptable. They found that "the number of incorrectly calculated doses based on the patient's body weight or age represented a more serious deficiency. More than one third of the prescriptions with dosage specified contained an error."[52] Children deserve a lot better. So summon up your courage the next time your doctor presents you with a prescription for your youngster and ask how she calculates dose. As we already discussed, even with something as comparatively safe as aspirin, there can be tremendous variability between doctors. If they know you care they will make an extra effort.

Although we have advocated therapeutic nihilism when it comes to giving drugs to children, we have to admit that many medications have made a huge difference in speeding up recovery from serious illness. Antibiotics are invaluable when used appropriately—they cure ear infections and prevent deafness for thousands of youngsters each year. They knock out urinary-tract infections fast and zap strep throats and pneumonia with ease. You can take an active part in your children's health care by learning how to take a throat and urine culture. And you can learn about the medicine the pediatrician prescribes. There is a short list of commonly used drugs at the end of this chapter which will give you an idea of the kinds of questions you should ask when they're prescribed. We regret the list can't be more complete.

So mom and dad, stop worrying about constipation or diarrhea, a stuffy nose, or a little cough. Accidents kill far more children than do these illnesses. You would do your children the biggest favor in the world if you scrapped a lot of the drugs in the medicine chest and invested in a sturdy child safety seat for the car. And every time you drive *anywhere* (even around the corner) strap them in. In fact, if you want to do your friends and relatives a great favor, buy the new babies a car seat instead of a toy. It could save a child's life! And remember, while you can take responsibility for your own health care, your children depend on your good sense, at least until you can train them to defend themselves against an advertiser's seductive sell. Children need to learn to recognize which symptoms require medical treatment, but they also need to learn that drugs aren't always the answer. If you help your children learn how to cope with minor problems when they're young there is hope they will turn into knowledgeable consumers when they get older.

A Children's Pharmacopeia

(NOTE: OTC stands for "over the counter." Rx stands for "prescription.")

ACETAMINOPHEN (Tylenol, Tempra, Liquiprin)   OTC

Usual dose: Under 3 years of age—ask doctor; 3 to under 4 = 160 mg; 4 to under 6 = 240 mg; 6 to under 9 = 320 mg; 9 to under 11 = 400 mg; 11 to under 12 = 480 mg. These doses are slightly higher than those on medication bottles but were established by the Food and Drug Administration for administration every four hours to a maximum of 5 doses in 24 hours.

There has been an extraordinary debate raging in medical circles as to whether acetaminophen is better than aspirin. They are basically similar in ability to lower a fever or relieve pain. Children who are allergic to aspirin or sensitive to stomach irritation may do better with acetaminophen.

Caution: An overdose with acetaminophen can be extremely dangerous. Liver damage can lead to severe toxicity. Because symptoms may not occur for 24 to 48 hours after a poisoning don't wait to contact your local poison-control center.

ASPIRIN (Bayer Children's Aspirin, Congestrin   OTC
        Chewable, St. Joseph Aspirin for Children
        Chewable Tablets)

Usual dose: See pages 328–331. Aspirin is generally safe and effective for most children. However it can cause stomach irritation and bleeding in sensitive individuals. Always follow chewable tablets with a generous amount of liquid to reduce this possibility. Kids who are allergic may develop asthma or hives.

Caution: An overdose of aspirin is much more serious for a child than for an adult. Keep *all* medications in child-proof containers and locked out of reach. Symptoms of an overdose include headache, dizziness, ringing in the ears, confusion, drowsiness, thirst, nausea, vomiting, and serious metabolic changes. Requires emergency treatment!

AMPICILLIN (Amcill, Omnipen, etc.) Rx

Dose: Physician is responsible for appropriate dosage information. A couple of general formulas are: (1) For respiratory tract infections 50 mg/kg per day divided in four equal doses or if the child weighs more than 44 pounds, 250 mg every six hours. (2) For gastric or urinary-tract infections, 100 mg/kg per day divided in equal doses every six hours, or if the child weighs more than 44 pounds, 500 mg every six hours.

Ampicillin has become one of the most popular antibiotics because of its broad-spectrum effectiveness. It is used for ear infections, croup, urinary tract infections, and other ailments. Diarrhea is the most common side effect but nausea and vomiting are also possible. Skin rash is another adverse reaction to be alert for—contact doctor immediately.

Caution: anyone allergic to penicillin must avoid ampicillin!

AMOXICILLIN (Amoxil, Larotid, Polymox, Trimox, Rx
etc.)

Dose: Physician is responsible for appropriate dosage information. One general formula is 9 milligrams per pound of body weight per day divided into 3 equal doses every eight hours. Best absorbed on an empty stomach with a large glass of water as a chaser.

Amoxicillin is growing in popularity though still not prescribed as often as **ampicillin.**

The most common side effects include indigestion, nausea, vomiting, diarrhea, and rash.

Caution: Anyone allergic to penicillin must avoid amoxicillin!

CHICKEN SOUP   OTC

Dose: Mothers are responsible for appropriate dosage information—as much and as often as necessary.

This "antibiotic" works for lots of ailments and is especially good for viral infections (such as colds). As far as we know, there are no side effects.

Caution: If home-made and delicious this remedy could be habit-forming.

CORTISPORIN   Rx
OTIC DROPS (Hydrocortisone, Neomycin Sulfate and Polymyxin-G)

Dose: Two to three drops 3 to 4 times per day in the bad ear. This medicine will relieve the awful pain of an external-ear infection. It contains a steroid to relieve the inflammation and two antibiotics to help clear up the infection. If it is used too long other beasties could begin to grow and cause a fungal infection. If there is any itching, burning, or stinging **stop** using the medicine and call the doctor.

ERYTHROMYCIN (Bristamycin,   E-Mycin,   Rx
Erythrocin, E.E.S., Robimycin)

Dose: Physician is responsible for appropriate dosage information. The range can run from 30 to 50 mg/kg over the course of a day divided into equal doses. Much depends upon the illness and its severity.

This drug is especially useful for children who are allergic to penicillin. It can be combined with a sulfa drug called **GANTRISIN** (sulfisoxazole) when an ear infection is resistant to cure with **ampicillin.**

Be on the lookout for nausea, vomiting, cramps, and diarrhea. If fever, rash, or jaundice occur call the doctor pronto!

PENICILLIN V (Pencillin VK, Pen-Vee-K, Robicillin,   Rx
V-Cillin-K, etc.)

Penicillin is still an old standby—dose range is wide depending upon the severity and type of illness. Your doctor has this information down cold so trust her.

This kind of Penicillin is best absorbed well before meals (at least one hour before and up to two hours after). No matter what, make sure your child finishes out the full course of treatment even if he starts to feel better after two or three days. You don't want that infection to come back stronger, so kill it dead! KEEP THE MEDICINE IN THE FRIDGE.

Side effects include indigestion, nausea, and diarrhea. If your child develops a rash, hives, or has difficulty breathing call the doctor immediately! HE OR SHE COULD BE ALLERGIC TO PENICILLIN.

STEROID CREAMS (Aristocort, Kenalog, Mycolog,
Hydrocortisone, Cort-Dome,   Rx/OTC
etc.)

What would doctors do without cortisone-type creams? These lotions work like magic to relieve itching, redness, rashes, and all sorts of skin irritations. These drugs should not be taken for granted and used continuously for long periods of time. Products that contain triamcinolone (such as Aristocort or Kenalog) should not be used on the face. Prolonged use can cause thinning of the skin and some people may develop acne. Use sparingly on the skin since large amounts may not only be wasteful but may increase the danger of systemic side effects.

SULFISOXAZOLE (Azo Gantrisin, Gantrisin, etc.)   Rx

Dose: Physician is responsible for appropriate dosage information.

This sulfa antibiotic is very useful for urinary tract infections or ear infections. But it can cause skin rash, itching, indigestion, and during the summer may make the skin extra sensitive to the sun and lead to a bad burn.

Caution: Avoid vitamin C when taking sulfa antibiotics. Fever, sore throat, or malaise should be reported immediately to the doctor.

THEOPHYLLINE (Elixophyllin, Somophyllin, S10-   Rx
                  Phyllin, Theodur, Theolair, Theolix-
                  ir, Theophyl, etc.)

Dose: Physician is responsible for appropriate dosage information. Asthma symptoms are so different from one person to another that it is hard to define a general dose.

There has been a tremendous resurgence of enthusiasm for this asthma medicine and we heartily agree that **theophylline** is an excellent•drug for treating asthma and used aggressively can really do the job.

Side effects can include stomach upset, nausea, vomiting, diarrhea, nervousness, and insomnia. Children who have heart, kidney, liver, or thyroid disease must be monitored with great care. Anyone with an ulcer or glaucoma should probably not receive the drug unless circumstances warrant.

TRIMETHOPRIM/   Rx
SULFAMETHOXAZOLE (Bactrim, Septra)

Dose: Physician is responsible for appropriate dosage information. A general guideline is: 8 mg/kg Trimethoprim and 40 mg/kg sulfamethoxazole per day in two divided doses.

This combination has been demonstrated to be very effective in treating urinary-tract infections and ear infections. The drugs can cause serious blood disorders, especially if used for a long period of time, so parents should be on the lookout for telltale signs— rash, fever, sore throat, sensitivity to bruising, unusual bleeding, jaundice, pallor, swelling around the eyes, aches and pains, and itching. If any of these symptoms occur contact the doctor immediately. Other side effects include nausea, vomiting, and diarrhea.

REFERENCES

1. Committee on Drugs. "Requiem for Tetracyclines." *Pediatrics* 55:142–143, 1975.

2. Rays, Wayne A.; Federspiel, Charles F.; and Schaffner, William. "Prescribing Tetracycline to Children Less Than 8 Years Old." *JAMA* 237:2069–2074, 1977.

3. Ibid.

4. Ibid.

5. Rays, Wayne A.; Federspiel, Charles F.; and Schaffner, William. "The Mal-Prescribing of Liquid Tetracycline Preparations." *Am. J. Pub. Health* 67:762–764, 1977.

6. D.L.A. "Prescribing of Tetracycline to Children Less Than 9 Years Old." *1978 Yearbook of Drug Therapy,* p. 37.

7. From the NIH. "Research Findings of Potential Value to the Practitioner." *JAMA* 237:635–636, 1977.

8. Mitchell, Edgar W. "The Cosmetic Treatment of Tetracycline-Stained Teeth." *Pharmacy Times* 45(7):34–35, 1979.

9. Ibid.

10. Hill, R. M., et al. "Drug Utilization During Prenatal Period." *Pediatric Res.* 11:417, 1977.

11. Udkow, Gail. "Pediatric Clinical Pharmacology." *Am. J. Dis. Child.* 132:1025–1032, 1978.

12. Brackbill, Yvonne. "Obstetrical Medication Study." *Science* 205:732–734, 1978.

13. Kolata, Gina Bari. "Behavioral Teratology: Birth Defects of the Mind." *Science* 202:732–734, 1978.

14. Ibid.

15. Kolata, Gina Bari. "Scientists Attack Report That Obstetrical Medications Endanger Children." *Science* 204:391–392, 1979.

16. Kolata, Gina Bari. "Drugs and Children (Special to the *Washington Post*)." *Durham Sun,* December 7, 1978, pp. 7–9.

17. Brackbill, op. cit.

18. Vorhees, Charles V.; Brunner, Robert L.; and Butcher, Richard E. "Psychotropic Drugs As Behavioral Teratogens." *Science* 205:1120–1125, 1979.

19. Committee on Drugs. "Effect of Medication During Labor and Delivery on Infant Outcome." *Pediatrics* 62:402–403, 1978.

20. Cormier, John F., and Bryant, Bobby G. "Cold and Allergy Products." In *Handbook of NonPrescription Drugs* 6th ed., L. Luan Corrigan, editor. Washington, D. C.: American Pharmaceutical Association, 1979, p. 84.

21. Ibid.

22. Committee on Drugs. "Camphor: Who Needs It?" *Pediatrics* 62:404–406, 1978.

23. Over-the-Counter Drugs. "Establishment of a Monograph for OTC

Cold, Cough, Allergy, Bronchodilator and Antiasthmatic Products." *Federal Register* September 9, 1976, p. 3836.

24. Package Insert for "Save-The-Baby," Vetree Products, Ltd.

25. Committee on Drugs. "Camphor: Who Needs It?" *Pediatrics* 62:404—406, 1978.

26. Medicaps. "FDA to Consider Banning OTC Camphor Products." *Drug Topics,* August 17, 1979, p. 58.

27. Ibid.

28. News. "Big Cough/Cold Winter." *Drug Topics* August 17, 1979, p. 20.

29. Bristol-Myers Co. Advertisement in *Drug Topics,* August 17, 1979, pp. 11—12.

30. Committee on Drugs. "Use of Codeine and Dextromethorphan-Containing Cough Syrups in Pediatrics." *Pediatrics* 62:118—122, 1978.

31. Committee on Drugs. "Inaccuracies in Administering Liquid Medications." *Pediatrics* 56(2):327, 1975.

32. Cormier, op. cit., p. 91.

33. "Mom and Dad Take Good Throat Swabs." *Med. World News* Dec. 12, 1977.

34. "Patients Can be 'Pros' in Obtaining Throat Cultures." *Hospital Practice,* April, 1978, pp. 52—57.

35. Kluger, Mathew J. "The Evaluation and Adaptive Value of Fever." *Am. Scientist* 68(1), 1978.

36. Dinarello, Charles A., and Wolff, Sheldon M. "Fever." *Human Nature,* 1979, pp. 66—72.

37. Done, Alan K.; Yaffe, Summer J.; and Clayton, John M. "Aspirin Dosage for Infants." *J. of Ped.* 95:617—624, 1979.

38. Ibid.

39. Ibid.

40. Medical News. "The Changing Picture of Otitis Media in Childhood." *JAMA* 242:707—709, 1979.

41. Scheivele, David A., and Smith, Arnold. "Home Testing for Recurrent Bacteriuria, Using Nitrite Strips." *Am. J. Dis. Child.* 132:46—48, 1978.

42. Randolph, Martin F., et al. "Home Screening for the Detection of Urinary Tract Infection in Infancy." *Am. J. Dis. Child.* 133:713—717, 1979.

43. Pediatrics. "Effective Method of Testing Urine for Bacteria at Home." *Mod. Med.* March 30, 1978, p. 158.

44. Fennell, R. S. III, et al. "The Combination of Two Screening Methods in a Home Culture Program for Children with Recurrent Bacteriuria." *Clin. Ped.* 16:951—955, 1977.

45. DeAngelis, Catherine. *Pediatric Primary Care,* 2nd ed. Boston: Little Brown, 1979, p. 283.

46. Curtis, J. A., and Goel, K. M. "Lomotil Poisoning in Children." *Arch. Dis. Childhood* 54:222—225, 1979.

47. "Lomotil for Diarrhea in Children." *Med. Letter* 17:104, 1975.

48. Rutledge, Mary Louise; Willmer, Milton M.; and Clayton, John M. "Clinical Comparison of Calcium Polycarbophil and Kaolin- Pectin Suspension in the Treatment of Acute Childhood Diarrhea." *Cur. Ther. Res.* 23:443—447, 1978.

49. The Boston Children's Medical Center and Feinbloom, Richard I. *Child Health Encyclopedia.* Mount Vernon: Consumers Union, 1978, p. 148.

50. Committee on School Health. "Medical Emergencies and Administration of Medication in School." *Pediatrics* 61:115—116, 1978.

51. Wingert, Willis A., et al. "A Study of the Quality of Prescriptions Issued in a Busy Pediatric Emergency Room." *Pub. Health Rep.* 90(5):402, 1975.

52. Ibid.

Drugs and Older People

Drug companies see dollar signs • Doses can get complicated • Prescription safety checklist • Insomnia: Curse or blessing—DALMANE can be devastating • High blood pressure: When to worry and how to treat it—DYAZIDE, ISMELIN, ALDOMET, ALDORIL, RESERPINE, DIUPRES, DIURIL, HYGROTON, HYDROPRES, SER-AP-ES, SERPASIL, INDERAL, LOPRESS-OR, and many more • Watch out for potassium: LASIX and LANOXIN • Antibiotics and your kidneys • Searching for the fountain of youth: GEROVI-TAL • Staving off senility.

When I get older losing my hair,
Many years from now . . .
Will you still need me, will you still feed me,
When I'm sixty-four.

—The Beatles, 1967

Well friends, if you have to ask yourself the question posed in the Beatles' song and you think that no one else needs you when you're sixty-four, you can be cheered by one thing—the drug companies certainly do. You make up a huge part of their business and one of the most lucrative parts at that. There are twenty-three million Americans over retirement age. Now that in itself doesn't mean a lot. We know people who are burned out at forty. They act as if they would prefer to pack it all in and prepare for a rocking chair and a pension. But we also know some folks in their seventies and eighties who are going so strong that we can't come close to keeping up. Growing "old" is as much a state of mind as it is anything else. And chronic illnesses like high blood pressure and arthritis can strike middle-aged or even young people. Nevertheless, the older you get the more likely you will end up taking one drug or another pretty regularly. although people who have retired make up only about 11 percent of the population they receive one out of every four prescriptions that are dispensed.[1,2]

As we get older, the body machinery starts to wear down. The pipes clog up and the blood pressure may begin creeping upward. The old ticker may miss on a few cylinders and the joints often start to creak. When a doctor puts you on a drug for one of these problems there is a good chance that you will be taking it for the rest of your life—and that spells some big bucks for the pharmaceutical manufacturers. Four tablets a day every day for twenty years adds up to over 29,000 pills. An arthritis drug like MOTRIN (ibuprofen) could well cost over $4,500 at the end of that many years. And some newer anti-inflammatory agents may run more than thirty cents for each tablet. When you consider that there are actually some 50,000,000 (that's right, *fifty million!*) people with arthritis, you have some idea of how much money is involved. Add to that the fact that many older people have to take more than one drug at the same time and you can understand why drug companies see dollar signs when you reach $ixty.

This may come as a harsh shock, but there is surprisingly little known about how drugs affect people as they grow older.[3] What is known is that your body changes with age and is often much more susceptible to good as well as bad effects from drugs. The dosage requirements of a 68-year-old hundred-thirty-five pound grandfather are very different from those of a 42-year-old two-hundred-twenty-five pound six-foot-four inch bulldozer jockey. And yet drug companies often do not take these differences into account. Once upon a time the pharmacist formulated a dose to meet the doctor's specific recommendations, which were tailored as much as possible to the patients' requirements. Today that is rare. Instead, the physician has to rely upon what is available from the pharmaceutical manufacturer and that may not correspond to the tremendous variability in patient needs.

Drugs behave differently in older people. Older bodies have less muscle and relatively more fatty tissue. Kidney function may not be what it once was. As a result of these changes, drugs may not be eliminated as quickly or effectively from the body. If doctors don't take these factors into account and reduce the dose accordingly, too much of the drug could accumulate in the body and adverse reactions become more likely.

Take good old George, for example. When he was fifty-one his doctor put him on a heart drug called LANOXIN (digoxin) at a dose of 0.5 mg and a diuretic called LASIX (furosemide) at 80 mg. This was just right and George never had any problems. Today George is seventy-four. He has faithfully continued to take his medicine exactly the same way he did twenty-three years ago and his doctor has never changed the dose. But George is different now. He only weighs 140 pounds and his arthritis has slowed him down so he doesn't get much exercise anymore. In addition, he never has much of an appetite and sometimes he's nauseated and has diarrhea. His muscles often cramp up and ache and his eyesight isn't what it used to be. His vision gets blurry and he may see yellow spots before his eyes. George feels droopy and tired much of the time. He's also bothered by a dry mouth. He's thirsty a lot and finds that he has to go to the bathroom so often it's embarrassing.

George has chalked up all these "minor" complaints to old age. He hates to bother his new physician (old Doc Hicks died a few years back) because the young whipper always has an office full of patients and is generally rushing around like a chicken without a head. He never has time to chat. Well, George is in mighty big trouble. Every single one of the problems just enumerated is caused by an overdose of his two drugs. The level that once was just right is now far too high. The LANOXIN is causing the loss of appetite, nausea, and diarrhea as well as the changes in eyesight. The LASIX has depleted too much potassium from his body and this in turn has produced the fatigue, dry mouth, and muscle pains. If someone doesn't adjust the dose of his drugs soon George could end up in the hospital with potentially fatal heart irregularities. George had better discuss his symptoms with the doctor and have some blood tests run.

George is not unique. Older people tend to be far more patient than they should be.[4] They often chalk their symptoms up to aging and if the doctor tells them not to worry or does not take time to explain what side effects to watch out for they may fail to take dangerous warning signals seriously for far too long.

Doctors prescribe too many drugs to older people. Although medicine can ease pain, limber up stiff joints, calm nerves, cure infections, and help the heart, when over-used it can also turn elderly folks into zombies. Dr. Peter Lamy, an expert on prescribing for the elderly, has outlined the depth of the problem:

> **Drug prescribing for the elderly is extraordinarily high, and it has been reported that more than 85% of elderly ambulatory patients and almost 95% of elderly institutionalized patients receive drugs, 25% of which may well be ineffective or unneeded. In addition, the use of nonprescrip-**

tion drugs is surprisingly high among this population and more than 70% of one elderly study population used nonprescription drugs without knowledge of the primary care provider.[5]

This problem is probably most severe in nursing homes, where nearly every patient receives several drugs, and mistakes may easily be made in administering medication.[6] But the problems of drug-caused disability or death are just as ominous for other folks. It is important for anyone and *crucial* for the older person to make sure the doctor knows all the other drugs you are taking, even those like laxatives, cigarettes, or coffee or tea, which you might forget or take for granted because they are habits of long standing. All of these substances can have important influences on the action of other drugs.

Side effects and overprescribing are not the only problems for older folks. There is always the bitter pill of price. Doctors are often oblivious to how much the drugs they prescribe cost their patients. Either they don't take the time to check or they just don't care. (In medical school such practical matters are rarely discussed in pharmacology classes.) And older people usually don't get a lot of help with their bills. One survey showed that 87 percent of their drug costs were paid directly out of pocket.[7] If a doctor writes a new prescription that is supposed to carry a patient for a few months and then the person discovers that he can't tolerate the medication because of a side effect—well, too bad! The pharmacy won't take back the "used" bottle of pills and the patient is stuck with an expensive bottle of useless medicine. The doctor's solution usually is just to write another prescription. A lot of older people living on fixed incomes are being pinched in the pocketbook. And doctors bemoan the fact that their patients don't always take the medicine they prescribe.

A few years ago the American Association of Retired Persons surveyed its membership about this issue. Among the responses was one from a widow in California: "One drug I take is quite expensive so instead of taking four a day as prescribed I take two." A woman from Plymouth, Michigan reported: "If a prescription is needed to be filled, then a bill must let go for awhile to buy the medication. This all makes me feel very depressed at times..."[8]

It makes us depressed too. Doctors need to be more sensitive to their patients' needs, and that includes economic needs. Many older people are too proud to ask for a less-expensive medicine. Instead of relying upon the never-ending promotions that spew forth from the drug companies, doctors should consider equivalent drugs that cost less. Just consider high blood pressure medicine. Anyone with hypertension will probably have to take these drugs for the rest of their lives in order to reduce the risk of heart attacks, strokes, or damage to the kidneys. But if a doctor prescribes an expensive medication, someone on a fixed income may not be able to get the prescription filled every month and may not be able to take her/his pills regularly. For example, **HYDRODIURIL** is a commonly prescribed diuretic (water pill) that is often used to treat mild high blood pressure. One hundred tablets (50 mg) cost anywhere from $6.50 to $8.00. The generic equivalent, hydrochlorothiazide, is usually about half as much—$3.75 per hundred tablets.

If the doctor opts for a potassium-sparing diuretic like **ALDACTONE** (spironolactone) the price can really soar. One hundred (25 mg) tablets could cost the consumer close to $16.00. Thirty days of treatment with **ALDACTONE** (100 mg each day) may run the patient almost $19.00, whereas a month of treatment with hydro-chlorothiazide (100 mg per day) should cost little more than $2.25. In our opinion the difference in price ($16.75) does not justify any advantages that might be obtained by preserving potassium. While it may be necessary to eat foods high in potassium, that certainly seems worth the effort. One expert on the use of drugs for high blood pressure, Dr. Ray W. Gifford, goes even farther. He believes that spironolactone (**ALDACTONE**) is "less potent, both as a diuretic and as an antihypertensive agent, than are the kaliuretic [potassium-depleting] drugs."[9] Another commonly prescribed potassium-sparing diruretic is called **DYAZIDE** (triamterene and hydrochlorothiazide). Even though it is available generically at a reduced price the brand-name product is prescribed in huge quantities with little consideration for the effect on people's pocketbooks.

Even more important than cost, however, is the problem of multiple prescriptions. While this is dangerous for anyone, it is particularly hazardous for older persons. A recent investigation of drug-taking by senior citizens in Albany, New York, turned up some frightening statistics. "Eighty-three percent of those sampled were taking two or more drugs. Fourteen percent were regularly using 7 to 15 drugs, and only 8 percent were completely medication-free."[10] What was especially disturbing was that "33 percent took one or more medications that they could not specifically name." That is dreadful! And it would appear to be the norm rather than the exception. Research on medication patterns in a group of older persons in Miami produced surprisingly similar data. "Eighty-eight point five percent of this total population was taking prescribed medications of some kind. Perhaps the most frightening revelations were that 22.6 percent of the 65+ population and 33.3 percent of the 75+ population were concurrently on four or more medications."[11]

When so many people are taking so many drugs at the same time and when they don't even know what they are taking, somebody is screwing up somewhere. The researchers who studied older people in Albany, New York, made a very important observation:

> **Many of the most commonly used drugs and substances mentioned in our data are cited to have interaction effects. In clinical practice it is not uncommon that subsequent drugs are prescribed to treat the side effects caused by previously prescribed drugs, frequently leading to the vicious cycle of polypharmacy. Additional medical risk from polypharmacy derives from the fact that many drugs interfere with the results of diagnostic laboratory tests, thus delaying or masking accurate diagnosis.[12]**

You don't believe doctors can make such mistakes in diagnosis very often? We wish that were true. But in a report to the *Workshop of Pharmacology and Aging,* sponsored by the National Institutes of Health, Dr. James Cooper reported that "in 100 consecutive nursing home admissions 64 percent of the patients' primary diagnoses were inaccurate; 84 percent of the secondary diagnoses were either lacking or inadequate."[13]

How can this sort of thing happen? Well, for one thing, medical students rarely receive specialized training for dealing with older people. When it comes time to prescribe a drug they just forge ahead the best they know how, which may be none too good. Take VALIUM (diazepam) for example. The manufacturer (Eli Lilly) makes it very clear on the brochure which accompanies the drug that there are important precautions doctors must be aware of: "In elderly and debilitated patients, it is recommended that the dosage be limited to the smallest effective amount to preclude the development of ataxia [incoordination] or oversedation (2 mg. to 2.5 mg. once or twice daily, initially, to be increased gradually as needed and tolerated.)"[14] Now nothing could be clearer, right? Wrong, at least as far as doctors' comprehension was determined in one study. As we mentioned in Chapter 1, a group of medical students, interns, residents, and supervising psychiatrists at a major teaching hospital in New York were tested for their knowledge of VALIUM. Astonishing as it may seem, more than two-thirds of these doctors were unaware that older people are at a greater risk of central-nervous-system depression if given VALIUM. And 80 percent had problems devising rational dosage schedules based on their knowledge of the action of VALIUM.[15] Unbelievable! It's no wonder some health workers use the term 'spaced-out Grandma syndrome' to denote the over-chemicalization of older persons using both prescription and nonprescription drugs."[16]

It's time to call a halt to this madness. We need a lot more sensitivity, cooperation, and communication from health providers. In an extraordinary plea to his colleagues that "Somebody *DO* Something... about the mistreatment of elderly patients," Fred B. Charaton, M.D., really put everything into perspective:

> **I'm angry about the aged; specifically, I'm angry about the way many of my colleagues treat their elderly patients. Can't you recall colleagues' comments, from medical school on, as if they were convinced they'd never grow old? Fogey, crock, geezer, and biddy are a few of the derogatory terms I've heard them use. I've also witnessed some of the following "treatments":**
>
> 1. *Impatience or not-so-benign neglect.*
> 2. *Parroting "It's just your age," with nary an attempt to find the underlying cause of symptoms, whether somatic (physical) or psychosocial.*
> 3. *Feeding the elderly patient a new drug for each new symptom. In time, the patient may be taking over a dozen drugs, with correspondingly increased risks of side effects and incompatible drug interactions.*
>
> **It's strange, really, that there should be so much overt and covert negative feeling towards the elderly. After all, an old person deserves some credit just for surviving to a good age, apart from credit due for his or her contributions to the community over many years... So, let somebody do something.[17]**

Amen! Let's start right now. We are all getting older. That's so obvious it may seem silly to mention it. But the temptation to run away from that simple fact of life is overwhelming for many people and it would seem that doctors suffer the same psychological hang-ups about aging as we less-exalted mortals. While we can't change doctors' attitudes overnight, at least we can establish some guidelines to help prevent the over-chemicalization of older people and perhaps cut down on the number of adverse reactions that occur with alarming frequency. We have worked out a checklist that we hope will assist in navigating the rough water of the pharmacological maelstrom. It may help to have some navigational charts which can aid you in avoiding the sinkholes.

Prescription Safety Checklist

1.   **Why is the drug being prescribed?**

     Is it really necessary? What is the cause of the symptoms and will the drug actually cure the underlying problem or will it only provide temporary relief?

2.   **Was the dose tailored to your body's needs?**

     Did the doctor take your sensitivity to medicine into account when computing dosage and was it the lowest level possible to achieve a therapeutic effect? Will the dose have to be changed in the future?

3.   **Do you understand the effects of the drug?**

     Did the doctor discuss the special characteristics of the new medicine—how to take it, undesirable effects, precautions, and expectations for benefits? Do you know under what conditions to discontinue the drug or call the doctor?

4.   **How long should the medicine be taken?**

     Does the drug have to be continued indefinitely? If it can be suspended are there any special instructions about tapering off gradually? When should the drug regimen be reviewed?

5. Were you provided with written instructions?

   Did the doctor take the time to write out legible, understandable directions? Did you receive a list of precautions, warnings, and side effects? Was a friend or relative advised of any special or complicated information in order to facilitate the treatment?

6. Did the doctor ask about your other drugs?

   When you visited the doctor's office did you take a list of everything you are taking including over-the-counter medications? Did someone check a reference book to make sure there were no incompatability interactions? Are you sure you aren't taking any duplication of similar kinds of medicine?

7. Did the doctor check the cost of the drug?

   Can you afford to pay for the new prescription, and if not, is there a cheaper alternative that will do the job? Did you shop comparatively?

8. Did you get a sample prescription?

   Were you given a free sample to test for side effects? If not, did the doctor provide two prescriptions—one small one for a short trial run and a regular one if all systems are Go? You don't want to get burned paying in advance for a large prescription for medicine you can't tolerate.

9. Did the pharmacist supply an easy-off cap?

   If you suffer sore fingers or arthritis did you receive a reversible lid on your prescription container? There are some nifty new caps that have two sides—one can be unscrewed with ease and when the grandchildren visit you can reverse it and create a child-proof top.

10. Do you know the expiration date of the drug?

Did the pharmacist type on the label the date when your medicine is no longer good? Never keep old bottles hanging around. Drug deterioration can lead to health problems.

11. What about non-prescription drugs?

Did you read the label or check with the pharmacist about any over-the-counter remedies you may have purchased? Are they safe and effective? Do you have a health condition that might make these drugs dangerous? Do you remain skeptical of miracle cures and drug commercials on television and radio?

12. Do you follow your doctors' instructions?

Once you understand why it's important to take your medicine do you follow through? Drugs save lives, but in order to work effectively you have to use them according to the doctor's directions. The only way blood-pressure pills can prevent the complications of hypertension (stroke, heart attack, kidney disease, etc.) is if you take them.

Now we grant you, this checklist seems like an awful lot of trouble for the doctor who has to answer all the questions, but we sincerely believe that it is well worth the effort. When you take an airplane trip you expect the pilot and crew to check the equipment out carefully. They have to make sure the plane has enough fuel, the tires are sound, the emergency gear is in working order, and that they have a clear idea of the flight plan and the weather conditions ahead. And you as the passenger want to know exactly where the plane is going. Their checklist may be complicated, but since you put your life in their hands when you fly you want to be sure they do their job well. The same thing holds true when you visit your doctor's office and put your life in his hands. A five-minute review of our "Prescription Safety Checklist" will help you know your drug destination and make your "trip" safer.

Okay, now that you've got a chart let's put it to work. There are quite a few drugs that older persons need to be especially careful with. If these medications aren't used wisely and cautiously, they can cause disaster. And sad to say, it is surprising how poorly informed doctors generally are about which drugs can be hazardous. The VALIUM case we mentioned earlier is hardly an isolated instance. So if you believe that forewarned is forearmed, hunker down and pay close attention. In the next few pages we will tell you which medications to regard with special vigilance. And you will learn of some early warning signals that can alert you to potential danger.

We will also bring you up-to-date on the elusive "Fountain of Youth." People are still looking for some way to stay young forever, but instead of searching for the legendary magical waters beyond the horizon they have turned instead to pills and injections. We will try to put some current treatments into perspective. In addition, you will learn about *treatment* for senility and some of the drugs that are being promoted for "confusion" and "forgetfulness." Even if you don't suffer any of these disorders yet, chances are pretty good that you know someone who does and in just a few years you're going to be there yourself. That doesn't mean you should anticipate problems, but it never hurts to "be prepared." Used properly and with respect, medications can relieve a lot of suffering and get you back in the ball game. Used casually or without adequate information, they can sideline you permanently.

INSOMNIA: CURSE OR BLESSING

Although you will learn everything you never wanted to know about sleep in Chapter 11, it is important for older people to be familiar with the drugs that are used to treat insomnia. For reasons that are not entirely clear, sleep patterns change as we get on in years. The newborn child sleeps somewhere between sixteen and eighteen hours every day. A young adult spends about seven-and-a-half to eight hours in the sack. And older people seem to require significantly less sleep—about four-and-a-half to six-and-a-half hours per night is the average. No one understands why some people flourish on just a few hours of sleep and others complain bitterly if that's all they get. One sleep researcher tells about a "happy, healthy 70-year-old Alabama grandmother who sleeps for an hour or so every two or three days."[19] But for every person who takes advantage of those extra hours there are hundreds of thousands if not millions who toss and turn.

It is not unusual for an older person to wake up at three or four o'clock in the morning and be unable to get back to sleep. This does not mean the person suffers from insomnia, just that the body may no longer require as many ZZZ's as it used to. But the medical profession seems to have allowed its collective brain to become stuck in a rut. Normal is often defined in terms of people between the ages of twenty and forty. If one strays from the accepted eight hours, it must be pathological and the solution to the "problem" should be a pill. Instead of counseling older people not to worry and encouraging productive activity, out comes the prescription pad.

The bottom of the bird cage on all this sleeping-pill stuff is these drugs are not very effective and can be darn dangerous, especially for older people. A special report on sleeping pills by the Institute of Medicine of the National Academy of Sciences recently concluded that:

> **The elderly are likely to remain relatively refractory, in many cases, to pharmacologic efforts. Taking any medication for sleep may add new hazards to their already complicated drug regimens.**[20,21]

An article in *Science* magazine summarized the Institute of Medicine report and its relevance for this segment of the population:

> **The significance of this whole chain of events, the panel notes, is felt particularly by the elderly, who experience insomnia as a natural development of aging. Currently, they receive 39 percent of all sleeping pill prescriptions; among nursing home patients alone, the prescription rate may be as high as 94 percent. The practice is almost entirely unwarranted, the panel suggests. Moreover, the diminished alertness caused by long-acting pills, such as DALMANE, may be confused with irreversible senility or dementia and lead to a host of other inappropriate treatments.**[22]

DALMANE (flurazepam) is the doctors' favorite prescription sleeping pill. A close relative of VALIUM and LIBRIUM, it is sold in enormous quantities. One reason it's so popular is that it works, at least for a while. Unlike many other prescription sleeping pills which begin to lose their effectiveness or may actually produce insomnia after a few nights, DALMANE is much longer-acting. And that, dear friends, is the rub, especially for older people. A breakdown product, or metabolite, of DALMANE also had sedative properties and tends to remain and accumulate in the body. "The consequence is that a patient using it on consecutive nights has a gradually increasing amount of the drug in his system; by the seventh night, patients have four to six times the amount present in their systems after the first night. The effects of the drug thus are increasingly felt during the day, contributing to greatly diminished alertness and hand-eye coordination, which may be important for driving."[23] What all that means is that after a few days the drug insidiously starts to build up and influence your ability to function while awake. And driving isn't all that can be affected. For someone getting on in years, regular use of this sleeping pill could cause mental confusion and even worse might cause difficulty in walking, which in turn could lead to a nasty fall, the last thing an older person needs.

We were so freaked out by the conclusions drawn by the Institute of Medicine that we decided to talk to the chairman of the committee under whose direction the report was written. William G. Anlyan, M.D., is what you would call a honcho in the world of medicine. He is Vice-President for Health Affairs at Duke University School of Medicine. He is also recognized internationally as an authority on medical education. In an interview for the *Journal of the American Medical Association* he stated, "The medical profession needs to clean up its own house."[24] This declaration intrigued us, so we traveled to Duke University to ask him directly what he thought about the drug education of doctors and in particular their understanding of DALMANE. Here is what he said:

> Our educational system of physicians is not geared to keep us from sliding into misuses. I've always been one of these people who hardly had aspirin in our home. Don't even have a thermometer. I hate to give anything to a patient unless they absolutely need it. On the other hand, I think that we're in a rut in terms of medical practice, particularly at the internship and residency level where it's just too common to find the admission orders include a hypnotic or sedative of choice ... I think there is a problem in many areas—for instance I worry about the misuse of antibotics ... I don't think we're up to snuff in clinical pharmacology in many areas ...

> I would want to make sure that the physician knew everything possible about DALMANE before he gave a prescription. As a matter of fact I've been amazed at the number of people who do prescribe DALMANE and VALIUM and who don't know the long term effects, particularly on elderly people.[25]

To reiterate: sleeping pills are not very effective, and they can be dangerous. Many fine doctors don't really want to prescribe drugs like DALMANE, DORIDEN (glutethimide), MILTOWN (meprobamate), NEMBUTAL (pentobarbital), and QUAALUDE (methaqualone). But. they get forced into it. Some patients put up such a fuss and feel so cheated if they don't receive a prescription that some doctors give up and say "to hell with it."[26] Out comes the prescription pad and off goes a patient with a potential problem.

What can you do if you aren't getting eight hours of sleep and sleeping pills aren't the answer? First, remember that there is no law that says "Thou Must Sleep Eight Hours." If you feel all right during the day, maybe its just your body giving you some bonus time for good behavior. But if you feel draggy and wiped out during the day, perhaps you are missing out on some needed sleep. There are a few tricks that may help. Since we are big fans of home remedies we were delighted to receive a letter from a great-grandmother in Knoxville, Tennessee. It sounded sensible enough to pass along. She and her husband "have learned that a drink of warm milk made with instant breakfast mixed with a spoonful of malt will give us the best sleep, for the longest time. And exercise is also necessary. We walk at least a mile every day and always do some gentle calisthenics before climbing into bed. We are 176 years old—each of us is 88—and still going strong."

While we cannot guarantee that this remedy will work for everybody, it is really quite logical. Sleep researchers have discovered that L-Tryptophan, an essential amino acid found in food, can have a natural sedative effect. When taken in tablet form, one or two grams is usually recommended. Unfortunately, it is expensive when purchased in health-food stores or your local pharmacy. However, milk and malt are high in tryptophan, and carbohydrates can enhance its effect. So great-grandmother's suggestion has scientific credibility. Adding a cookie or a few crackers to the warm milk will supply the carbohydrates and you may be surprised how much this diet will help. And exercise has almost always been shown to be beneficial in reducing insomnia. Other possibilities that may make falling asleep easier include a nice hot bath before bedtime and satisfying sex. But remember, even if you have trouble dropping off to dreamland, there is no reason to worry. Most people suffer some sleeplessness from time to time and experience no ill effects.

HIGH BLOOD PRESSURE

High blood pressure, also called hypertension by doctors and snobs, is everywhere. According to the people who make it their business to keep such records, at least 35 million Americans suffer from elevated blood pressure (defined as greater than 160/95) and another 25 million have borderline hypertension (defined as greater than 140/90).[27] This makes a combined total of 60 million Americans, and believe it or not the figures may even be conservative. To say high blood pressure is prevalent in epidemic proportions would be an understatement.

There is a lot of controversy surrounding the whole issue of high blood pressure and how vigorously it should be treated. Some British doctors believe that Americans get too carried away in their efforts to bring everyone down toward the so-called normal 120/80.[28,29] For example, one professor of geriatric medicine at the University of Edinburgh stated that "Every physician who is especially interested in old age will probably agree that he has seen more ill effects than benefits from hypotensives [blood pressure medicine] in this age group. The indications for lowering blood pressure in the over 70s are few . . ."[30]

But some recent investigations in the United States indicate that even moderate elevations deserve rigorous treatment. So it looks as if you "pays your money and takes your chances." This is still a hot potato and the total picture has yet to be painted. Until we know more the decision should be up to you and your doctor as to when to begin treatment. We will, however, provide you with some early warning signals that may tip you off to medication troubles.

One of the most common and unpleasant problems associated with high blood pressure treatment is something called "orthostatic hypotension." This occurs more often with ISMELIN or ESIMIL (guanethidine) but may also be a problem for folks taking Methyldopa (ALDOMET, ALDORIL, and ALDOCLOR). Other drugs that can cause this condition include L-DOPA, DARVON, SINEMET, PAR-LODEL, PRAZOSIN, and THORAZINE. Paradoxically, orthostatic hypotension is a problem of low blood pressure that accompanies changes in posture or position. Now wait just a minute—that sounds ridiculous. How can low blood pressure be a problem if a person is being treated for high blood pressure? Okay, we grant you it does seem impossible, but what this means in practical terms is that if you stand up suddenly, blood rushes to your feet and you feel faint. The medicine has knocked out some normal reflexes that help pump blood back up to your brain. The result is that you can pass out or get so dizzy that you fall over. Just think of those British honor guardsmen who must stand at rigid attention, even on very hot days. They keel over from exactly the same problem—blood pools in the veins of their legs and their head gets woozy. For an older person, this drug-induced postural low blood pressure can be particularly bad when you get out of bed in the middle of the night to go to the bathroom or when you arise first thing in the morning. If you feel giddy when you stand up or if your legs give way, chances are you have "orthostatic hypotension." Throw that term at your doctor next time you see him and we guarantee that you will get a rise out of him!

There are some things you can do to minimize the symptoms. Avoid sudden changes in posture, especially after a warm bath or upon arising in the morning. Get up very slowly and carefully, and if you feel faint, lie down again and hold on to something the next time you try. Support stockings, worn both day and night, can help prevent blood from pooling in the legs and may make a big difference. But if the symptoms persist and make life difficult, it would be an excellent idea to review your drugs and dose with your doctor.

Drugs that contain reserpine (DIUPRES, HYDROPRES, HYDROTEN-SIN, NAQUAVIL, RAUDIXIN, RAU-SED, RAUZIDE, REGRROTON, SAL-UTENSIN, SANDRIL, SER-AP-ES, SERPASIL, etc.) can cause chronic stuffy nose, stomach irritation and ulceration, and psychological depression. There has also been considerable controversy and concern about a potential cancer link.

ISMELIN (guanethidine) has a host of side effects too numerous to mention. One of the undesirable results may be inability to ejaculate in intercourse. Doctors often assume that elderly men no longer have an interest in sex and so prescribe ISMELIN. But as many of you know better than I, older people have sexual desires too, and it is outrageous that physicians often fail to inform a patient about this sexual side effect. Other adverse reactions to be alert for include diarrhea, dizziness, weakness, dry mouth, and fluid retention.

INDERAL (propranolol) and LOPRESSOR (metoprolol) are kissing cousins—that is, they are pharmacologically close relatives, having much the same action upon the body. INDERAL has become extremely popular of late and has been used for a number of ailments, including angina pectoris, high blood pressure, irregular heartbeats, and migraine headaches. Unfortunately, older people may be more susceptible to side effects because the drugs seem to be eliminated from the body more slowly once you reach sixty.[31] Side effects to be aware of include tiredness, weakness, light-headedness, stomach upset, diarrhea, wheezing or difficulty in breathing, decreased heart rate (some slowing of the pulse is to be expected), and congestive heart failure (symptoms include shortness of breath and cough after lying down at bedtime, fatigue after mild exertion, sensitivity to cold, severe cough, and sudden weight gain due to fluid retention and edema).

These drugs can be very effective for lowering blood pressure, but it is imperative that the dose be adjusted to meet each person's individual needs. Given the wide range of medications available to treat hypertension today there is no reason for someone to suffer unpleasant and dangerous side effects. A physician should be patient enough and happy to experiment with various agents in different doses until he finds just the right combination for you.

WATCH OUT FOR POTASSIUM

Almost inevitably, an older person will end up taking a diuretic, or water pill, at some time or another. This is because these drugs are the first line of attack in treating high blood pressure and are important in the control of heart failure. But one of the big problems with many diuretics is that they force potassium out of the body. Drugs like ALDORIL (methylodopa and hydrochlorothiazide), DIUPRES (chlorothiazide and reserpine), DIURIL (chlorothiazide), ESIDRIX (hydrochlorothiazide), ENDURON (methyclothiazide), HYDRODIURIL (hydrochlorothiazide), HYDROPRES (hydrochlorothiazide and reserpine), HYGROTON (chlorthalidone), and LASIX (furosemide) can really foul up your electrolyte balance. ("Electrolyte balance" is the fancy way of talking about keeping water and such important minerals as potassium, sodium, and chloride where they belong in the body so that your cells—particularly the muscle cells in your heart—can work properly.)

The early warning signals of a problem include muscle pains or cramps, muscular fatigue, dryness of the mouth, thirst, weakness, drowsiness, reduced urine flow, increased heart rate, and nausea and vomiting. The most serious problem of potassium loss occurs if you are also taking a digitalis heart medication like LANOXIN (digoxin) or digitoxin. Lack of potassium makes the heart extremely sensitive to the toxic effects of digitalis. Irregular or premature heartbeats and palpitations are a red flag that you could be in trouble. Make sure you have regular blood tests no matter what diuretic you take so that there will never be a problem with inadequate potassium. There are many ways to keep your levels up and the list of foods we have provided on page 105 should be invaluable. If it's necessary to take a potassium supplement please discuss all aspects of this therapy with your doctor before you blast off on an uncharted course.

As bad as too little potassium can be, too much may be even worse. Some folks take matters into their own hands and figure that they can just hop into the nearest health food store and stock up on some potassium tablets. Or perhaps you are one of those people who is being careful about how much salt (sodium chloride) you take in. You have purchased one of the "light" salts or potassium-chloride salt substitutes at the grocery store just to be on the "safe" side. Well, if you're not careful, this unsupervised supplementation can be a problem. In fact, too much potassium could be a killer, especially if you are taking a diuretic that preserves potassium. Now, that may be confusing. We've mentioned that a great many water pills deplete the body of potassium, and here we are saying that some others "spare" or help you retain potassium. Well, that's show business. Drugs like ALDACTAZIDE and ALDACTONE which contain an ingredient called spironolactone and DYAZIDE and DYRENIUM which contain triamterene can lead to a build-up of potassium. Be sure to find out whether your diuretic "wastes" potassium or whether it helps the body conserve it. Ignorance in this regard may have serious consequences.

Excessive potassium can be lethal. And unfortunately, early warning symptoms are few and not very specific: numb or tingling feelings on the face, scalp, tongue, hands, or feet; muscle weakness; poor respiration; and irregular heartbeats.[32] It takes an electrocardiogram to see really clear signs of toxicity and by then you are skating on some very thin ice. Older people are particularly sensitive to this condition (called "hyperkalemia" in medicalese). According to Dr. Hershel Jick, one of the leading authorities on drug-induced illness, 4 to 6 percent of elderly people experience potassium toxicity.[33,34] The only way to prevent this from happening is to go in for regular blood tests and make sure you don't overdo with a potassium supplement.

DIGITALIS HEART MEDICINE

LANOXIN is big number one! The Burroughs Wellcome drug company has really snowed the docs on this one and so their brand-name preparation outsells the generic digoxin hands down. Well, we won't quibble. The price isn't too bad and they do have a fine quality control record. We do object to the scare tactics that have been used to make people believe that generic versions are inadequate or dangerous, but that is a whole other matter. No matter what the name of the drug is—digoxin, digitoxin, LANOXIN, ACYLANID, CEDILANID, CRYSTODIGIN, DIGITALINE, GITALIGIN, PURODIGIN, or whatever— you could get into big trouble if you don't keep an eye out for what is commonly called "digitalis intoxication." These symptoms could be your lifeline to safety: loss of appetite, nausea and vomiting, changes in vision (problems with blurring of colors, especially yellow), fatigue, weakness, palpitations, increased salivation or dry mouth, bad dreams, nervousness, hallucinations, and increased pain of angina pectoris. Any of these symptoms should make you hot-foot it in to see your doctor quickly, before you get fatal heart disturbances and she or he should order an immediate blood test to check out your blood levels of the drug.

There are some very thought-provoking research reports coming out of Britain these days. Some investigators believe that "many patients are taking **Digoxin** unnecessarily as long-term treatment."[35] If you have a "normal" heartbeat which doesn't need **Digoxin** to stay normal, we recommend that you talk to your physician about some alternatives. Ask him or her to read the following articles and evaluate your particular situation:

> Editorial. "Digoxin in Sinus Rhythm." *British Medical Journal,* vol. 1, p. 1103, April 28, 1979.

> Abramowicz, Mark, ed. "Drugs in the Elderly." *Medical Letter on Drugs and Therapeutics,* vol. 21, no. 10, pp. 43–44, May 18, 1979.

> Halberstam, Michael, J. "Digoxin: Is Less More?" *Modern Medicine* vol. 47, no. 13, pp. 11–15, July 15–August 15, 1979.

Dr. Michael Halberstam sums up the most recent research in his article this way:

> **... All the authors—including those contributing to the letters column—stressed that it was in elderly patients that DIG [digitalis drugs] might be most readily stopped. Elderly patients are most prone to DIG toxicity as well, and the theraputic margin of the drug, never great, gets even narrower in the elderly, the frail, the**

forgetful, and kidney-damaged ... Given the
narrow therapeutic margin of the glycosides
[digitalis drugs], the multiple and subtle
manifestations of digitalis toxicity, and the
failure of serum levels to discriminate absolutely between "toxic" and "therapeutic" doses, it
is possible that we might all need to reevaluate
use of these drugs.[36]

ANTIBIOTICS

For reasons that are not entirely clear, both patients and physicians
tend to let down their guard with antibiotics. The great usefulness of
the drugs sometimes clouds our puny little brains and we forget that
they can be overprescribed and that they have side effects. You have
already read what Dr. Bill Anlyan had to say about the misuse of
antibiotics. Well, for older persons whose kidney function just isn't
what it used to be, antibiotics can pose a special problem. Even when
there is no out-and-out kidney damage, there may be subtle
reductions in efficiency, and drugs can build up to toxic levels instead
of being eliminated promptly. Drugs which require extra caution
include tetracycline (ACHROMYCIN V, MYSTECLIN-F, PANMYCIN,
ROBITET, SUMYCIN, TETRACYN, TETREX, etc.), gentamycin
(GARAMYCIN), kanamycin (KANTREX), and STREPTOMYCIN. Even an
old favorite like AMPICILLIN (AMCILL, OMNIPEN, PEN A, PENSYN,
POLYCILLIN, PRINCIPEN, and TOTACILLIN) can make waves. It is
"one of the most common causes of skin rash in this age group."[37]
Other side effects to be alert for include itching, severe diarrhea,
"hairy" tongue, sore throat, and fever.

Okay, we have just taken you on a whirlwind mystery tour of drugs
and older people. All these medications have a place, even the
sleeping pills (used infrequently for an occasional sleepless night
they rarely cause trouble). When prescribed carefully and used wisely
with full knowledge of potential adverse reactions there is every
reason to believe that anyone can benefit from these medications.
However, if you are unprepared or uninformed, you are courting
disaster, especially when you pass fifty-five.

THE FOUNTAIN OF YOUTH

GEROVITAL: RIP-OFF OR RINGER?

Ah, to be young and beautiful again! What a joy! Nonsense! One
can be beautiful at any age. And trying to recapture one's "glorious"
past with a drug is ludicrous. Of course many of us wish we could live
forever in perfect health and harmony. But folks, it ain't gonna

happen any time soon, so stop holding your breath. Unfortunately, there are quite a few unscrupulous, unethical, and downright selfish stinkpots out there who would like nothing better than to convince you that their special formula will rejuvenate and restore eternal youth. There are wonder serums and special gland formulations and, yes, even hormone-replacement therapies. A book appeared not too long ago called *Feminine Forever* that touted the benefits of estrogens. We now know that this foolish fad led to a dramatic increase in cancer of the uterine lining of women who were talked into the treatment, often on the recommendation of their doctors. Well, we may have learned about hormones but that doesn't mean we have become any smarter. The current fad is GEROVITAL (procaine plus?). Let's take a look at the evidence and see whether this product is worth the attention it has received.

GEROVITAL is supposed to be a miraculous rejuvenator. Professor Ana Aslan of the Bucharest Institute of Geriatrics has been touting the marvelous benefits of this "wonder" drug for over thirty years. Now before you get all excited, perhaps we should tell you what the mystery drug actually is. Procaine or NOVOCAIN should be familiar to anyone who has ever visited a dentist's office. It is a local anesthetic, injected to "deaden" nerves. Now it's true that this injectable procaine has been modified slightly because in its regular form it deteriorates rather rapidly. But GEROVITAL H3, as it is called, is really nothing more elegant than a local anesthetic and has been available for years.

Does it work? Well, the claims are extraordinary, to say the least. Its advocates say it will prevent or relieve arthritis, arteriosclerosis, angina pectoris, deafness, neuritis, senile psychosis, wrinkling of skin, psoriasis, anxiety, peptic ulcer, impotence, Parkinson's disease, high blood pressure, and depression. Some people even assert that GEROVITAL will bring color back into your glorious locks. That's right—you can become a brunette again, or a blond or a whatever ... And best of all, the drug can add years to your life. The Rumanian National Tourist Office claims that the Aslan Clinic has treated "certain world-renowned actors, actresses, writers and statesmen who have the secret of eternal vigor and youth."[38] We've been told that Nikita Khrushchev, Ho Chi Minh, and President Sukarno of Indonesia all made the pilgrimage in order to be rejuvenated.

But, to repeat our question: Does it work? Well, we hate to be party poopers, but we do have some bad news. Dr. Adrian Ostfeld, from the Department of Epidemiology and Public Health at the Yale University School of Medicine, recently reviewed data from 285 articles and books that described the treatment in more than 100,000 patients in the past 25 years. Her conclusions: "Except for a possible antidepressant effect, there is no convincing evidence that procaine (or GEROVITAL of which procaine is the major component) has any value in the treatment of disease in older patients."[39] There is some evidence that the drug can act as an antidepressant, but there are other, more effective medications for that purpose. For another evaluation read what the experts from the *Medical Letter on Drugs and Therapeutics* have to say. They have no axe to grind and inevitably tell it like it is: "GEROVITAL H3 has not been shown to be of value in retarding the aging process, or for the treatment of any disorder in the elderly."[40] Although side effects are relatively rare, some people are allergic to procaine and this could cause serious problems. Symptoms may include low blood pressure, breathing difficulty, flushing, itching, skin rash, and convulsions.

Where do we go from here? As the eminent geriatric specialist, Dr. William Davison, recently said:

> **Drugs for eternal youth? No, not yet! No practical knowledge from gerontological studies has appeared to make any impact in terms of drug treatment on the aging process; claims to the contrary tend to be based on inadequate evidence . . . To achieve a normal, disease-free old age the best advice is the adoption of a more healthy lifestyle with plentiful vigorous physical exercise and a more frugal diet. When things go wrong timely and appropriate medical intervention has a lot to offer.[41]**

We apologize for bringing the sad news. It would be lovely to announce a wonder drug that would cure everything that ails you. But we assure you, if such a miracle existed, you would hear about it quickly—and the doctors would probably be the first to hop on the bandwagon. There are a lot of old dudes in the medical profession who would love nothing better than some snazzy rejuvenator so they could keep doing their thing. The secret would be out of the bag instantly, especially since there would be some big bucks to be made by all concerned. So dear reader, don't give up hope, but don't expect a miracle anytime soon. Do your best to stay healthy, enjoy your life, and keep on truckin'.

SAVE US FROM SENILITY

We all have problems with memory at some time or another. How many times have you said, "Where did I leave my keys, what happened to my glasses, where's my wallet, who stole my pocketbook?" If any of that sounds familiar, relax, it happens to everyone with great regularity. But maybe you are worried that your memory is getting worse than just routine forgetfulness. Well, senility, or as it has recently been dubbed, organic brain syndrome (leave it to the doctors to sanitize and confuse an understandable word), may affect approximately 5 percent of the elderly population. Many people assume that this is a natural part of aging. But what is not realized is that quite often symptoms of senility may be caused by some underlying factor. And prescription medication may be one of the most common and unrecognized parts of the problem. Sleeping pills, sedatives, tranquilizers, anti-anxiety agents (like VALIUM) and a host of other nervous-system depressants can cause confusion and lead to memory loss. In fact, a group of specialists on aging gathered by the National Institute of Health's Institute on Aging reported that 300,000 to 600,000 people who show some symptoms of reduced mental capability may be mislabeled "senile" all because the underlying cause has gone unrecognized. Dr. Richard Besdine of Harvard Medical School and author of the committee's draft report brings the problem into painful focus: "The prospect of 300,000 doomed people in the United States today who could have been restored to useful life by appropriate evaluation and treatment is staggering and demands action."[42] According to the experts, one of the most important causes of "false senility" was drug intoxication — remember the "spaced-out Grandma syndrome" we mentioned earlier in this chapter?

Tranquilizers are not the only medicines that can affect mental stability. Blood-pressure drugs that produce psychological depression can add to the dilemma. One geriatric psychologist, Dr. Robert Kahn from the University of Chicago, claims that depression itself makes people think they have trouble with their memory even though they score well on memory tests. There are also a number of easily missed diseases that can contribute to reversible senility. They include heart disease, thyroid gland problems, infections (pneumonia can be a real problem for an older person), diabetes, and even nutritional deficiency.[43] So if you are afraid that you are losing that edge, perhaps it's time to have a thorough physical examination with special attention devoted to reviewing all your medications, just in case a combination of drugs is turning you into a zombie.

But what if the memory loss is real and isn't due to any drug or underlying condition? Is there anything that can help? The answer is yes and no. There have been some pretty impressive claims and some unpleasant disappointments. Let's try to bring you up to date on what is the current thinking among geriatric specialists. The most heavily promoted drugs to reverse the mental problems of aging are the Hydrogenated Ergot Alkaloids. Popular brands include **HYDERGINE**, **DEAPRIL-ST**, and **CIRCANOL**. Medical journals often carry very slick and appealing color ads for these products. Picture the perfect grandparents—they're bright and cheerful and off on vacation just having a grand old time. Not a care in the world and **HYDERGINE** is the reason. Here's an example of the promotion to doctors:

> **They're in their late sixties, the beneficiaries of more liberal retirement laws and more enlight- ened attitudes toward the elderly. They're lead- ing socially productive lives. But recently, without any clear cause, they had each begun to experience mild episodes of symptoms such as confusion, mood-depression, and dizziness. Their ability to function could have been jeo- pardized. That's then they became the benefici- aries of oral HYDERGINE.**[44]

As promising as that may seem, there is actually relatively little evidence to support such enthusiastic claims. Although there may be small improvement for some persons, the benefits have been far from dramatic and most authorities remain skeptical. The experts consulting for the *Medical Letter* concluded that "There is no convincing evidence that dihydrogenated ergot alkaloids are effective for treatment of 'Idiopathic Cerebral Dysfunction' or any other disorder of elderly patients."[45] Does that mean the drugs should never be tried? Absolutely not! They are relatively innocuous with few side effects. There may be some temporary nausea or stomach upset, but that is about all. If you suffer from confusion, depression, and dizziness, as described in the drug ads, it may be worth giving the ergot alkaloids a whirl for a month or two, but don't expect miracles, especially not for your memory. Quite sincerely we believe that a little love, attention, and social support from friends, family, and neighbors will go a lot farther than any pill ever can. There are even many physicians who agree.[46]

But what about memory? Alright already, we haven't forgotten the question! We are not always nay-sayers. There have been some tantalizing research reports that have surfaced lately regarding a drug called **CHOLINE**. Actually, it isn't a true drug, but rather a constituent of food like egg yolks, fish, lecithin, and so on. It is a building block for an important chemical called acetylcholine, which is found in the brain and is thought to play an important role in memory. Anything that increases acetylcholine levels (such as CHOLINE, and a drug called physostigmine) may be able to improve memory.[47,48] Unfortunately, the work is purely preliminary and will require much closer scrutiny before you can count on it. Choline is available (as is lecithin) from many pharmacies and health food stores.

Perhaps the most exciting research involves a drug called vasopressin (PITRESSIN). Although its benefits for memory loss in senility have been somewhat questionable, there have been some extraordinary case reports mentioned in the medical literature. Although we tend to be doubtful about "testimonial" reports because they are so unscientific, we feel it might be worth sharing some of the stories with you because we found them so fascinating:

> ...A man aged 55 had had a serious car accident six years previously. On leaving the hospital a year after the accident, he was still mentally impaired with considerable defects of memory, especially remote memory. Vasopressin treatment was started by nasal spray. After the first five days of treatment, progress was remarkable: his mood improved (he became more lively and regained a taste for reading) and his memory returned (he could recall the date of the accident, date of his wedding, the age of his wife and his daughter, the different jobs he had had). When seen on day twenty-eight, this improvement had been maintained at the daily dose of 15 I.U.

> ...A man aged 21, presented with severe retrograde amnesia after a car accident six months previously (coma for 15 days). He could remember nothing of the three months before the accident and the three and a half months after it. Vasopressin was given by nasal spray. After one day the patient could recall several features of the accident, and his memory rapidly improved... Improvement progressed continuously, and by day seven he had completely recovered his memory.[49]

There have been other case reports of rather astonishing success with Vasopressin and animal studies also appear encouraging.[50–52]

But, and that is one humongous BUT, please don't take these very preliminary reports too seriously. Follow-up research could quite easily contradict and deflate initial enthusiasm. There is an awful lot more work that must be done before anyone can give a stamp of approval to this treatment. If that sounds like we are being overly cautious, you bet your booties we are. The drug is not harmless. It can constrict blood vessels and in sensitive persons might cause an angina attack. It might also be a problem for people with heart failure, asthma, epilepsy, or migraine. People who are allergic to vasopressin (PITRESSIN) may experience sweating, tremor, vertigo, difficulty in breathing, pounding in the head, nausea, and gas. Despite these words of caution we are excited about the possibilities and hope that new research will give us some definitive answers in the near future.

LET'S TAKE IT ON HOME

We have covered a lot of territory. You have learned why drug companies are enamored of older people. You have been cautioned that dosage requirements change with age. Multiple prescribing, or polypharmacy as it is called by the insiders, can be a horrendous problem for people when they pass fifty-five. And cost can prevent some folks from purchasing needed medicine. We have provided a checklist and some navigational charts that should guide you along your pharmacological journeys. We hope we steered you past the rapids of sleeping pills and around the sinkholes of high blood pressure. We put up some sign posts for potassium, digitalis, and antibiotics. And last but not least, we tried to keep you from drowning in the fountain of youth.

REFERENCES

1. Loh, Lilah. "Drug Misuse in the Elderly: Those Hurt Most Are Least Able to Prevent It." *Am. Pharmacy* 18(7):32–33, 1978.

2. Vestal, Robert E. "Drug Use in the Elderly. A Review of the Problems and Special Consideration." *Drugs* 16:358–382, 1978.

3. "How Does Aging Affect Drug Metabolism?" *Duke University Medical Center Intercom* 25(22):2, 1978.

4. Editorial. "Drugs in the Elderly." *Br. Med. J.* 1:1168, 1978.

5. Lamy, Peter P. "Considerations in Drug Therapy of the Elderly." *J. of Drug Issues* 9(1):27–45, 1979.

6. Exton-Smith, A. N. "Hazards in Old Age" (book review). *Br. Med. J.* 2:267–268, 1979.

7. Wegner, Fred. "Needed: A Comprehensive Drug Benefit for the Elderly." *Am. Pharmacy* 18(7):29, 1978.

8. Ibid.

9. Gifford, Jr., Ray W. "Drugs for Arterial Hypertension." *Drug of Choice* 1978—1978. Walter Modell, ed.; St. Louis: C. V. Mosby, 1978, p. 424.

10. Piao Chien, Ching; Townsend, E. J.; and Townsend, A. R. "Substance Use and Abuse Among the Community Elderly. The Community Aspect." *Addictive Disease: An International Journal* 3(3):357—372, 1978.

11. Solomon, Jeffrey R. "The Chemical Time Bomb: Drug Misuse by the Elderly." *Contemporary Drug Problems* 6(2):131—143, 1977.

12. Piao Chien, Op. cit., p. 367.

13. Cooper, Jr., James W. "Drug Therapy in the Elderly: Is It All It Could Be?" *Am. Pharmacy* 18(7):25:26, 1978.

14. Huff, Barbara B., ed. *Physicians Desk Reference,* 33rd edition. Medical Economics Co., Oradell, N. J., 1979, p. 1469.

15. Gottlieb, R. M.; Naapi, T.; and Strain, J. J. "The Physician's Knowledge of Psychotropic Drugs. Preliminary Results." *Am. J. of Psychiatry* 135: 29—32, 1978.

16. Green, Grent. "The Politics of Psychoactive Drug Use in Old Age." *The Gerontologist* 18(6):525—530, 1978.

17. Charatan, Fred B., "Somebody *DO* Something ... About the Mistreatment of Elderly Patients." *Mod. Med.* 46(5):35, 1978.

18. Cohen, Sidney. "Sleep and Insomnia." *JAMA* 230:875—876, 1976.

19. Wartik, Louise D., ed. "Doctor, Why Can't I Sleep?" *Faces of Penn State* 2(2):2—3, 1976.

20. Solomon, S., et al. "Sleeping Pills, Insomnia and Medical Practice." *New Eng. J. of Med.* 300:803—808, 1979.

21. *Medical News.* "Physician Prescribing Practices Criticized; Solutions in Question." *JAMA* 241:2353—2360, 1979.

22. Smith, R. Jeffrey. "Study Finds Sleeping Pills Overprescribed." *Science* 204:287—288, 1979.

23. Ibid.

24. *Medical News,* op. cit.

25. Personal interview at Duke University School of Medicine with Dr. William Anlyan, June 14, 1979.

26. *Medical News,* op. cit.

27. Robert Levy, M.D., Director Division of National Heart, Blood and Lung Institute (National Institutes of Health). (Personal Communication).

28. Green, Kenneth G. "Optimised Blood-Pressure." *Lancet* 11:33, 1979.

29. Stewart, I. McD. G., "Optimised Blood-Pressure." *Lancet* 11:33, 1979.

30. Williamson, J. "Prescribing Problems in the Elderly." *Practitioner* 220:749—755, 1978.

31. "Drugs in the Elderly." *Med. Letter* 21(10):43—44, 1979.

32. Robinson, Corinne H., and Lawler, Marilyn R., *Normal and Therapeutic Nutrition.* New York: Macmillan Publishing Co., 15th ed., 1977, p. 131.

33. Hershel Jick (Boston Collaborative Drug Surveillance Program). (Personal Communication).

34. Lawson, D. H. "Adverse Reactions to Potassium Chloride." *Quart. J. Med. News Series* 43:433, 1974.

35. Editorial. "Digoxin in Sinus Rhythm." *Br. Med. J.* 1:1103, 1979.

36. Halberstam, Michael J. "Digoxin: Is Less More?" *Mod. Med.* 47(13):11—15, 1979.

37. Ward, Morton, and Blatman, Morris. "Drug Therapy in the Elderly." *Am. Family Physician* 19(2):143—150, 1979.

38. "Gerovital H3." *Med. Letter* 21:4, 1979.

39. Ostfeld, Adrian, et al. "The Systemic Use of Procaine in the Treatment of the Elderly: A Review." *J. of the Am. Geriat. Soc.* 25:1—19, 1977.

40. "Gerovital H3." op. cit.

41. Davison, William. "Drugs for Eternal Youth: Scientific Attempts to Combat Aging." *J. of Drug Issues* 9(1):91—104, 1979.

42. Cohn, Victor. "Up to 600,000 Elderly Americans are Mistakenly Labeled as Senile." Washington Post- L. A. Times News Service. *Durham Sun*, p. 7- A, Aug. 2, 1978.

43. Ibid.

44. Sandoz Hydergine Advertisement. *JAMA* 241:2704—2705, 1979.

45. Reichel, William. "Family Practice and Care of the Elderly" (guest editorial). *Am. Family Physician* 20:85—86, 1979.

46. "Deapril- ST for Senile Dementia." *Med. Letter* 19(15):61—62, 1977.

47. "Stimulants and Other Drugs for Treatment of Mental Symptoms in the Elderly." *Med. Letter* 20(7):75, 1978.

48. News. "Choline May Curb Memory Loss." *Am. Family Physician* 19(4):196, 1979.

49. Oliveros, J. C., et al. "Vasopressin in Amnesia." *Lancet* 1(8054):42, 1978.

50. LeBoeuf, Alan, et al. "Vasopressin and Memory in Korsakoff Syndrom." *Lancet* 2(8140):1370, 1978.

51. Legros, J. J., et al. "Influence of Vasopressin on Learning and Memory." *Lancet* 1(8054):41, 1978.

52. Pfeiffer, W. Dean, and Borkin, Howard D. "Vasopressin Antagonizes Retrograde Amenesia in Rats Following Electroconvulsive Shock." *Pharmocol. Biochemistry Behavior* 9:261—263, 1978.

10

Arthritis: from A (aspirin)
to V (vinegar)

The amorphous disease. Charlatans and folk remedies, placebos and acupuncture. The amazing tale of angina. Arthritis treatments tried and true: **Aspirin**, MOTRIN, NAPROSYN, CLINORIL, NALFON, and TOLECTIN • A cost comparison of **Aspirin** and prescription arthritis drugs • Bringing out the heavy artillery: INDOCIN and BUTAZOLIDIN • There's more to gold than just glitter • Malaria drugs for arthritis • Last but not least: **Cortisone**, CUPRIMINE, and LEVAMISOLE.

Arthritis is a bummer. It affects around fifty million Americans, of whom about twenty-two million require treatment. According to the Arthritis Foundation, the money lost in wages, taxes, and disability payments each year amounts to over eight billion dollars. Another four billion is spent on some form of medical care.[1] In economic terms the cost of arthritis is staggering. In human terms the cost is immeasurable. Arthritis can be so painful and disable you so badly that you can't get around. Just getting in and out of a car can be pure agony. Trying to climb up into a bus can be like tackling Mount Everest and take almost as much courage to conquer. Accompanying the pain is the frustration and depression of reduced activity. All in all, arthritis stinks!

One of the main problems about arthritis is its name. It's a catch-all term that encompasses a large number of distinct ailments that range from mild to severe. There's osteoarthritis (the most common form), rheumatoid arthritis, ankylosing spondylitis, systemic lupus erythematosus (lupus for short), bursitis, gout, and a number of other inflammatory diseases. There is even "Lyme arthritis" named after a small town in Connecticut.[2] It is hard enough to pronounce many of these ailments, let alone understand them. And quite honestly, we are barely out of the Dark Ages as far as our comprehension of what these common conditions are all about. Despite what you may read in

379

the papers about miracle cures and fantastic breakthroughs, the "experts" are still feeling their way along one step at a time.

Although we may not understand very much about what causes arthritis or why some people are more susceptible than others, that does not mean the arthritis sufferer has to toss in the towel. Pain and inflammation can be reduced and it is possible to avoid disability. The key to proper treatment is correct diagnosis. Because aches and pains come on gradually and because almost everyone has a touch of the "rheumatism" now and again, a lot of people self-diagnose and self-medicate and delay a trip to the doctor. And unfortunately, some doctors themselves may be unprepared to distinguish adequately between all the various types of arthritis.

For example, osteoarthritis is generally mild and rarely deforming. It comes on as joints slowly degenerate with age. If we all lived long enough everyone would probably experience some degree of this kind of arthritis. While there may be some pain and stiffness associated with osteoarthritis, signs of inflammation (redness, heat, and swelling) are not common or long-lasting and anti-inflammatory drugs are not usually necessary. Moderate doses of aspirin or acetaminophen (TYLENOL, DATRIL, NEBS, TEMPRA, etc.) can reduce the pain and help you keep on truckin'. More on these drugs later. Rheumatoid arthritis, on the other hand, can produce severe inflammation and if not handled correctly can cause serious disability. It often requires powerful anti-inflammatory agents to halt the destructive process.

If you want to get a handle on this complicated subject we highly recommend an excellent book titled *Arthritis, A Comprehensive Guide,* written by Dr. James F. Fries, Director of the Stanford Arthritis Clinic (Addison-Wesley Publishing Company). It will help you understand the various forms of this amorphous disease and enable you to comprehend what your doctor is talking about when she starts throwing around those complicated-sounding medical terms.

ARTHRITIS CURES BEYOND BELIEF

Besides the pain and frustration of the disease itself, one of the hardest crosses to bear with arthritis is that there are so many rip-off artists out there just waiting to exploit your suffering for their own profit. The waters are filled with leeches and sharks. If the leeches don't suck you dry first, the sharks will eat what's left. They offer tantalizing cures that promise fast relief. That kind of promise is hard to ignore, especially if you are hurting. Greed is a powerful motivator and with so many potential victims praying for help these unscrupulous operators realize that they can clean up. The experts for Consumers Union note that millions of arthritic Americans "are a prime target for hucksters, miracle-cure promoters, and charlatans. According to the Arthritis Foundation, a nonprofit national health organization, the annual bill for unproved or quack arthritis remedies totals an estimated $950-million."[3]

A recent review of ridiculous treatments was documented in *Consumer Reports:*

> **Among the most popular devices were vibrators. One model for arthritics came with five attachments, including one guaranteed to banish dandruff ... For a while, radiation was in. Arthritis victims could pay for the privilege of sitting in an abandoned uranium mine to absorb the "healing radiations." If they were too poor or crippled to take advantage of this sovereign remedy, they could still buy mitts or pads supposedly containing low-grade radioactive ore. A typical one, the marvpad, cost $30 and was filled with gravel.[4]**

Not only was this remedy ineffective, long enough exposure to even low-level radiation might increase the likelihood of cancer many years later. Fortunately, most of these patently ludicrous devices have disappeared, but there are always new fads to replace old ones. And newspaper tabloids know that arthritis stories sell papers. The tabloids continually run headlines of the latest cure in two-inch-high print on their front page. It's hard to ignore these rags when you stand in the line at the check-out counter of your supermarket. The other day we came across one for a doctor's wonder serum—"It can cure arthritis, it may beat cancer, it boosts your sex life." According to the article, a physician in France had discovered "The Fountain of Life." It "has halted crippling arthritis, rheumatism and skin diseases. And kept the horrors of old age at bay." As if that weren't enough, another benefit of this treatment "is virility: sex!"

Nothing drives a pharmacologist bananas faster than this sort of baloney. Okay, we can hear you saying, what's the big deal? Why get so hot and bothered over some "sensational" newspaper report? Well, if this stuff really has been tested and is effective we should all be packing our bags and heading for France (or wherever) in order to cure our ills, improve our love life, and stay young forever. But as usual, there were no scientific tests and no valid controlled evaluations. This kind of story represents the worst kind of exploitation there is. Not only does it play upon people's misery and pain but it can generate false hopes. Many folks feel cheated because they think that somewhere a cure exists that will solve all their medical woes. A few desperate souls, following the example of Ponce de Leon, might even pack up and travel in search of the wonder drug. Not only will they be blowing hard-earned money, they might discontinue other treatments that were beneficial.

Wait just one minute, Mr. Smart Guy!, you may be thinking about now. If all these claims are pure bunk, why do they survive? Someone must be getting better from them or else it would be like trying to sell smog in Los Angeles. Okay, you have a point. Some folks do actually feel better after the treatment, whether it be some new and mysterious injectable serum, a copper bracelet, or an old Vermont doctor's vinegar-and-honey recipe. We would be the first to admit that many folk remedies do help and that "modern" medicine does not hold all the answers. People who benefit from bone meal, alfalfa tea, or cherry juice should count their blessings because these are much safer solutions than potent anti-inflammatory drugs. But without sound scientific testing it is hard to separate the psychological expectations of the patient (or the practitioner) from the actual curative powers of the remedy. In order to accurately gauge effectiveness you would have to perform a "double-blind test" where neither the investigator nor the subject knew if the actual substance or an inactive placebo (sugar pill) was being used. The mind behaves in strange and incalculable ways. It often responds to suggestion and, yes, the good old-fashioned placebo. We understand so little about placebos and the relationship between the mind and body that it is sinful. Most patients and doctors disdain this approach but it can be an important therapeutic tool. It is amazing what can happen if you believe hard enough.

Does that mean that arthritis is all in the mind and that a bogus therapy will work for everyone? Absolutely not! Unfortunately, arthritis is all too real. But so is the debilitating heart disease called angina and it too responds in a most extraordinary way to placebo treatment. Please bear with us for a moment while we digress and describe the power of the mind to alleviate physical symptoms. Dr. Herbert Benson, Associate Professor of Medicine at Harvard Medical School, and a renowned expert on the relationship between mind and the body recently published a most impressive article in the *New England Journal of Medicine* titled "Angina Pectoris and the Placebo Effect."[5] Dr. Benson reviewed once-respected medical procedures for the treatment of angina that have fallen into disfavor because careful testing proved them ineffective. However, at the time, there was an overall improvement in over 80 percent of the patients treated with the various inactive remedies. People were able to increase their exercise, reduce their reliance upon **Nitroglycerin** and their electrocardiogram actually showed improvement!

In one of the most famous and somewhat unethical placebo experiments ever performed, two groups of surgeons performed sham operations. They wanted to compare an actual coronary artery surgery procedure that was gaining favor in the mid-1950s with a placebo. The only way that they could think to carry out the investigation was to fake surgery in one group of patients in order to create the placebo effect. Under anesthesia they actually made a small incision that looked for all intents and purposes like the real thing. The patients thought they had gone through an operation, when in reality all they had received was a cosmetic scar. Another group of patients actually did go under the knife and had their coronary artery operated upon.

Well what happened? The answer is astounding! In the group that received the fake surgery, every single person (100 percent) had a decreased need for their **Nitroglycerin** medicine and had a greater ability to exercise. Of the patients who had the real surgery, only 76 percent experienced these benefits.[6] Hard as it is to accept, the placebo treatment was actually more effective. All of the patients who had received the fake operation maintained their improvement for more than six weeks and some were still better in six months. If anything demonstrates the power of the mind to affect the body, these experiments did so. Dr. Benson concluded his article with some important observations:

> **Although the placebo effect is commonly believed to be of limited duration, several of the studies indicate relief for a year or more. The placebo effect will most likely persist as long as the psychological context in which it was evoked remains unchanged. Patient and physician belief in efficacy of the therapy and a continuously strong physician-patient relation should maintain the effects for long periods. Conversely, a poor physician-patient relation or patient or physician doubt about the therapy would quickly abolish the placebo effect . . . The placebo effect has been viewed primarily as a confounding, bothersome artifact. However, the placebo effect has always been one of the**

physician's most potent therapeutic assets.
Even with inactive procedures, physicians in
the past have consistently achieved marked
symptomatic improvement in approximately 80
percent of patients with angina pectoris. This
remarkable efficacy should not be discouraged
or ridiculed. After all, unlike most other forms
of therapy, the placebo effect has withstood the
test of time and continues to be safe and
inexpensive.[7]

So what? Does all this angina stuff have any relevance to arthritis?
You bet your belly button it does. Now you know why so many
questionable treatments work. Take acupuncture for example. This
therapy has been widely recommended for all sorts of maladies,
including arthritis. Despite widespread enthusiasm there have been
few well-controlled experiments to test the effectiveness of acupuncture. The results of one study that was carefully planned were
published in the *New England Journal of Medicine*. The researchers
wanted to discover whether acupuncture could truly relieve the pain
of osteoarthritis. One group of patients received a sham treatment by
having needles placed in "placebo points" that did not correspond to
traditional Chinese acupuncture points. The other group went
through a regular course of therapy. It should come as no surprise to
learn that both groups of patients experienced benefits. And by now
you should be prepared for the punch line: the improvement wasn't
significantly different between the two groups. There are a couple of
different explanations for this outcome. First, the arthritis might have
improved whether or not the experiment had been done. Second,
sticking needles in someone is so dramatic that it may produce a
placebo response whether it's genuine acupuncture or not. But more
likely than not there is something else going on and the doctors who
did the research offer the following factors:

The patient's expectations and desire for relief
from pain; the physician's expectation of
therapeutic results; the interpersonal relations
between patient and acupuncturist, as well as
physician evaluators; the desire of patients to
contribute to scientific experimentation and
advance scientific knowledge; and the possible
suggestive factor engendered by widespread
publicity in the media about the alleged effectiveness of acupuncture in relieving pain. In

addition, when patients appeared regularly for
evaluation, evaluators and acupuncturists were
attentive to the patient's complaints.[8]

Does all this mean that placebos should never be used for arthritis?
Not on your life. Go to Jail, do not pass GO and do not collect $200.
Reread what Dr. Benson said. As long as treatment is safe and
inexpensive, great. What we object to is paying a lot of money for air.
No one should get rich at someone else's expense.

ARTHRITIS TREATMENTS: TRIED AND TRUE

Well, what can be used that really does work—no ifs, ands, buts, or
placebos? There are a large number of "legitimate" medications that
are available to the arthritis victim that truly can make life bearable
and prevent deformity. Whether you suffer from gout, rheumatoid
arthritis, or just aches and pains, there is a lot you can do (including
non-drug treatment) to improve your condition. First, find out from
your doctor exactly what kind of arthritis you have. If it's
osteoarthritis (the most common kind) you will probably be able to
get by with aspirin. Acetaminophen (TYLENOL, DATRIL, etc.) may
help relieve pain but it can't reduce inflammation. If you experience
more pain than these drugs can handle you may want to add
something a little stronger. Some doctors are free with the pain pills—
they will load you up on TALWIN (pentazocine), DARVON, or
DARVOCET (propoxyphene plus acetaminophen), DEMEROL, (me-
peridine), or PERCODAN (oxycodone, aspirin, phenacetin, and caffeine) to name just a few commonly prescribed analgesics. If you
use these medications so that you can continue to function you are
making a big mistake. It is a little like sending a football player back
into the game with a broken foot, a concussion, and a crushed rib by
doping him up to the point where he can't feel the pain. Obviously,
greater damage will be done to an already battered body.

On the other hand, there are doctors who believe in stoicism and
urge their patients to tough it out with just plain aspirin or TYLENOL.
We feel that the middle road is more appropriate. We don't believe in
suffering, but we also believe that pain is a good warning sign that is
trying to tell you something. If you continue to use an inflamed joint
you will do it additional damage. Rest is necessary and if you do take
the warning seriously we see no reason why additional relief should
not be obtained occasionally by adding a little codeine to the aspirin
or acetaminophen. When the pain has subsided, you can forgo the
codeine. If you're allergic to codeine have your doctor prescribe an
equivalent analgesic. During painful periods rest is important. But

when you are feeling better it is helpful to keep those joints and muscles active. Skip the skiing, horseback riding, handball, or any other exercise that will increase pain or inflammation. Slow, steady movement, on the other hand, such as swimming, walking, or biking can be excellent for joints. As long as you don't overindulge you will make progress.

If you have rheumatoid arthritis, you have a lot of inflammation and that will cause the pain. Relief depends upon interrupting the inflammatory process. Fortunately, many drugs have been introduced over the last decade that can do a pretty fine job if they are used wisely. Unfortunately, these medications also have the potential to cause a number of undesirable effects, some of which are quite hazardous. In order to use them effectively you have to be on your toes to make sure the remedy won't cause more problems than the ailment.

ASPIRIN

Without a doubt aspirin truly is a miracle drug. Every year over nineteen billion doses are sold.[9] At regular doses (two tablets) it is an excellent pain reliever and in high doses (ten to twenty-four tablets over a day) it is also a fine anti-inflammatory agent. It has been used for seventy-five years and has an admirable track record. For it to be useful for rheumatoid arthritis you have to take a whopping big dose that your doctor should determine. At these levels stomach irritation can be a real problem. Other side effects to watch out for include ringing in the ears (tinnitus), nausea or stomach pain, and paradoxically, headaches. According to Dr. James Fries (author of *Arthritis, A Comprehensive Guide,* that excellent reference book we mentioned earlier in the chapter) these symptoms do not mean that you have to panic and give up on aspirin. He claims that "most patients receiving aspirin for anti-inflammatory purposes will have some ringing in the ears and some nausea. This is just a reason to slow down a little bit and to establish what dose is the exactly correct one for you. If you don't know this principle, you are going to give up too soon on a superb drug and you won't get better."[10]

Another physician who agrees with Dr. Fries is John L. Decker, Chief of the Arthritis and Rheumatism Section of the National Institute of Arthritis, Metabolism and Digestive Diseases. He claims that aspirin's side effects "have been very much overrated. American physicians do not use enough aspirin, simply because they don't like the idea of handing the patient a bill for $50 and then advising him simply to take aspirin."[11] You really do have to give aspirin at least two weeks at a high dose in order to experience much relief from inflammation. But if you do stick with it, you will be amazed at how excellent this everyday take-it-for-granted medicine really can be for relieving arthritis pain.

Despite the fact that aspirin is both cheap and effective, let's not forget that it can cause complications. The most common undesirable effects of large doses are gastric upset and bleeding. Ulcers are a major concern and anyone with a history of peptic ulcer should be exceedingly careful and probably avoid aspirin altogether. There are some tricks of the trade that can make taking aspirin easier. Although food may reduce absorption somewhat, it can also reduce irritation. So if you are having problems, take your aspirin during meals or snacks. One of our favorite techniques for lessening the likelihood of digestive upset is to take a mouthful of milk and while holding it in your mouth pop in two aspirin tablets. Then chew with the milk and swallow the glop down. Follow that mess with a full eight ounces of milk and you should diminish some of the symptoms. In addition, the aspirin should get into your bloodstream faster. If chewing sounds too terrible (we guarantee that it isn't that bad) you could always purchase aspirin already in powdered form. These are old-fashioned remedies, but they have some merit. Some doctors recommend that you take your aspirin with an antacid or in a buffered formula in order to reduce gastritis. ASCRIPTIN, ATHRITIS PAIN FORMULA, ARTHRITIS STRENGTH BUFFERIN, and BUFFERIN have huge sales for this very reason. They all contain aluminum and magnesium antacids. Unfortunately, you pay a price for decreased irritation. Antacids increase the alkalinity of the urine and this in turn speeds elimination of the drug from your system. The end result is that you will get lower blood levels and less benefit from the aspirin. One study found blood concentration decreased by 30 to 70 percent when antacids were taken simultaneously.[12] For additional information on other drugs that may interact with aspirin, we highly recommend that you turn to pages 113—115 in the chapter on drug interactions.

One final word of caution. Some people are allergic to aspirin and may not know it. This is especially true if you are susceptible to asthma and tend to be allergic to ragweed and other pollens. The symptoms of aspirin allergy include wheezing, abdominal pain, and difficulty in breathing. It can precipitate a serious asthma attack and in some cases could even be life-threatening. If you have nasal polyps (if you've got them you'll know what we mean; if you don't, forget it) be extra careful, the chances are greater that you will have a sensitivity to aspirin allergy.

Despite all the discussion of side effects, aspirin really is one of the safest drugs you can use for arthritis. We have had many years of experience with it and unlike some of the new and much more expensive medications that have recently arrived on the medical marketplace, there is little likelihood of unpleasant surprises down the road. In addition there is one very important potential bonus with aspirin. Research keeps taking place that seems to indicate this drug will help prevent heart attacks and strokes. The most recent report we've seen had some encouraging news:

> **Previous studies showed that an aspirin a day can decrease the number of heart attacks and strokes that occur in people who have already been afflicted. The new study, however, suggests that aspirin may prevent heart conditions from ever occurring.**[13]

The final story on this is not in, but all the preliminary data look good. We have yet to learn what is the optimum dose and there is some concern that too much aspirin might actually reverse the effect. Stay tuned for latest developments.

One final word of advice. Do not be hoodwinked by fancy advertising. Aspirin is aspirin is acetylsalicylic acid, whether it be in ANACIN, ARTHRITIS PAIN FORMULA, EMPIRIN COMPOUND, EXCEDRIN, VANQUISH, or whatever. Don't waste your money on expensive brands, and believe us, they are expensive. Remember, you are paying for all that high-priced advertising when you go the brand-name route. But before you buy the el cheapo house brand, sneak a whiff. That's right, open the bottle and smell it right in the store. If you detect an acidy, vinegar-like odor don't buy that product because it has started to deteriorate. When aspirin goes bad it breaks down to acetic acid (vinegar) and while not dangerous, you won't be getting your money's worth. If you truly can't tolerate regular aspirin, however, you might want to buy a special kind that is coated (enteric form) and does not dissolve in the stomach. It won't dissolve until it reaches the small intestine where there will be less problem with irritation. ECOTRIN is one brand that has received favorable reports, but it is a little more expensive than regular old aspirin, and should be reserved for people with particular sensitivity.

By now you should have a pretty good overview of aspirin. It is cheap and effective and generally considered the drug of first choice by the majority of doctors. However, in recent years we have seen the introduction of new "anti-inflammatory agents" such as MOTRIN (ibuprofen), NAPROSYN (naproxen), CLINORIL (sulindac), NALFON (fenoprofen), and TOLECTIN (tolmetin). Doubtless there will be more in the near future given the tremendous economic incentive the arthritis "market" provides. Drug companies promote the dickens out of these new medications. They are introduced amid great fanfare and promise. Television reports and newspaper articles herald the "breakthrough" in arthritis treatment. Because of the publicity many patients immediately call their doctor, seeking a prescription for the long-awaited "new cures to end crippling pain for millions."[14] But are these drugs really more effective than simple aspirin for relieving inflammation? Although this may come as a shock to many people, the answer appears to be no.

Does this mean that these drugs (some of which are a hundred times more expensive than aspirin) aren't more effective than good old acetylsalicylic acid? Yes, that is just what we are saying. But please don't take our word for it. Listen to what a random sampling of experts have reported: Writing in *Resident and Staff Physician,* Dr. Louis A. Healey, Clinical Professor of Internal Medicine at the University of Washington School of Medicine, compared MOTRIN, NAPROSYN, NALFON, and TOLECTIN and concluded that, "All are about as effective in treating the inflammation of rheumatoid arthritis as aspirin. Whether they are more effective, as effective, or less effective is debatable, but clearly any differences are small."[15] Dr. John R. Lewis, Senior Scientist in the AMA's Department of Drugs, had this to say about NALFON, NAPROSYN, and TOLECTIN in *JAMA:* "Their efficacy is comparable, but not superior, to that of aspirin in usual oral doses."[16] Dr. Arthur L. Scherbel, head of the Department of Rheumatic Diseases at the Cleveland Clinic, makes the important point that "Nonsteroids, in general, are better tolerated than full doses of aspirin and are *almost* as effective."[17] (Italics mine.)

All right already, ease up! The point has been made. But remember, we are talking about BIG money—"about $690 million a year is spent on prescription anti-arthritic drugs, and $575 million on non-prescription drugs to treat the disease."[18] (And that doesn't take into account visits to the doctor which the Arthritis Foundation estimates at close to $900 million annually.) If a person can tolerate aspirin, why should he pay one hundred times as much per pill for some high-falutin' new arthritis medicine—unless he believes it's more effective? What's that, you say? You heard it—ONE HUNDRED TIMES MORE! The house brand of aspirin on sale can cost as little as thirty cents per hundred. CLINORIL (sulindac), a new anti-inflammatory agent, can run over thirty-three dollars per hundred.

But wait. We can hear the drug companies yelling foul. They will remind us that, to be fair, you have to take therapeutic doses into account. You only need two CLINORIL tablets to equal the effect of sixteen aspirin tablets. But even taking that into account, aspirin is a whole lot cheaper. The makers of BAYER ASPIRIN have it all figured out on the basis of the average pharmacy cost for thirty days of treatment.

COST COMPARISON OF ASPIRIN AND PRESCRIPTION ARTHRITIS DRUGS

MEDICATION	CLAIMED EFFICACY	ECONOMY (average cost per month)
MOTRIN (ibuprofen 400 mg)	Comparable to aspirin*** (osteo & rheumatoid arthritis)	$19.20*
NALFON (fenoprofen 300 mg)	Comparable to aspirin*** (osteo & rheumatoid arthritis)	$15.90*
NAPROSYN (naproxen 250 mg)	Comparable to aspirin*** (rheumatoid arthritis)	$20.10*
TOLECTIN (tolmetin 200 mg)	Comparable to aspirin*** (rheumatoid arthritis)	$25.50*
CLINORIL (sulindac 150 mg)	Comparable to aspirin*** (osteo & rheumatoid arthritis)	$20.10*
BAYER ASPIRIN (acetylsalicylic Acid 325 mg)	Aspirin—the standard	$ 5.29**

*Average pharm. cost; 30 days of therapy.

**Average retail cost; 12 tablets a day; 30 days of therapy. 100 tablet size package.

***Please note that the package circulars of MOTRIN, NAPROSYN, TOLECTIN, and CLINORIL claim effectiveness only *comparable to aspirin in controlling signs and symptoms of the types of arthritis disease activity set forth above. (No comparison was made with aspirin in connection with the additional indications for CLINORIL.)*

This above cost comparison was prepared by the makers of Bayer Aspirin, Glenbrook Laboratories, Division of Sterling Drug, Inc. on May 1, 1980.

And nothing says you'd have to take BAYER, when the less-expensive house brands of aspirin work just as well.

Now before you throw out those expensive prescription medications there is, of course, a flip side of the coin. While these drugs are no "stronger" than aspirin for relieving arthritis problems, they may cause fewer adverse reactions. For someone who cannot tolerate aspirin, especially because of stomach upset, these new drugs do represent an important step forward. Dr. Louis Healey puts their use into perspective:

> **What, then, is the role of the new drugs in rheumatoid arthritis? The patient with mild to moderate disease who is not helped by aspirin or who finds the tinnitus [ringing in the ears] or indigestion intolerable may receive sufficient benefit to make the additional cost worthwhile.[19]**

Although these new medications are less likely to cause aspirin's possible side effects for many patients, that doesn't mean they don't produce problems of their own. In the following section we will briefly outline what you can expect from various arthritis drugs.

MOTRIN (IBUPROFEN)

For reasons that are not entirely clear, MOTRIN has the inside edge on all other anti-inflammatory agents. It is prescribed more often by more doctors than anything else. We consulted various physicians to try and get a handle on this amazing popularity and pretty much drew blanks. One doctor suggested that it was due to intense promotion by salespeople for the drug company (Upjohn). Another thought that it was high on the hit parade because it was the first of the new-generation drugs and doctors had a little more experience with it. And another doctor volunteered, "It's a bright orange, pretty pill." Whatever the reason, MOTRIN sure is raking it in for Upjohn. And we have received more questions about this drug than any other.

It is certainly true that MOTRIN does cause less gastric upset than aspirin, but according to one reliable source, it is only equal to aspirin if doses in the range of 1,600 mg to 2,400 mg are used each day (four to six tablets).[20] And Dr. Fries seems to think that it may be a little "weaker" than other drugs in its class.[21] While it causes fewer stomach problems than aspirin, that does not mean that it won't do a number on your tummy. Approximately 4 to 14 percent of the people who use this drug will experience some gastrointestinal problems.[22] There have been cases of peptic ulcer and even severe bleeding of the stomach. Fortunately, such instances have been rare. If you take your pills with meals you may be able to prevent symptoms of nausea, heartburn, diarrhea, abdominal pain, and vomiting that sometimes occur with MOTRIN. If these undesirable effects remain, check with your doctor about an alternative medication.

Dizziness, skin rash, hives, and itching may occur in about 3 to 9 percent of the patients who use this arthritis drug, so be alert for such symptoms. Most important of all, note any changes in vision. MOTRIN can cause blurring of vision or the appearance of "colored lights." While rather rare, these symptoms demand immediate attention. If you notice ANY alteration in your sight STOP taking this medicine and have an eye examination. We received a sad letter from one reader who was never informed about the potential problems of MOTRIN:

> Prior to taking MOTRIN I had 20/20 vision. Four to six months later I was told I had the beginning of a cataract. During that time I questioned the doctors about my vision going bad, but was told that something else was causing the problem and not MOTRIN and to keep on taking it four times a day. I was operated on for cataracts about a year later and will have to retire at age 53 because of my eyes.

> —A veteran in North Carolina

If you are using MOTRIN successfully, and not experiencing any stomach upset or visual problems, wonderful! The high price is probably worth the benefit you are obtaining.

NAPROSYN (NAPROXEN)

This arthritis drug is gaining in popularity after almost being banned by the Food and Drug Administration. In 1976 it was discovered that testing done under contract to the manufacturer (Syntex) "failed to follow accepted laboratory procedures and therefore must be invalidated."[23] An expert for the FDA found that "some of the rats on which the drug was tested were decomposed and destroyed without full tissue evaluation; the dates of some animal deaths weren't accurate; some animals died and were replaced with other animals given the same code number, and some findings of tumors in the test animals weren't reported to the FDA by Syntex."[24] Fortunately for Syntex, their sixty-million-dollar-plus NAPROSYN baby did not get thrown out with the bathwater. Subsequent testing did not show any cancer potential and so, after quite a scare, the drug company is back in business.

One of the advantages of NAPROSYN is that it lasts longer than aspirin or some of the other arthritis drugs in the body. The result: you don't have to take as many pills. Usually, two a day will do the job. As with most of these kinds of anti-inflammatory agents, NAPROSYN can cause stomach upset. According to the manufacturer about one out of seven patients will experience heartburn, nausea, indigestion, abdominal pain, and so forth. While uncommon, peptic ulceration can occur. About one in twelve folks will notice headache, drowsiness, dizziness, incoordination, or difficulty in concentrating. And about one in twenty will develop a skin problem such as itching, sweating, or a rash. Occasionally there may be fluid retention. All in all this medicine is similar to MOTRIN and many of the other new arthritis drugs.

CLINORIL (SULINDAC)

The introduction of CLINORIL to the American public was made amid great fanfare. If we had been living in the days of King Arthur and the Knights of the Round Table you would have heard the trumpets blaring day in and day out for weeks. Doctors got really ticked off because the drug company (Merck Sharp & Dohme) announced this fantastic new "breakthrough" drug to the common riffraff before giving the doctors a look at it. This monumental blunder cost the drug company a lot of good will with the physicians and there were a surprising number of nasty letters that appeared in medical journals, such as the following one in the correspondence section of the *New England Journal of Medicine:*

> *To the editor:* **Recently, a new non-steroidal anti-inflammatory agent produced by Merck Sharp and Dohme was promoted heavily to the public via the media of television, radio and newspaper. Most physicians, including rheumatologists, were not prepared for the onslaught of telephone calls and patient inquiries concerning this new drug, SULINDAC. Most physicians practicing primary medicine had no knowledge of this compound; 10 primary physicians in our area who were polled had neither heard of the drug before news releases were made in the media nor seen any advertisements in medical publications. All physicians polled had received several telephone calls from their patients concerning the "new wonder drug." ... Patients with arthritis have enough difficulty**

> dealing with the widespread quackery available
> to them in this day and age. They should not
> have to be exposed to "blitz" attacks by drug
> companies.[25]

We have had ample time to take a look at this "new cure" as the tabloids called it, and while a small step forward, CLINORIL sure ain't no miraculous breakthrough. Like NAPROSYN, CLINORIL is a long-acting medication and you need take only two tablets each day. But it is also very expensive. Considering that it is probably no more effective than aspirin, the convenience of fewer pills may not be worth the extraordinary difference in cost (about five cents for a day's dose of aspirin compared to over sixty cents for CLINORIL).

The company brags that this drug works in a unique fashion. Instead of the chemical exerting an anti-arthritic effect of its own, your body transforms the drug from an inactive state to an active form. The "pro-drug" or precursor effect doesn't impress us a whole bunch because the final outcome is the same. But in the highly competitive drug market a manufacturer must take advantage of every promotion angle and Merck is in there fighting and scratching with the best of them.

As far as side effects are concerned, again we are faced with much the same situation you have with the other drugs of this class: stomach upset, nausea, heartburn, pain (about one in ten users), diarrhea, constipation, and gas. Dizziness and headache occur in about 3 to 9 percent of the patients and some folks will notice ringing in the ears. As usual, be prepared for a rash or itchy skin in some cases All in all, CLINORIL is on a par with the other arthritis drugs like MOTRIN or NAPROSYN. It does cost more, however, and certainly did not live up to its initial billing. One word of caution—do not take aspirin while you are on CLINORIL; the aspirin prevents the nifty conversion of the inactive drug to the active form so it will not be as effective.

NALFON (FENOPROFEN)

There isn't much new that we can say about this drug. The dose is one or two 300-mg capsules three or four times a day. This makes it somewhat less convenient than NAPROSYN or CLINORIL, but otherwise it's in the same ball park. Some side effects to be alert for include indigestion (about one in seven will experience this problem), constipation, nausea, vomiting, abdominal pain, heartburn, bloating, gas, itching, skin rash, fluid retention, fatigue, confusion, ringing in the ears, blurred vision, headache, etcetera, etcetera. If you had trouble with one of the other anti-inflammatory agents you may be able to get by with NALFON but don't expect miracles. There is nothing that makes NALFON super-special or stand out from the other drugs of this group. And if you start on NALFON and have trouble you may want to try one of the others, but they won't be more effective. It may take six weeks for you to see the maximum benefit of NALFON, but if you haven't seen any improvement by the end of the first week it is unlikely additional exposure will produce extra help.

TOLECTIN (TOLMETIN)

And here we have still another "new" anti-inflammatory agent. TOLECTIN, like many of the other arthritis drugs, reduces inflammation. It requires a dosage of between six and eight 200-mg tablets per day. If you are one of the unlucky ones you may experience heartburn, nausea, indigestion, diarrhea, constipation, gas, blurred vision, changes in color perception, skin rash, headache, fluid retention, and fatigue. Some people do better on this medication than others and there is no way to predict in advance whether you will respond favorably. If any side effects occur contact your physician immediately, which is sound advice no matter what arthritis drug you are taking.

By now you probably realize that these five arthritis drugs (MOTRIN, NAPROSYN, CLINORIL, NALFON, and TOLECTIN) are fairly similar both in the benefits they provide and the side effects they may produce. Don't get us wrong, however, for there are subtle differences and if a person doesn't respond to MOTRIN or NAPROSYN it might be worth giving TOLECTIN a try. This also holds true for undesirable effects. Someone who develops a headache or dizziness from one of these drugs may not have problems with another. But don't expect miracles. While less irritating to the digestive tract than aspirin, these drugs can all cause stomach symptoms in sensitive persons. Everyone is different and it's hard to predict in advance who will respond how to what. No matter what drug you and your doctor select, keep in mind that if you don't notice improvement after two or three weeks it is unlikely that this new medicine is for you. And remember, none of these new-fangled, expensive arthritis drugs will provide greater relief than aspirin.

INDOCIN (INDOMETHACIN)

Okay, let's now move up the therapeutic ladder. If none of the drugs already discussed do much to relieve inflammation, maybe it's time to check out something a little "stronger." INDOCIN (indomethacin) has been around since 1963, which makes it an old/new anti-inflammatory agent. It has been used to treat rheumatoid arthritis, ankylosing spondylitis, psoriatic arthritis, and gout. Some doctors even prescribe the drug to relieve tennis elbow or washerwoman's knee. While it may be a shade more effective it is also significantly more toxic. (When you've got arthritis you hardly ever get something for nothing and the price you pay for greater relief often takes the form of more serious side effects.) About 35 to 50 percent of those people who receive INDOCIN will develop some nasty side effects, and ultimately about one out of every five who start on the drug will have to give it up.[26]

The main problem with this arthritis medicine is, as usual, irritation of the gut. Other common complaints include loss of appetite, indigestion, heartburn, nausea, pain, diarrhea, and gas. Most serious of all the side effects are ulcers with bleeding and occasionally the complication of perforation. You may be able to diminish the gastric irritation by taking the drug with or immediately after meals, but all in all it's a pretty unpleasant picture. But that's not all. As many as 50 percent (one out of every two) of the people who take INDOCIN may develop an incredible headache. This can be accompanied by a spacey feeling along with dizziness, incoordination, and confusion. It should be obvious that driving is *verboten* when these reactions occur and working is not a good idea either, especially if you have to use any kind of machinery. With luck, these adverse side effects might disappear after a couple of weeks, but if you haven't noticed any improvement or your head still feels like a watermelon after three weeks, you should definitely switch medications. Less common but nevertheless bothersome complaints may include fatigue, depression, blurred vision, and ringing in the ears.

Despite this bleak picture, INDOCIN does have a place. Oh right, just like Russian roulette (especially after reading the case history on pages 18–20). It may sound strange, but not everyone runs into trouble. About 25 percent of those who take this drug will have good to excellent results with it. We don't believe it should ever be considered a first-choice drug. But if aspirin and rest don't help and the other non-steroidal anti-inflammatory agents don't get you moving, then it may be worth considering.

BUTAZOLIDIN (PHENYLBUTAZONE) AND TANDEARIL (OXYPHENBUTAZONE)

BUTAZOLIDIN is a problem. It's an oldie, but not necessarily a goodie. This drug has been around since 1949 and was one of the first high-powered non-cortisone treatments for rheumatoid arthritis. It's still in demand at race tracks where unethical trainers give "Bute" to horses in order to ease inflammation in those expensive thoroughbred legs and keep the nags running. The Big B has some benefits. After more than thirty years we've had plenty of experience with it and time and there shouldn't be any surprises hidden in the Cracker Jack box. It is also available generically under the name phenylbutazone (or AZOLID) and that means $avings which is more than you can say for some of the newer drugs on the market. It is about comparable to INDOCIN in terms of anti-inflammatory effects, though some people with spinal arthritis may do a little better on BUTAZOLIDIN than some of the other drugs available.

The good thing about this medication is that it is quite effective, especially for acute flare-ups or temporary problems like tennis elbow. It is also excellent for treating a short attack of gout. But watch out for long-term use! The drug can be a killer. Although very rare, there have been cases of fatal aplastic anemia or agranulocytosis. These are as serious as the names suggest. In either case, the bone marrow goes haywire and stops making blood cells the body needs; this reaction may be irreversible. Fortunately, short-term use rarely leads to this disaster. Like all the other drugs we have discussed, BUTAZOLIDIN can mess up your guts. Watch out for nausea, indigestion, heartburn, abdominal pain, vomiting, diarrhea, and worst of all, peptic ulcer. If you experience gastric upset and aren't careful you could develop a bleeding ulcer and perforation. It's possible to diminish the likelihood of these problems if you take the medicine with food or with an antacid (BUTAZOLIDIN ALKA comes formulated with aluminum and magnesium antacids already included). A close relative of BUTAZOLIDIN, TANDEARIL (oxyphenbutazone), might cause a little less upset for some folks and may be worth consideration.

Besides the blood disorders and stomach irritation there are a few other important undesirable effects to be alert for. STOP these medicines at once if you become excessively fatigued or develop a sore throat, mouth ulcers, and difficulty swallowing, especially if you also have fever and chills. These symptoms can possibly be the signs of aplastic anemia (sometimes mistaken for the common cold). Get in touch with your doctor *right away;* also reach for the phone if you suddenly notice shortness of breath, skin rash or itching, gain in weight, blackish stools, or jaundice. A low-salt diet is advisable when you are on this drug because fluid retention is not uncommon. Anyone who receives BUTAZOLIDIN should have a blood test every week or two for the first few months to monitor for the development of aplastic anemia. Unfortunately, some cases are not detected before they have become irreversible. Ideally, these medications "should be limited to short-term therapy of not more than 1 week during any one treatment period."[27] They probably should not be used in older persons since the toxic effects are more common in this group. It is especially hazardous in combination with other prescription drugs, such as anti-coagulants, aspirin, diabetes medicine, or DILANTIN.

MORE TO GOLD THAN JUST GLITTER

The time has come to consider even heavier artillery. If an arthritis sufferer has gone through the non-steroidal anti-inflammatory agents and still has not obtained any measurable relief, then many practitioners will bring on the **gold.** Now that sounds ridiculous. How can gold be a drug? It does seem odd, but gold has been established as an important therapeutic tool in treating arthritis since the 1930s and its track record is reasonably strong. But what about the cost? Relax. It's not pure gold and you don't take that much. You receive injections of a water-soluble gold solution on a weekly basis. The two most common gold preparations are SOLGANAL (gold sodium thioglucose) and MYOCHRYSINE (gold sodium thiomalate). There is some evidence that SOLGANAL is less toxic and better tolerated.[28] The price to your doctor for each injection only runs about $1.25 to $1.50 so you don't have to be afraid to question whether he is goosing the price.

The usual practice is to start out with a small test dose of 5 to 10 mg. If no bad reactions occur the dose is boosted to 50 mg once a week until there is some improvement in the arthritis (about two to three months). Thereafter a shot is usually given about once a month, though under ideal conditions your doctor will individualize the dose to suit particular needs. If there hasn't been any benefit after six months the gold should probably be stopped since there is little hope it will ever do much of anything. If it was working almost imperceptibly, you would know because once it's stopped you would feel worse.

Gold shots generally help about 60 to 70 percent of the people who go through the series of injections.[29] (Some enthusiastic doctors report that 80 percent of their patients benefit from gold.)[30] When it works, it works well! A few lucky people improve so dramatically that there is almost complete relief from pain and inflammation. The best results usually occur if gold is started before the disease has progressed too far (less than a year). As usual, there are side effects.

As many as 30 percent who start the treatment will have to stop because of an adverse reaction.[31] Most commonly an itchy skin rash will occur after about ten to twenty injections. Unless it gets really bad the injections are often continued in spite of the red blotches. They may disappear spontaneously after three or four months. Another unpleasant side effect may be irritation of the mouth in the form of ulcers.

Of a more serious nature, gold can damage the kidneys and for this reason it is always a good idea to have a urinalysis every two weeks. (If your doctor wants to save you money he will provide you with some test strips that will enable you to do this test at home—see page 269). A blood test should also be performed periodically to make sure the bone marrow is not being affected. Jaundice or nausea are two other symptoms to be alert for because they may signal damage to the liver or digestive tract. Fortunately, these problems are rare. Even if it becomes necessary to discontinue gold therapy because of a rash or even kidney problems, some doctors find that if the treatment is started again cautiously, after the symptoms have disappeared, it can be tolerated better the second time around. By the way, no one really knows how gold works, it just does.

BRING ON THE MOSQUITOES

An unexpected bonus from the anti-malarial drugs, chloroquine (ARALEN, AVLOCLOR, RESOCHIN, and generics), and hydroxychloroquine (PLAQUENIL) is relief when taken for rheumatoid arthritis. Some doctors will even go to these drugs before trying the gold shots. (A good argument could be made both ways.) The advantages of these drugs are that they can be taken orally and much less monitoring for toxic effects is necessary. As with gold, it may take three to six months to see much improvement. The good news is that side effects are relatively rare but watch out for damage to the eye. If undetected, blindness could result. For this reason you should have an eye examination before the treatment is started and then every six months during therapy.[32] PLAQUENIL may be a little less likely to cause vision problems but it is also five times the price of generic chloroquine. These drugs may also cause a mild skin reaction and some people develop stomach upset. However, compared to other treatments it can truly be said that the anti-malarial drugs are significantly safer and reasonably effective.

PENICILLAMINE

We have now reached still another level of treatment. Don't let the name fool you. CUPRIMINE (penicillamine) is not an antibiotic and is very different from good old penicillin. This is a very potent drug for the treatment of severe rheumatoid arthritis. Although it has been around since the 1950s, only in the last few years has this drug gained acceptance in the treatment of arthritis. It's a tough drug to handle but the new "go slow — go low" philosophy has made it much more acceptable.[33] First the good news; about 80 percent of those people who use this medicine will feel a lot better, though it may take two to four months to start working. The bad news is there are some heavy-duty side effects associated with CUPRIMINE.[34] Of those who start using it, 30 to 50 percent will have to give it up. For openers, you might lose the senses of smell and taste and along with that your appetite. Fortunately, these problems usually disappear after a few months. Nausea, indigestion, skin rash, and ulcers inside the mouth may also cause problems, though in the low-dose regimen they are less common.

The really big worry with CUPRIMINE is that it can cause serious blood disorders and damage the kidney. For these reasons blood and urine tests are an absolute must every two weeks during the first four months of treatment. (You can do your own urinalysis at home with your doctor's cooperation.) Once you make it over the initial hurdles, these tests can probably be continued once a month. Here's one hot tip that your doctor may forget to mention. The more water you drink the less drug you will have to take and the fewer side effects you will encounter. And we do mean *drink!* Short of drowning yourself, really flood the system. Before you go to sleep at night put down a pint and if at all possible get up and drink another pint in the middle of the night.

WARTS, WORMS, CANCER, AND ARTHRITIS . . .

It's a bird, it's a plane, it's a wonder-drug! LEVAMISOLE looks good. It's new and exciting—so new, in fact, that at this writing the drug has still not been approved for use in the United States. Although we are always skeptical of enthusiastic reports that have not yet stood the test of time, there is some reason to pay close attention to this drug. It was first used as a wormer in animals and in fact is available in this country for veterinary use. In time, a few imaginative doctors began experimenting with LEVAMISOLE for the treatment of warts. The drug can stimulate the immune system and the hypothesis was that warts that refused to go away with any other treatment were probably the result of weak immunity. Because the immune system was involved, suspicions were aroused that this medicine might be important for treating some kinds of cancer. If you could goose the person's natural immunological response, it was thought, there was a good chance the cancer might give up and go away. Finally, some experimenters in England discovered that LEVAMISOLE could help people who were suffering from severe rheumatoid arthritis.[35, 36]

We hesitate to go into any detail on a drug that has not yet been approved for use by the Food and Drug Administration, but we believe that LEVAMISOLE could represent an important step forward and deserves mention. In the few experiments that have been tried, 30 to 80 percent of those treated experienced benefit. There are serious side effects, however, and like so many other arthritis medicines there may be a skin rash to contend with. In addition, mouth ulcers can be very serious and a flu-like illness usually has been reported. Of greater concern are blood and kidney disorders that would require very careful monitoring. Even with these problems there is reason to anticipate that this new and potentially useful drug will soon be approved for experimental trials in the United States.

CORTISONE — LAST BUT NOT LEAST

CORTISONE is the highest rung on the ladder of arthritis treatments. When CORTISONE was first introduced in the 1950s many people thought we had a miracle drug on our hands. There was real hope that arthritis would be a disease of the past. Strong anti-inflammatory action led to prompt relief of pain and swelling. Unfortunately, as is so often the case, initial optimism has slowly been replaced with grave reservations. We now know that steroids like ARISTOCORT, DECADRON, HYDROCORTONE, PREDNISONE, and PREDNISOLONE can cause serious side effects in just about every user if they are used long enough in high doses. Some of the adverse reactions noted include stomach ulcers, susceptibility to infection, psychological disturbances (psychosis, depression, and euphoria), water retention, and electrolyte imbalance. There is often loss of muscle tone which causes weakness. Depletion of calcium from bones makes them fragile and can make people susceptible to breaks, which is about the last thing someone with arthritis needs. As if this weren't enough, cataracts are an additional complication if the drug is taken over a long time. CORTISONE-type medications MUST be tapered off slowly to allow the body to get its own production back in business.

While these drugs do have an important place in treatment programs, there has been widespread abuse. Some particularly outraged physicians wrote to the *Journal of the American Medical Association* (*JAMA*) the following:

We believe that the indiscriminate use of corticosteroids can be appropriately labeled "quackery," even though the providers are licensed physicians. Certainly, patients travel to Mexicali [Mexico] for the same reasons that they purchase copper bracelets, follow unproved faddist diets, or spend hours sitting in mine shafts. Unfortunately, these forms of quackery are difficult to control. But the indiscriminate use of corticosteroids is potentially dangerous.[37]

Appropriate use of CORTISONE requires that the doctor and patient follow certain general principles. Here are a few that we believe will make these drugs much safer:

1. **Use corticosteroid therapy only when a diagnosis has been established and when less harmful forms of therapy have failed.**

2. **Use the smallest therapeutically effective dose.**

3. **Use alternate-day therapy whenever possible. (Single daily dose of up to 15 mg of PREDNISONE may have less deleterious impact on the adrenal gland when given in the morning).**

4. **Increased dose is required during "stresses." A higher dosage might well make all the difference between a return to health and further deterioration.[38, 39]**

When used wisely and carefully, steroids can make life bearable and even comfortable. The prevention of serious complications, however, requires close communication between doctor and patient.

PLAY IT AGAIN, SAMANTHA

We have come a long way since Grandmother's day. Arthritis doesn't have to be a crippler anymore. There are so many alternatives and so many different levels of treatment that most sufferers will be able to lead healthy and productive lives. Knowledge is the key to success—along with a patient physician who will guide you through the maze of therapeutic agents cautiously and wisely. With appropriate exercise, rest, and drug therapy you have every reason to be optimistic.

And what about the future? It looks brighter still. Intensive research is leading investigators down some promising paths. We are being tantalized by theories that rheumatoid arthritis may be a response to an infectious process. Some researchers have implicated bacteria, some think that viruses may be responsible, and some believe that a protozoan parasite could be the guilty party. [40-42] If some nasty beastie is triggering off the immune system in a prolonged and pathological way there is hope that we might be able to isolate and kill it as we have other infectious plagues of the past.

And finally, experiments involving the immune system's own defenses are yielding impressive results. Experimenters have removed blood or lymph from a patient's body, put it through an extraction process, and then returned the concentrated nutrients to the patient. Dramatic improvement has been seen even for people who have not benefited from potent drug treatment.[43] So there is plenty of hope. Not only can we brag about our accomplishments right now, the future looks bright indeed.

Here is a list of fine books that will really help you understand about as much as we currently know about arthritis:

> *Arthritis. A Comprehensive Guide,* by James F. Fries, M.D. Addison-Wesley, Reading, Mass., and Menlo Park, Calif., 1979, $6.95.

> *The Arthritis Handbook—A Patient's Manual on Arthritis, Rheumatism and Gout,* by Darrell C. Crain, M.D., Arco, New York, 2nd edition, $6.50.

> *Arthritis—Complete, Up-to-Date Facts for Patients and Their Families,* by Sheldon P. Blau, M.D., and Dodi Schultz, Doubleday, Garden City, N.J., 1974, $5.95.

> *Beyond the Copper Bracelet: What You Should Know About Arthritis,* by Louis A. Healey, M.D., Charles Press, Bowie, Maryland, 2nd Edition, 1977, $5.95.

> *Living with Your Arthritis,* edited by Alan M. Rosenberg, M.D., Arco, New York, 1979, $8.95.

There may be many more books on the subject and each year you will find additions to the list. There are also many rip-offs. Let your common sense be your guide.

Special arthritis centers which can provide expert assistance and care are listed below. For information on the specific programs that are available call the public information office at the center closest to you:

University of Michigan, Ann Arbor, Mich.

Johns Hopkins University, Baltimore, Md.

Medical University of South Carolina, Charleston, S.C.

Robert B. Brigham Hospital, Boston, Mass.

Indiana University Foundation, Indianapolis, Ind.

University of Arizona, Tucson, Ariz.

Washington University, St. Louis, Mo.

Stanford University, Stanford, Calif.

Louisiana State University, Shreveport, La.

Boston University, Boston, Mass.

University of Alabama, Birmingham, Ala.

University of Texas, Dallas, Tex.

Dartmouth College, Hanover, N.H.

University of California, San Francisco, Calif.

Louisiana State University, New Orleans, La.

REFERENCES

1. The Arthritis Foundation. "Arthritis the Basic Facts." Atlanta, 1976.

2. Kaslow, Richard A. "New England's Own Arthritis." *JAMA* 238:330−335, 1977.

3. "The Mistreatment of Arthritis." *Consumer Reports* 44(6):340−344, 1979.

4. Ibid.

5. Benson, Herbert, and McCalle, David P. "Angina Pectoris and the Placebo Effect." *New Engl. J. Med.* 300:1424−1429, 1979.

6. Diamond, E. G.; Kittle, C. F.; and Crockett, J. E. "Comparison of Internal Mammary Artery Ligation and Sham Operation for Angina Pectoris." *Am. J. Cardiol.* 5:483−486, 1960.

7. Benson, op. cit.

8. Gaw, Albert C.; Chang, Lennig W.; and Shaw, Lein-Chun. "Efficacy of Acupuncture on Osteoarthritis Pain." *New Engl. J. Med.* 293:375−378, 1975.

9. Progress Report: "The OTC Drug Review." *FDA Consumer* 13(1):18−22, 1979.

10. Fries, James F. *Arthritis. A Comprehensive Guide.* Addison Wesley, Menlo Park, 1979, p. 97.

11. Medical News, "New Drugs May Soon Supplement Aspirin in Treating Arthritis." *JAMA* 229:505−507, 1974.

12. Levy, Gerhard, et al. "Decreased Serum Salicylate Concentrations in

Children with Rheumatic Fever Treated with Antacids." *New Engl. J. Med.* 293:323–325, 1975.

13. News. "Aspirin May Prevent Heart Attacks." *Am. Family Physician* 19(6):183, 1979.

14. Harris, Rosa. "Arthritis: A Super Drug Brings Relief." *Midnight Globe* 26(16):9, 1979.

15. Healey, Louis A. "More on the New Arthritis Drugs." *Resident and Staff Physician* 23(2):109–110, 1977.

16. Lewis, John R. "New Antirheumatic Agents." *JAMA* 237:1260–1261, 1977.

17. Scherbel, Arthur L. "Nonsteroidal Antiinflammatory Drugs New Alternatives for Rheumatic Disease." *Postgrad. Med.* 63:69–74, 1978.

18. Gorman, Trisha. "Arthritis: Is There New Hope for Relief?" *Drug Topics* 22(3):47–69, 1968.

19. Healey, Louis, op. cit., p. 110.

20. "Ibuporfen, Motrin." *Med. Letter* 16:109, 1974.

21. Fries, op. cit., p. 103.

22. *Physician's Desk Reference,* Medical Economics Co., Oradell, N. J., 33rd edition, 1979, p. 1766.

23. "A Bitter FDA Pill for Syntex to Swallow." *Bus. Week* Aug. 30, 1976, pp. 21–22.

24. "Studies of Syntex Drug Done by Testing Lab Draw FDA Questions." *Wall Street Journal* July 20, 1976, p. 33.

25. Solomon, Sheldon D., et al. "Complaint About Promotion of New Anti-Arthritic Drug." *New Engl. J. Med.* 300:203, 1979.

26. Woodbury, Dixon M., and Fingl, Edward. "Analgesics—Antipyretics, Anti-inflammatory Agents, and Drugs Employed in the Therapy of Gout." in *The Pharmacological Basis of Therapeutics.* 5th ed., Louis S. Goodman and Alfred Gillman, eds., MacMillan, N. Y., 1979, p. 342.

27. Op. cit., p. 340.

28. Rothermich, N. O., et al. "Chrysotherapy: A Prospective Study." *Arthritis Rheum.* 19:1321–1327, 1976.

29. Williams, Ralph C. "Rheumatoid Arthritis." *Hospital Practice* 14(6):57–63, 1979.

30. Johnson, James S., et al. "Chrysotherapy for Drug-Refractory Rheumatoid Arthritis." *Mod. Med.* 43(6):84–88, 1975.

31. Decker, John L. "The Management of Rheumatoid Arthritis." *Resident and Staff Physician* 24(8):50–56, 1978.

32. Lightfoot, Robert W., Jr. "Therapy of Rheumatoid Disease." *Am. Fam. Physician* 19(3):186—196, 1979.

33. Colin, Andrei. "Rheumatoid Arthritis." *Am. Fam. Physician* 18(1):89—94, 1978.

34. Bunch, Thomas W. "How to Use D-Penicillamine in Rheumatoid Arthritis." *Mod. Med.* 47(7):78—80, 1979.

35. Multicentre Study Group. "Lavamisole in Rheumatoid Arthritis." *Lancet* 2:1007—1012, 1978.

36. El-Ghobarey, Ahmey E. el at. "Clinical and Laboratory Studies of Lavamisole in Patients with Rheumatoid Arthritis." *Quart. J. of Med.* XLVIII:385—400, 1978.

37. Kirkpatrick, Richard A., et al. "Corticosteroid and Arthritis." *JAMA* 231:(letter) Feb. 24, 1975.

38. Streeten, David H. P. "Corticosteroid Therapy." *JAMA* 233:944—947, 1975.

39. Klinefelter, Harry F., et al. "Single Daily Dose of Prednisone Therapy." *JAMA* 241:2721—2723, 1979.

40. Editorial. "Rheumatoid Arthritis and the Gut." *Br. Med. J.* 1:1104, 1979.

41. Bingham, Robert. "Rheumatoid Disease: Has one Investigator Found its Cause and its Cure?" *Mod. Med.* 44(4):38—47, 1976.

42. Brown, Thomas McP. "Rheumatoid Inflammation: Part II." *Inflo: News of Inflammation Research and Therapy* (The Upjohn Company). 12(1):2—3, 1979.

43. Williams, Ralph C. "Rheumatoid Arthritis." *Hospital Practice* 14(6):57—63, 1979.

11

Drugs and Your Head: The Care and Feeding of Your Psyche

The billion dollar boondoggle • Modern "cures" for modern anxieties: VALIUM, LIBRIUM, ELAVIL, MILTOWN, EQUANIL, MELLARIL, TRANXENE, TRIAVIL, THORAZINE, SERAX, DORIDEN, TUINAL, QUAALUDE, and PLACIDYL • Shoring up social support • Insomnia, real and imagined—Scalped by sleeping pills. Simple home remedies • Psychological depression can be devastating: ELAVIL, ENDEP, LIMBITROL, TRIAVIL, TOFRANIL, IMAVATE, AVENTYL, NORPRAMIN, and SINEQUAN. • MAO inhibitors: useful but dangerous • **Lithium**: Bringing down the highs • Schizophrenia: Biochemical theories and medications: THORAZINE, MELLARIL, STELAZINE, COMPAZINE, and HALDOL • Getting unstuck without coming unglued.

We live in stressful times. In case you haven't noticed, it's tough out there, baby. Everyone feels pushed to the wall these days. If it's not the pressure on the job, it's the pressure at home. While we may wistfully wish for the good old days when prices were lower and life was simpler there is no clear evidence that the demands placed on our parents or grandparents were any less difficult for them than today's demands are for us. There is one huge difference, though, and it's how we cope with our modern-day stress. Over the last twenty years the slogan "Better living through chemistry" has won the hearts and minds of the American public. We have drugs to relieve anxiety, drugs to lighten depression, drugs to put you to sleep, to wake you up and get you going. What we lack is social support.

Our parents and our grandparents may not have had "tranquilizers," "sedatives," "hypnotics," "anti-anxiety agents," or any other mood-altering molecules but they did have family and friends.

They had a large group of people they could count on to care—people who would come running when they were needed. To be sure, life had its ups and downs in those days, but they were easier to handle when there were lots of folks around who were more than happy to help shoulder the burdens, share the sorrows, and celebrate the triumphs.

Today most people are out there on their own. There's Mom and Pop and the two kids. The grandparents are off somewhere else, perhaps Sun City or Miami. The brothers, sisters, aunts, uncles, and cousins are scattered all over the map and friendships are fleeting. Twenty percent of our population moves every year—which is to say, the average American family packs up the house and changes location lock, stock, and barrel every five years. That kind of mobility doesn't lend itself to strong support networks. And divorce isn't just a way of life, it's an institution. Single-parent families make up more than 30 percent of all households these days. Is it any wonder that Americans spend more than $1,000,000,000 (one billion) on tranquilizers each year and that VALIUM has been the most frequently prescribed drug in this country since 1972? Instead of sharing our anxieties with friends and relatives and seeking support and guidance we subdue our fears with drugs.

Hoffman-La Roche, the parent company that makes VALIUM, guards sales figures as if they were the crown jewels. Actually the drug may be worth more. During an interview with Robert B. Clark, President of Hoffman-La Roche, on the TV show "Sixty Minutes," host Mike Wallace asked about the difference between the cost to produce the drug and the price that is charged the pharmacist:

> *Mr. Wallace:*
> **Why this astronomical mark-up on Valium, talking about the budget?**
>
> *Mr. Clark:*
> **What astronomical mark-up?**
>
> *Mr. Wallace:*
> **According to the British Monopolies Commission, the active ingredients in Valium cost you about $50 a kilo (2.2 pounds), which you then sold to your British subsidiary for $23,000 a kilo, and they sold to retailers for the equivalent of $50,000 a kilo. From $50 a kilo to you people, active ingredients. British subsidiary, $23,000 a kilo. To retailers at double $50,000 a kilo. That's what I mean by astronomical mark-up.**[1]

Every year Americans spend approximately half a billion dollars on almost 60 million prescriptions for VALIUM (diazepam).[2] If the average number of pills per prescription is about fifty, that would amount to around three *billion* tablets—about fourteen for every man, woman, and child in the country. Now add approximately 13 million prescriptions for DALMANE (flurazepam), 10 million for LIBRIUM (chlordiazepoxide), 9 million for ELAVIL (amitriptyline), 8 million for MILTOWN or EQUANIL (meprobamate), 7 million for PHENOBAR-BITAL, 6 million for MELLARIL (thioridazine), 6 million for TRANX-ENE (clorazepate), 5 million for TRIAVIL (amitriptyline and perphenazine), 4 million for THORAZINE (chlorpromazine), 3 million for SERAX (oxazepam), and then throw in a few million more for DORIDEN (glutethimide), NEMBUTAL (pentobarbital), SECONAL (secobarbital), TUINAL (secobarbital and amobarbital), QUAALUDE (methaqualone), and PLACIDYL (ethchlorvynol).[3] Now do you begin to get some idea of how much head medicine is being used in this country?

We can conservatively estimate that each year more than 120 million prescriptions are written for drugs that will lift you up, put you down, level you off, or lay you out, and that doesn't even include the prescriptions written for hospitalized patients. That represents so many billions of pills that it's mind-boggling in more ways than one. In one small survey carried out in Minneapolis, the researchers found that in a suburban community there were, "on average, 12 drugs per household ... Ninety-five per cent of the households had on hand one or more drugs acting on the central nervous system."[4]

Most doctors really care about their patients' welfare. But when someone comes into the office with a case of "nerves" it is much easier for them to reach for the prescription pad than to try to seek other solutions to the problem. Few doctors have the time, training, or inclination to "talk things out" with an upset client and chances are that no attempt will be made to find a supportive self-help environment where that can be done. At best there may be a referral to a psychiatrist who will be expensive and will also reach for the prescription pad. Yet the evidence is strong that what people really need is people. Social support is not only crucial for mental health, it is necessary for physical well-being too. Drs. Lisa Berkman and Leonard Syme found that "social isolation may lead to depression, which might, in turn, predispose to suicide and accidents; the absence of social networks may produce physiological changes in the body which increase general susceptibility to disease, whereas the presence of social support systems may actually decrease physiological susceptibility."[5,6]

What this means is that people who feel lonely and isolated may be more likely to suffer heart disease, cancer, mental illness, and other physical complaints. People who belong to self-help groups, who have a commitment to others, who maintain an active religious affiliation, or who nourish a strong network of friends and family will be less likely to suffer from fear, anger, anxiety, depression, and overall illness. A member of *our* support group, Dr. Tom Ferguson, reminded us of a wonderful old children's song that sums it all up beautifully:

> *Make new friends*
> *But keep the old.*
> *One is silver,*
> *The other, gold.*

We have put forth what we hope is a strong alternative to drug therapy. But if you think we are always opposed to head medicine you'd be very wrong. Sometimes anti-anxiety agents are useful. For someone who has experienced a terrible personal tragedy and is so distraught that rational action is impossible, these drugs can assist in getting past the acute crisis. For an executive who has to meet an impossible deadline and is so desperate that he experiences "butterflies," palpitations, sweaty palms, and diarrhea, a sedative could enable him to establish his equilibrium long enough to make it over the hump. And for some people, life is a constant state of panic—they're afraid to go anywhere, they have the "shakes," feel dizzy, are apprehensive, and have difficulty sleeping. A drug which calms them down long enough for a therapist to help them "unlearn" the anxiety can be a powerful tool.

The point here is that in the short run there are times when drugs like VALIUM, LIBRIUM, DALMANE, TRANXENE, ATIVAN, AZENE, SERAX, MILTOWN, and EQUANIL are useful and appropriate. If a person who is feeling terribly tense and fearful on a new job takes advantage of an anti-anxiety agent to temporarily reduce the fear long enough to master the new situation, the medication can be beneficial, as long as it is phased out gradually when confidence has been gained. Dr. Joseph Strayhorn describes it this way: "By using the drug we have set up an intermediate step, a rung on the ladder low enough to be grasped but high enough to give access to the next rung."[7] But whatever drug is used, it must be treated with respect and recognized for what it is—a temporary patch to hold the line until a permanent solution to the problem can be found.

Unfortunately, too many doctors and patients take these medications for granted. Instead of using them as a ladder for attaining personal growth they become a permanent crutch. Instead of short-term therapy the drugs are used year in and year out. Open-ended renewable prescriptions are a matter of course. Instead of telling people how to phase out sedatives the doctor may actually encourage their continuation. The safe use of drugs like VALIUM, LIBRIUM, and TRANXENE requires a complete understanding of side effects, precautions, and most important of all, a knowledge about how to get off them.

Adverse reactions to anti-anxiety agents and "muscle relaxants" are not common but they do occur, so everyone should be aware of the potential problems. Drowsiness, fatigue, and incoordination are the most common side effects associated with these medications. Advertisements appearing in medical journals for these drugs can lull doctors into believing otherwise; that could be disastrous for patients. For example, the makers of TRANXENE tell doctors: **"Anxiety symptoms dispelled yet not drowsy by day,"** in bold letters at the top of one ad. However, on the next page in tiny print, under the heading "Adverse Reactions," we discover that "The side effect most frequently reported was drowsiness. Less commonly reported were dizziness, various gastrointestinal complaints, nervousness, blurred vision, dry mouth, headache, and mental confusion."[8] A physician who doesn't take the time to check the fine print might forget to advise a new patient to avoid drinking, operating equipment, or anything else that might require mental alertness.

The possible complications associated with most anti-anxiety agents like VALIUM, LIBRIUM, LIBRITABS, LIBRAX, ATIVAN, SERAX, TRANXENE, VERSTRAN, and MOGADON are similar: drowsiness, fatigue, incoordination, skin rash, itching, nausea, headache, dizziness, light-headedness, confusion, slurred speech, depression, irritability, impaired sexuality, blood disorders, constipation, menstrual irregularities, troubled breathing, and jaundice. Fortunately, most people do not experience these problems. Even when drowsiness or unsteadiness is a problem in the beginning, it often disappears after a few days of treatment. But even though adverse reactions are rare people should know what to expect. Older people and those who are debilitated will be especially sensitive to side effects and must receive the lowest therapeutic dose possible.

Before anyone receives a prescription for one of these kinds of drugs the doctor should take time to emphasize what should by now be common knowledge: *Avoid Booze* and any other drug that might add to nervous system depression. Even with all the publicity that this problem has received, many people still think that they can get away with downing just one or two drinks after work, especially if they've had a grueling day at the office. What they don't realize is that this kind of combination can impair motor coordination so much that getting into a car to drive home is almost like playing Russian roulette with all chambers loaded.

DALMANE is particularly insidious in this regard. It is often used at night to relieve insomnia. Few doctors or patients realize that the drug lingers in the body so that after a few days enough has accumulated in the system to impair judgment and affect driving ability. A person who is unaware that the drug has been building up may not think that the sleeping pill they took last night at 11:30 could still have any effect by 6:30 the next evening. They could easily down a few beers or cocktails and not realize the danger. The result could easily be an accident. Even a simple allergy or cold medicine could have disastrous results when combined with a sedative because antihistamines can add to nervous-system depression.

One final caution: even though pregnancy may be a time of anxiety for some women, they should avoid minor tranquilizers if at all possible since there is concern that these drugs can affect the fetus in an adverse manner, especially during the first trimester. And because they also get into the breast milk a nursing mother should try to steer clear of these compounds.

What we have said up to now pales in comparison with what comes next. The real problem with VALIUM and all its chemically related cousins is not so much the side effects while you *take* the medicine (which are relatively rare) but what happens when you *stop* taking the medicine. For years doctors believed that these drugs could not produce dependency and that people could discontinue their VALIUM whenever they chose to. *Wrong, Wrong, Wrong!* Go back and read the letter on page 18 for a personal account of what happened to one person after long-term VALIUM use.

Dr. J. Richard Crout, Director of the Bureau of Drugs for the FDA, recently testified before a congressional committee about the addiction potential of anti-anxiety agents. His comments were summarized in *The Nation's Health,* the newspaper of the American Public Health Association:

> **Although it has been clear for some time that these drugs produce psychological dependency, more recently it has been recognized that they produce physical dependence and can cause withdrawal symptoms such as agitation, insom-**

nia, sweating, tremors, abdominal and muscle
cramps, and even convulsions . . Crout stated
that people who take the drug for longer than
four months are most at risk of becoming
dependent. [9]

Most people believe that only junkies get into trouble with drugs
like VALIUM and then only after they take large doses for long periods
of time. However, recent letters in the medical literature tell a
different story. Writing in the *Journal of the American Medical
Association* (*JAMA*) Drs. Arthur Rifkin, Frederic Quitkin, and
Donald Klein reported "a severe withdrawal reaction on a therapeutic dose of diazepam" (VALIUM):

> The patient was a healthy, 23-year-old man who
> suffered from moderate anticipatory anxiety
> mainly related to fear of poor performance at
> work. Treatment with diazepam, 10 mg three
> times per day, brought considerable relief.
> After three months of drug treatment he went
> to an army base to fulfill his reserve duty
> obligation. At this time, he abruptly disconcin-
> ued use of diazepam. Five days later he had two
> grand mal convulsions within three hours.
> Physical and neurological evaluation in a
> hospital (including electroencephalogram) did
> not show any abnormalities. He was not placed
> back on any drug regimen, and there were no
> further adverse reactions.
> *Comment.*—We reported this reaction to the
> manufacturer, who stated that there had been
> previous reports of seizures on withdrawal from
> therapeutic doses of diazepam given for several
> months but none on as low a dose as our patient
> for this period of time.
> Considering the vast use of benzodiazepenes
> [Valium-like drugs], the incidence of with-
> drawal seizures must be low. However, it is our
> recommendation that if these drugs are given
> continuously for months, benzodiazepines
> should be withdrawn gradually. [10]

The most insidious condition arising from this kind of drug
dependency is that withdrawal of the medication can produce many
of the same symptoms it was supposed to eliminate—insomnia,
feelings of nervousness, trembling, poor appetite, numbness, faint-

ness, weakness, irritability, nausea, lack of energy, headache, and muscle cramps.[11,12] A person might start using an anti-anxiety agent to get through a temporary crisis only to find that every time he tried to stop the drug he would feel so anxious he would have to start up again, even though the original problem was long gone.

What is the solution to this madness? Our psychiatric consultants advise patience. When it's appropriate to discontinue the sedative it must be done slowly, especially if the drug has been used for more than six months. If the dose is cut back by thirty to fifty percent a week over the course of six weeks the withdrawal symptoms should be minimal. For example, if someone were taking three 5 mg tablets of VALIUM every day, they could start by eliminating one dose every other day during the first week. During the second week they could try to use only two tablets daily. During the third week another tablet could be phased out. And in the fourth week they should try to make do with only one. If at any time side effects start to become uncomfortable a small temporary increment in the dose should eliminate the discomfort. Finally, the pills can be cut in half and then in quarters until eventually the person is weaned entirely. Along with the gradual reduction in dosage, the person should increase exercise and daily outdoor activities while simultaneously learning other ways to reduce stress. Mental relaxation techniques or biofeedback training has been helpful in this regard. Ultimate success will depend upon the person's ability to identify those situations which are stressful and anxiety-provoking in order to begin to deal with them in a more appropriate manner.

SCALPED BY SLEEPING PILLS

Everyone has trouble falling asleep now and then. A late-evening cup of coffee can cause insomnia and so can a reprimand from the boss. The excitement of a new love affair can keep you awake and so can jet lag after a trip across the country. Anxiety and psychological depression are often underlying causes of insomnia, and some people are so convinced they won't get a good night's sleep that they don't. Many sleep researchers report that chronic insomniacs commonly think that they get less sleep than they actually do. I can personally testify to that fact. Having conducted sleep research myself I had the dubious pleasure of staying awake all night monitoring sophisticated recording equipment while the insomniacs slept. In the morning they would fill out a questionnaire and almost inevitably they would report a miserable night. One of our subjects claimed that he didn't sleep a wink and yet his sleep records clearly demonstrated he consistently got in a good seven hours. Although none of the "insomniacs" ever slept less than six hours, and most slept significantly more, they almost always complained that their sleep was inadequate. Why some people are bothered more by their perception of lost sleep than others is a mystery.

The doctor's solution to insomnia, no matter what the origin, is almost always a prescription. The most reliable estimate of how many drugs are prescribed each year is made by the people who conduct the National Prescription Audit. They concluded that:

> **38 million prescriptions for sleep medications averaging 30 doses each are written by American physicians each year. Total number of pills prescribed: one billion. Combined with over-the-counter [non-prescription] sleep medications, the number of pills consumed each year rises to 3 billion.**[13]

One of the leading sleep researchers in this country, Dr. Ernst Hartmann, estimates "that at least 10 percent of the entire adult population in the United States uses sleeping pills at least once each year."[14] If you include the use of drugs like VALIUM, LIBRIUM, and other anti-anxiety agents that are also employed to relieve insomnia, the numbers would be much higher. And about half of the 33 million people admitted to hospitals each year automatically receive prescriptions for hypnotics. Hard as it may be to believe, nurses have been known to wake people up in order to give them their sleeping medication.

Perhaps you're wondering, so what's the matter with sleeping pills? Plenty! Doctors have no business prescribing these drugs with such enthusiasm. Please don't take my word on this. Listen to what a group of distinguished physicians and sleep researchers had to say about their colleagues' prescribing patterns. A special report was recently prepared by the Institute of Medicine (IOM) of the National Academy of Sciences, and the conclusions are unassailable:

> **The committee finds that, although hypnotics [sleeping pills] are widely prescribed, most physicians receive little training in their use . . .**
>
> **The beneficial effect, if any, of a hypnotic drug upon sleep measures is typically to reduce the time needed to fall asleep by 10 to 20 minutes and to lengthen the night's total sleep time by 20 to 40 minutes . . .**

> It is difficult to justify much of the current prescribing of sleeping medication. As a class of drugs, hypnotics should have only a limited place in contemporary medical practice.
>
> The committee believes that, until long-term safety and efficacy of regular hypnotic use is established, physicians should rarely, if ever, prescribe hypnotic drugs for periods longer than two to four weeks for patients who have not yet become reliant on regular use of hypnotics.[15,16]

The Institute of Medicine report was a strong indictment of doctors' knowledge and use of these medications. Instead of trying to track down the cause of a patient's sleeping distress and attempting other alternatives the most common first-line treatment has been a prescription. And that can lead to trouble. Even though most drugs become less effective as sleep inducers after a few days they continue to interfere with normal sleep patterns. They are especially good at depriving people of dreaming sleep. When the drugs are discontinued the body demands that the dream "debt" be paid back in full and the result is often so many unpleasant nightmares that the insomniac hops right back on the drug bandwagon. Sleep Researchers at Stanford University have reported that "40 percent of their patients who complain of insomnia actually lose sleep because of the very drug they are taking to 'treat' insomnia."[17] And even when medications really do help insomniacs get a little more sleep at night there is doubt that this leads to any "improvement in various dimensions of daytime mood or performance."[18,19]

So what can you do if the insomnia blues have got you down? Well, first, give your body a chance to do its own thing. Usually, insomnia is self-limiting. If you had trouble getting in the ZZZ's last night, the chances are pretty good that you will make up for it tonight, as long as you got up early and haven't taken any naps during the day. Exercise is a great way to insure a good night's sleep. There are very few lumberjacks or farmers who suffer from insomnia. If you can get in a good hour of vigorous activity during the day you'll be surprised what a difference it can make at bedtime. A nice hot bath before bed is good for relaxing the old bod. And mother's old favorite, a glass of warm milk, can also make a big difference. It turns out that a naturally occurring amino acid called **L-Tryptophan** which is found in food may act as a natural sleep-inducing substance. The best way to insure that the greatest concentration of **L-Tryptophan** will reach the brain is to eat a snack that is high in carbohydrate and low in protein. Some crackers, toast or cookies along with a glass of malted milk and some enriched cereal powder (HORLICK'S) should do the trick quite nicely. And avoid caffeine like the plague. Once you are in bed try some relaxation techniques where you consciously loosen all the muscles in your body one by one. Satisfying sex is also an excellent way to shorten the time it will take to reach dreamland. And if everything fails remember that lack of sleep is not necessarily bad for you. Many people get by very nicely on four or five hours a night and never complain. If, however, the sleeping problems persist and you feel miserable during the day, better seek some professional help. One of the most common symptoms of psychological depression is insomnia.

DUMPING DEPRESSION

It's normal to feel depressed once in a while. You'd be more than a little odd if you weren't occasionally sad. A lost friend, a lost job, or a lost love could give anyone the blues. But most often the smell of the roses is stronger than the prick of the thorns. And even after some major disappointments or the death of a loved one, most people are able to bounce back and put the pieces of their life together again, especially if they can muster support from friends and relatives. Some folks, however, can't get themselves out of the briar patch no matter how hard they try. Every year over seven million Americans suffer terrible, overpowering bouts of depression and anywhere from 26,000 to 75,000 get so low they feel that they have to try and put an end to their lives.

Why? What is it that makes some folks turn to suicide as the only answer? Well-intentioned friends often think that a depressed person could get better if he or she only tried a little harder. "Snap out of it—pull yourself together!" is common advice, as if it were the individual's fault and all that is necessary is to turn on a little will power. But it's just not that simple. People who are deeply depressed are different from everyone else—different both genetically and biochemically. For one thing, they often feel bad when there is no "logical" reason for it. Even when there are no major problems at work or at home the person may have no appetite, have difficulty sleeping, lose interest in sex, always feel tired, and ultimately feel helpless and hopeless. This is what psychiatrists refer to as "endogenous" depression, which means that the sadness seems to well up from inside instead of occurring because of some external life event. This is not to say that environmental factors don't play a role— they do. But often what would be a minor upset for a normal person becomes a tragedy for someone who is susceptible to this illness. The loss of a pet, for example, may precipitate grief that lasts for months and months or a broken appliance might cause feelings of despair. Often the mornings are the worst time of the day and by afternoon there may be some slight improvement in outlook.

This kind of endogenous depression tends to run in families, which is why the current thinking has it that your genes may predispose you to this illness. Abnormal levels of brain chemicals neuro-transmitters may be responsible for long-lasting mood changes. Although researchers have measured and tinkered with all sorts of biochemicals over the last twenty years and have discerned differences between depressed patients and "normals," there are still more questions than answers. The brain is like a mysterious black box and it gives up its secrets grudgingly. But even though we don't have any real clues there is no need to despair either. Antidepressant medications have made life better than bearable for millions of people: they have made it worth living.

Doctors can choose between two basic classes of drugs—the *Tricyclics* and the *MAO Inhibitors* (MAO is short for Monoamine Oxidase). The tricyclics are by far the most popular and are considered the first line of defense. Some of the most commonly prescribed medications contain *amitriptyline*. They are ELAVIL, AMITRIL, ENDEP, ETRAFON, LIMBITROL, and TRIAVIL. Other tricyclics that are also routinely employed include *imipramine* (TOFRANIL, ANTIPRESS, IMAVATE, JANIMINE, and PRESAMINE); *nortriptyline* (AVENTYL, PAMELOR); *desipramine* (NORPRAMIN, PERTOFRANE); *protriptyline* (VIVACTIL); and *doxepin* (ADAPIN, SINEQUAN).

Although there may be subtle differences among these various drugs they all work in a similar manner and tend to have common side effects. Occasionally someone will do better on one particular tricyclic than on another, but more often than not it is the physician's familiarity with a particular brand that will determine which medication is selected. Although it often takes about two or three weeks for the antidepressant effect to begin to take hold, once it starts to work about 70 percent of the people who receive it will feel much better and often be able to resume normal activities. No one should feel that he or she has given a fair test to these drugs until at least six weeks have gone by since it may take that long to achieve the optimum benefit.

The most common side effects associated with the antidepressant medications include dry mouth, drowsiness, dizziness, constipation, blurred vision, eye pain, difficulty with urination, irregular heartbeat, fainting, shakiness, or increased appetite for sweets and weakness. Often the drowsiness will disappear after a few weeks but in the early stages of treatment driving or operating machinery can be quite hazardous. When dizziness or light-headedness are a problem they usually occur when someone stands up rapidly. By getting up slowly from a lying or sitting position the adverse reaction can be reduced.

The bothersome dry mouth that often accompanies the use of tricyclics may be diminished in two ways; Vitamin B_6 (pyridoxine) in a dose of 25 mg two to four times a day has been reported to be of some value.[20] Another alternative that will probably produce better results is a saliva substitute that was originally developed for patients who had to undergo radiation therapy for head and neck cancer. After treatment they too often experienced symptoms of a dry mouth. Physicians at Baylor College of Medicine and the Houston Veterans Administration Hospital tested this same saliva substitute (VA ORALUBE) on depressed patients and had surprisingly favorable results:

> **Xerostomia [dry mouth], a side effect of major tranquilizers and tricyclic antidepressants, is one of the most common drug side effects encountered in psychiatric practice... For patients with artificial dentures, most of whom are elderly, a chronically dry mouth becomes a rather serious problem. The tissues underlying the denture are constantly painful, there is pronounced tissue shrinkage leading to poor fit... In addition, the persistence of oral dryness tends to affect patient medication compliance adversely and thus may contribute to psychiatric treatment failure...**
>
> **We have employed a therapeutic mouthwash that not only relieves the painful soft tissue problems but also can remineralize tooth surfaces that have been damaged as a result of salivary deprivation.**
>
> **Relief of symptoms of dryness was immediate and complete. The duration of lubricant effect varied among patients but generally ranged from 1 to 3 hours. No adverse reactions were noted.[21]**

The way in which this saliva substitute is used is to place a few drops of the liquid in the mouth, swish it around, and then expectorate. Unfortunately, VA ORALUBE is only available through

Veterans Administration hospitals but an identical commercial product called XERO-LUBE should have much the same effect. Chances are that the local pharmacy won't have it in stock but they can order XERO-LUBE from Scherer Laboratories, Inc.; P. O. Drawer 400009; Dallas, Texas 75240.

All antidepressant drugs have the potential to interact in a dangerous way with many other medications. Alcohol, non-prescription cold and allergy medications, barbiturates, sedatives, blood pressure medicine, prescription pain relievers, sleeping pills, and other drugs for depression can all cause serious adverse reactions in combination with tricyclics. Before anyone combines one of the tricyclics with any other medication they should get the approval of their physician. And no one should abruptly discontinue taking an antidepressant without checking on that too. When it's appropriate to phase out the medicine the dose should be reduced gradually under professional supervision. These drugs do save lives!

MAO INHIBITORS

The development of the "monoamine oxidase inhibitors" has a fascinating history. The first drug of this class was IPRONIAZID. It was originally developed in 1951 to treat tuberculosis. Because the TB patients of those days were usually pretty psychologically down, doctors were amazed to see that after treatment with the new tuberculosis drugs these people were cheerful and in some cases actually dancing in the corridors of the sanitariums. It was such a contrast that it was hard not to figure out that something interesting was going on. Soon additional drugs were created and tested, and sure enough, they too had antidepressant activity. By blocking the enzyme monoamine oxidase certain neurotransmitters were built up in the brain (norepinephrine and serotonin) and elevated the mood of depressed patients. These neurotransmitters are the biochemical messengers used by nerve cells to communicate with each other. During severe depression the concentration of these chemicals in the brain apparently gets out of whack and the antidepressants attempt to re-establish the equilibrium.

In recent years MAO inhibitors have fallen into disfavor, mainly because they interact adversely with many common foods such as bananas, avocados, pickled herring, salami, beer, and wine (see the table in the drug interaction chapter for a more complete list). The result of this combination can lead to extremely hazardous elevations in blood pressure and a stroke could result. Other side effects include liver toxicity, insomnia, tremors, and agitation. The drugs may also cause dizziness, vertigo, headache, impaired sexuality, dry mouth, blurred vision, difficult urination, and constipation. When tricyclics have not been effective doctors often resort to MAO inhibitors and when used carefully with a restricted diet they can be helpful. The medications that are used today are MARPLAN (isocarboxazid), NARDIL (phenelzine), and PARNATE (tranylcypromine).

LITHIUM CARBONATE

For years lithium was an underground drug. Underground in the sense that the Food and Drug Administration delayed its approval and it was only available from a few selected research institutions. Some clinicians smuggled the drug into the country for their patients because it was available only overseas. Today, lithium has a solid place in the doctor's black bag. It is available generically or by brand name: ESKALITH, LITHANE, LITHONATE, and LITHOTABS.

Lithium is not generally used to treat people who just suffer from depression. Instead it is reserved for those persons who suffer the wild swings in mood called manic-depression. By knocking out the manic phase of the disease lithium apparently can interrupt the depressive phase as well. It is particularly interesting to watch the effects of lithium on sleep. When people who are manic really get going they hardly ever sleep. They are so wound up that they keep going almost twenty-four hours a day. Lithium can calm a person down and help her or him obtain a normal night's sleep.

The big catch with lithium is its toxicity. The therapeutic dose is close to the dose where side effects occur. It is imperative that anyone on lithium have periodic blood tests to make sure that the fine line between safety and danger has not been crossed. Side effects to be alert for include fatigue, shakiness, muscle weakness, drowsiness, slurred speech, nausea, vomiting, diarrhea, and a tremor of the hand. As long as the drug is monitored carefully it can be a valuable tool in preventing the return of devastating bouts of depression.

SCHIZOPHRENIA: THE UNSOLVED MYSTERY

Perhaps no other ailment known to man has stimulated so much confusion, fear, and mistreatment. In the past the mental outcasts of society were shunted to the back wards of mental institutions. Books like *One Flew Over the Cuckoo's Nest* are entertaining but they provide a better glimpse of society as a whole than they do of mental illness per se. Although psychiatrists are in theory the ones who are supposed to rehabilitate and retread our walking wounded the reality is that they are more gatekeepers than anything else. Psychoanalysis and psychotherapy have terrible track records when it comes to solving the riddle of psychosis.

One of our favorite psychiatrists, Dr. Hugh Drummond, spells out the way in which patients are often treated by his colleagues:

> The only consistent pattern is that the more the doctor likes the patient, which by and large means the closer they are in social class, the more likely he is to diagnose the patient as neurotic rather than psychotic. Poor people, Blacks and Hispanics are quickly labeled psychotic or character-disordered for the *same behavior* that earns white, middle-class patients the label neurotic (i.e. relatively healthy). To be called neurotic by a psychiatrist is a compliment.
>
> In one study, verbatim transcripts of normal speech were given to a group of psychiatrists who were asked to make a diagnosis. The speakers were identified as patients and were unknown to the psychiatrists. They were free of symptoms, led normal lives and had average scores on psychological tests. Forty percent of the psychiatrists chose "acute paranoid schizophrenia" to describe these examples of normal verbal behavior.[22]

In recent years attempts to uncover the causes of schizophrenia have taken on the character of the search for the holy grail. Almost every other year a new biochemical theory emerges that is supposed to explain why psychotic patients hear voices that aren't there and fear forces that the rest of the world cannot perceive. Dr. Drummond levels his sights on the proponents of these theories with the same ruthless candor he showed in analyzing the diagnostic methods of his colleagues:

> ... It is remarkable that so much genius is shown in trying to analyze the biochemical differences between patients and nonpatients ... That "the disease" is defined by fickle perceptions of conversational style has not prevented a whole juggernaut of chemical crusaders from searching for *the* defect as if it were the true cross.
>
> You know what happens when crusaders search for the true cross—they find it. So it is

not surprising that the psychiatric literature
has silted up with a number of breakthroughs in
biochemistry in recent years—all dramatic, all
unique and all washed away by subsequent
waves of researchers sniffing and snorting after
a Nobel Prize like pigs after truffles.[23]

Meanwhile the search continues for the biochemical causes behind
the delusions and hallucinations of schizophrenia. Currently, the
neurotransmitter dopamine is in the ascendency. The theory which is
most popular *today* suggests that nerve endings in the brain release
too much dopamine which in turn allows a surplus to build up.
Antipsychotic medications like THORAZINE (chlorpromazine),
MELLARIL (thioridazine), STELAZINE (trifluoperazine), COMPAZINE
(prochlorperazine), and HALDOL (haloperidol) are thought to counteract the disorganized thoughts, delusions, and hallucinations by
blocking the action of the excess dopamine which has accumulated at
the synapses. Whether this theory will stand the test of time is
anyone's guess, but one thing is clear, the drugs do have an effect.

There is a price that has to be paid for the benefits of these anti-
psychotic medications. Tardive dyskinesia is a complicated-sounding
side effect that is terribly disruptive. It manifests in uncomfortable
involuntary movements and muscle spasms—lip chewing, tongue
biting, neck twitching. Parkinson-like symptoms are also common
where the patient has a tremor that is impossible to control and a
shuffling walk. Other symptoms of anti-psychotic medications
include blurred vision, dry mouth, nasal congestion, difficult
urination, constipation, impaired sexuality, dizziness, fainting, increased sensitivity to sunburn, jaundice, and heartbeat irregularities.
Some of these side effects are quite common and as many as 40
percent of the people taking these drugs for any length of time will
develop tardive dyskinesia.

Even with all the drawbacks of the head medicines we have
discussed, they do work. Depression is dissipated and many suicides
are prevented. Delusions tend to fade into the background even if
they don't always disappear, and incapacitating anxiety becomes
something that can be handled successfully.

GETTING UNSTUCK WITHOUT BECOMING UNGLUED

Mental institutions are no longer snake pits, and straightjackets,
wet sheets, and padded cells are mostly a thing of the past. The
revolving-door policy adopted a few years back has attempted to get
the patients in and out as quickly as possible. In some ways that has

been a great leap forward, in other ways a terrible regression. If there is no support on the "outside" many of society's psychic invalids end up wandering the streets and living in lonely flophouses. The drugs do help many people successfully return to society, but they are not cures. Often the disordered thinking improves but the delusions are still there. They just don't seem quite as important.

The care and feeding of the psyche is a difficult task. It requires people who care and are willing to spend the time to look for the reasons behind the pain and suffering and then help the victim to do something to create meaningful change. Dignity and a sense of self-worth are essential to mental health. If you load someone up on tranquilizers and push him or her back into the same maelstrom of society you haven't accomplished a damn thing. Drugs can be useful but only if they are used as tools in a total treatment program. When they are the only response to psychological problems they can become a terrible trap.

REFERENCES

1. From a Transcript of an Interview from the CBS Television Program "*Sixty Minutes*," October 9, 1977.

2. Edmiston, Susan. "The Medicine Everybody Loves." *Family Health* 10(1):25—52, 1978.

3. Figures extrapolated from data provided by the National Prescription Audit via *Pharmacy Times* April, 1979, pp. 29—50.

4. Larkin, Jeffery K., and Wertheimer, Albert I. "Old Drugs At Home." *N. Engl. J. Med.* 298:857, 1978.

5. Ferguson, Tom. "Social Support Systems as Self-Care." *Med. Self-Care* 7:3—7, 1979.

6. Berkman, Lisa F., and Syme, Leonard S. "Social Networks, Host Resistance, and Mortality: A Nine-Year Follow-up of Alameda County Residents." *Am. J. Epidem.* 109(2):186—204, 1979.

7. Strayhorn, Joseph. "Using the Sedative-Hypnotic Drugs." Academic Press. In press.

8. Advertisement for Tranxene as it appeared in *JAMA* 243:303—304, 1980.

9. FDA Testimony. "Valium, Similar Drugs Physically Addicting." *The Nation's Health* 9(11):10, 1979.

10. Rifkin, Arthur; Quitkin, Frederic; and Klein, Donald F. "Withdrawal Reaction to Diazepam." *JAMA* 236:2172—2173, 1976.

11. Pevnick, J. S.; Jasinski, D. R.; and Haertzen, C. A. "Abrupt

Withdrawal from Therapeutically Administered Diazepam: Report of a Case." *Arch. Gen. Psychiatry* 35:995—998, 1978.

12. Editorial. "Benzodiazepine Withdrawal." *Lancet* 1:196, 1979.

13. "Some Facts and Figures on Sleeping Pills." *Med. Times* 107(6):23, 1979.

14. Ibid.

15. Solomon, S., et al. "Sleeping Pills, Insomnia and Medical Practice." *N. Engl. J. Med.* 300:803—808, 1979.

16. Medical News. "Physician Prescribing Practices Criticized; Solutions in Question." *JAMA* 241:2353—2360, 1979.

17. Frye, Janet. "Taking Sleeping Pills Worse Than Losing Sleep," reprinted in *Duke University Medical Center Intercom* 25(31):2, 1978.

18. Gillin, J. Christian; Mendelson, Wallace B.; Dement, William C.; and Solomon, Frederic. "Flurazepam and Insomnia." *Science* dd205:954—955, 1979.

19. Church, M. W., and Johnson, L. C. *Psychopharmacology* 61:309, 1979.

20. Adams, R. D. "Manic-Depressive Psychosis, Involutional Melancholia, and Hypochondriasis," in Wintrobe, M. M., et al. ed: *Harrison's Principles of Internal Medicine,* 6th ed., New York: McGraw-Hill, 1970, pp. 1876.

21. Fann, William E., and Shannon, Ira L. "A Treatment for Dry Mouth in Psychiatric Patients." *Am J. Psychiatry* 135:251—252, 1978.

22. Drummond, Hugh. "Dr. D. is Mad as Hell (Let's Increase His Thorazine)." *Mother Jones* December, 1979, pp. 50—61.

23. Ibid.

12

Saving Money in the Pharmacy

Chain store competitive prices versus old-fashioned apothecary care • Shopping for a pharmacist • A Guide to Prices of Frequently Prescribed Drugs.

It used to be that drug prices were remarkably inflation-proof. Even when the cost of living was rising at 8 or 9 percent a year drugs went up only 3 or 4 percent. And there were many products whose price didn't even change at all from one year to the next. Most people never bothered to shop comparatively for their medicine. It just wasn't good form to ask the price of a prescription in advance. Well, all that has changed. Although the cost of drugs may not have jumped as fast and as far as some consumer items it has been common to see increases of 9 or 10 percent in recent years. Checking prices has become a way of life for most folks these days, especially if they are on a fixed income. And it can pay off in big savings.

The cost of the same, identical medication can vary well over 100 percent from one pharmacy to another. This is like paying two dollars for a box of Kleenex in one store and eighty-nine cents somewhere else. And if you request a generic prescription the savings can be even greater. For example, a brand-name anti-anxiety agent like LIBRIUM can cost more than twice as much as its generic equivalent, chlordiazepoxide. Now before you rush off to the el cheapo chain store on the corner remember that saving money is not always the highest priority. The discount drugstores that sell motor oil, fishing tackle, stereos, and lawn sprinklers may be more committed to the hardware section than to the drug department. The pharmacy is often stuck away in a corner someplace where a few druggists are separated from the public either by a glass partition or some kind of tall barricade. There these assembly-line pill packers fill prescriptions as fast as their fingers can fly. Chain-store managers concerned about bottom-line profits may be more committed to the number of "scripts" filled in a day than communication with consumers. A clerk grabs your prescription and when it's filled takes your money. Unlike the days of the "mom and pop" type apothecary you may not even get close to a real live pharmacist.

If, on the other hand, you have a pharmacist who gladly finds the time to tell you everything you need to know about your medicine — how to take it, special precautions, and what the side effects are, you may want to pay a little extra for that kind of professional service. If he also keeps a patient profile of all the different medications you are on (including non-prescription remedies) in order to prevent dangerous drug interactions, then slightly higher prices are well worth what you pay. But if you aren't getting these benefits, by all means shop comparatively. And request generic equivalents whenever feasible. Pharmacists are highly trained professionals who set strict standards for all the medicines they stock. Ignore the fear campaigns waged by the major drug companies to discredit generic substitutions. You can save money and still obtain quality medications.

The following list of prices was obtained from Osco Drugs, Inc. This Chicago-based pharmacy chain has long maintained a commitment to comparative pricing information. You will find both the cost of brand name drugs as well as their generic alternatives in this table. These figures represent 1980 retail costs to the consumer. They can be expected to increase approximately 8 to 10 percent each year. Not all prescription products are available generically because the seventeen-year patent may not have expired. If this is the case you will find a dash (—) which means the generic equivalent has not yet been marketed.

GUIDE TO CHAIN-STORE PRICES OF FREQUENTLY PRESCRIBED DRUGS

BRAND NAME	GENERIC NAME	STRENGTH	QUANTITY	PRICE	PRICE OF GENERIC*
ACHROMYCIN-V	Tetracycline HCl	250 mg	40	$ 3.17	$2.23
ACTIFED	Triprolidine HCl	2 mg	100	5.80	3.59
	Pseudoephedrine HCl	60 mg			
ALDACTAZIDE	Spironolactone	25 mg	100	14.29	8.29
	Hydrochlorothiazide	25 mg			
ALDOMET	Methyldopa	250 mg	100	8.99	—— (patent)
ALDORIL	Hydrochlorothiazide	25 mg	100	13.99	—— (patent)
	Methyldopa	250 mg			
AMOXIL	Amoxicillin	250 mg	100	25.29	minor saving**
ATROMID-S	Clofibrate	500 mg	100	7.94	—— (patent)
BENDECTIN	Doxylamine succinate	10 mg	100	15.66	—— (patent)
	Pyridoxine	10 mg			

CLINORIL	Sulindac	150 mg	100	28.08	—— (patent)
COUMADIN	Warfarin Sodium	5 mg	100	6.13	minor saving**
DALMANE	Flurazepam HC1	30 mg	100	13.74	—— (patent)
DARVOCET-N 100	Propoxyphene napsylate	100 mg	100	12.99	—— (patent)
	Acetaminophen	650 mg			
DARVON COMPOUND-65	Propoxyphene HC1	65 mg	100	9.19	5.99
	Phenacetin	162 mg			
	Aspirin	227 mg			
	Caffeine	32.4 mg			
DIABINESE	Chlorpropamide	250 mg	100	14.47	7.77
DILANTIN	Phenytoin Sodium	100 mg	100	3.39	minor saving**
DIMETAPP EXTENTABS	Brompheniramine Maleate	12 mg	100	11.19	6.76
	Phenylephrine HC1	15 mg			
	Phenylpropanolamine HC1	15 mg			

GUIDE TO CHAIN-STORE PRICES OF FREQUENTLY PRESCRIBED DRUGS

BRAND NAME	GENERIC NAME	STRENGTH	QUANTITY	PRICE	PRICE OF GENERIC*
DIURIL	Chlorothiazide	500 mg	100	6.39	4.74
DYAZIDE	Hydrochlorothiazide	25 mg	100	10.45	—— (patent)
	Triamterene	50 mg			
ELAVIL	Amitriptyline HCl	25 mg	100	10.59	7.68
ERYTHROCIN	Erythromycin Stearate	250 mg	40	8.50	4.98
FIORINAL	Butalbital	50 mg	100	7.51	4.75
	Aspirin	200 mg			
	Phenacetin	130 mg			
	Caffeine	40 mg			
HYDRODIURIL	Hydrochlorothiazide	50 mg	100	6.40	4.99
HYGROTON	Chlorthalidone	50 mg	100	12.19	—— (patent)
INDERAL	Propranolol HCl	10 mg	100	5.09	—— (patent)
INDERAL	Propranolol HCl	40 mg	100	9.22	—— (patent)

Brand	Generic	Dose	Qty		
ISORDIL	Isorbide Dinitrate	10 mg	100	6.55	3.07
KEFLEX PULVULES	Cephalexin Monohydrate	250 mg	40	15.62	—— (patent)
LANOXIN	Digoxin	0.25 mg	100	1.69	minor saving
LASIX	Furosemide	40 mg	100	9.29	—— (patent)
LIBRAX	Clidinium Br Chlordiazepoxide HCl	2.5 mg 5 mg	100	11.13	6.99
LIBRIUM	Chlordiazepoxide HCl	10 mg	100	9.98	4.49
LOMOTIL	Diphenoxylate HCl Atropine sulfate	2.5 mg .025 mg	100	11.98	6.88
MOTRIN	Ibuprofen	400 mg	100	13.99	—— (patent)
NITROGLYCERIN (ALL)		all	100	1.51	1.51
ORINASE	Tolbutamide	500 mg	100	9.99	6.02
ORTHO NOVUM	Norethindrone Mestranol	1 mg 50 mcg	1 month	4.99	—— (patent)

GUIDE TO CHAIN-STORE PRICES OF FREQUENTLY PRESCRIBED DRUGS

BRAND NAME	GENERIC NAME	STRENGTH	QUANTITY	PRICE	PRICE OF GENERIC*
OVRAL	Norgestrol Ethinyl Estradiol	0.5 mg 50 mcg	1 month	5.39	—— (patent)
PAVABID TD	Papavarine HCl	150 mg	100	10.99	6.59
PERSANTINE	Dipyridamole	25 mg	100	12.29	7.59
POLYCILLIN	Ampicillin Trihydrate	250 mg	40	4.79	3.13
QUINIDINE SULFATE (LILLY)	QUINIDINE	200 mg	100	13.37	8.99
SER-AP-ES	Hydrochlorothiazide Hydralazine HCl Reserpine	15 mg 25 mg 0.1 mg	100	11.78	6.18
SLOW K	Potassium Chloride Slow-release tablets	600 mg	100	7.77	—— (patent)
TAGAMET	Cimetidine	300 mg	100	24.20	—— (patent)

THYROID 1 GRAIN	THYROID	1 grain	100	1.79	minor saving
TYLENOL NO. 3	Acetaminophen Codeine Phosphate	300 mg 30 mg	40	5.54	4.23
V-CILLIN-K	Potassium Phenoxymethyl Penicillin	250 mg	40	5.65	3.34
VALIUM	Diazepam	5 mg	100	10.89	—— (patent)
ZYLOPRIM	Allopurinol	100 mg	100	8.29	—— (patent)

*Whenever a drug is not available generically it will be designated with —— (patent). When a generic equivalent is available the prices can vary widely and will depend upon the particular distributor. These retail figures are only meant to serve as a guideline. Even greater savings may be available in your area.

**There are occasions when a brand name is so inexpensive that generic equivalents are hard pressed to beat it. AMOXIL, COUMADIN, and DILANTIN are priced so low that generic savings are hardly worth the effort. If your pharmacist can save you money, fine, but don't expect a significant difference in price.

AFTERWORD

People's Pharmacy-2 evolved in large measure as a response to the fantastic outpouring of mail we received from readers of *The People's Pharmacy*. We'd love to know your reaction to this book. Your comments, criticism and suggestions are extremely important to us and we always welcome new ideas for handy-dandy home remedies. Although we can't guarantee that we will be able to answer each and every letter personally, we will try.

Very best wishes for Good Health!

Address all cards and letters to:

The Graedons
People's Pharmacy-2
Avon Books
959 Eighth Avenue
New York, N.Y. 10019

Joe Graedon, who was born in 1945 in New York City, grew up in eastern Pennsylvania and graduated from Pennsylvania State University with a B.S. in 1967, became interested in pharmacology while doing research at the New Jersey Neuropsychiatric Institute in Princeton.

He later took a master's degree in pharmacology at the University of Michigan, then taught pharmacology at the medical school in Oaxaca, Mexico. He is a member of the Society of Neuroscience, the Association for the Psychophysiological Study of Sleep, the American Association for the Advancement of Science, and the New York Academy of Sciences.

Joe now lives in Durham, North Carolina, and writes a syndicated column, "The People's Pharmacy," on self-care drug information. He administers a course called "Pharmacology for People" in the continuing education program at Duke and serves as a consultant to the Federal Trade Commission.

Joe Graedon is the author of THE PEOPLE'S PHARMACY, and the Drugs Editor of *Medical Self-Care Magazine.* He is currently at work on a pharmacology textbook for professionals in allied health sciences.

Teresa Graedon, born in Nebraska in 1947, received her B.A. in anthropology in 1969 from Bryn Mawr, and her M.A. in 1971 and Ph.D in 1976 from the University of Michigan. Her research in both urban and rural Mexico led to her dissertation on community health and nutritional status and to the development of her specialization in medical anthropology.

While in Mexico, Teresa taught anthropology at the Universidad Autonoma "Benito Juarez" de Oaxaca. She later taught courses in health care and nutrition at the Duke University School of Nursing while she served on the faculty as Assistant Professor. As Adjunct Assistant Professor in the Department of Anthropology at

Duke, she helped develop a course on "Perspectives on Food and Hunger" and taught medical anthropology. With her husband Joe Graedon, she also taught a nutrition course at the Duke School of Continuing Education.

Teresa Graedon has presented papers on her research at anthropological conferences in the U.S. and Mexico, and is currently writing a book with co-author Joanne E. Hall entitled *Nursing Practice with Families.*

Index